METHODS IN MOLECULAR BIOLOGY™

Series Editor
John M. Walker
School of Life Sciences
University of Hertfordshire
Hatfield, Hertfordshire, AL10 9AB, UK

For other titles published in this series, go to
www.springer.com/series/7651

In Silico Tools for Gene Discovery

Edited by

Bing Yu

Department of Molecular and Clinical Genetics, Royal Prince Alfred Hospital, The University of Sydney, Camperdown, NSW, Australia

Marcus Hinchcliffe

Department of Molecular and Clinical Genetics, Royal Prince Alfred Hospital, The University of Sydney, Camperdown, NSW, Australia

Humana Press

Editors
Bing Yu, MD, Ph.D.
Department of Molecular & Clinical Genetics, Royal Prince Alfred Hospital
The University of Sydney
Camperdown, NSW 2050, Australia

Marcus Hinchcliffe
Department of Molecular & Clinical Genetics, Royal Prince Alfred Hospital
The University of Sydney
Camperdown, NSW 2050, Australia

ISSN 1064-3745 e-ISSN 1940-6029
ISBN 978-1-4939-6188-7 ISBN 978-1-61779-176-5 (eBook)
DOI 10.1007/978-1-61779-176-5
Springer New York Dordrecht Heidelberg London

Printed on acid-free paper

Humana Press is part of Springer Science+Business Media (www.springer.com)

Preface

The ultimate goal of the Human Genome Project is to understand the biology and underlying physiology of human health and disease. Functional genomics has become one of the major focuses in molecular biology in this post-genomics era. It is no longer difficult to initiate DNA variant screening at a genome scale by using massive parallel sequencing technologies. However, it remains a challenge to decode and understand hundreds, indeed thousands, of identified variants. Also, what constitutes a gene has been dramatically expanded by the discovery of widespread transcription beyond the protein coding unit. Therefore, we need more sophisticated tools to assist us in the identification of the functionality of undefined genes and the correlation of DNA variants with a particular phenotype.

In silico tools are pivotal along the journey of gene discovery. Although there is a wide spectrum of these tools, they are not well disseminated or easily applied by the end users. The scope of this volume of *Methods in Molecular Biology*^{TM} is to collect common and useful in silico tools. These tools have been arranged into three sections. The first section (**Chapters 1**, **2**, **3**, **4**, **5**, **6**, and 7) includes locus mapping information on linkage analysis, association mapping, integrative analysis, and exome analysis. Tools for DNA marker selection, in silico PCR, and statistical analysis are also provided in Section I. The second section (**Chapters 8**, **9**, **10**, **11**, and **12**) focuses on gene discovery from a defined locus. Included are in silico tools for knowledge tracking, application of gene ontology, phenotype mining, and in silico gene prioritization. Finally, in the last section (**Chapters 13**, **14**, **15**, **16**, **17**, **18**, **19**, **20**, and **21**), many useful in silico tools are presented for the functional characterization of genes, which includes DNA sequencing analysis, variant characterization, as well as RNA structure prediction. Detailed protocols are provided for the design and analysis of quantitative PCR, and the prediction of both transcriptional factor-binding sites and potential splice-affecting DNA variants. In silico tools are also assessed for the prediction of post-translational modifications as well as protein motif discovery and structure analysis.

Each chapter provides a brief introduction and clear instructions for the applications of a particular in silico tool. Furthermore, each chapter is supplemented with additional notes that provide insights into the working of the tool in question. These brief notes provide valuable keys that allow for successful application. Hopefully researchers in the field of gene discovery will find this series of articles resourceful and easy to follow. The applications of these in silico tools will facilitate locus mapping, accelerate gene identification, and help ascertain the functionality of DNA variation.

We would like to express our gratitude to all contributors of this book *In Silico Tools for Gene Discovery* for their collaboration and collective effort. We also thank our series editor, Professor John Walker, for his help and guidance throughout the process.

Bing Yu
Marcus Hinchcliffe

Contents

Contributors

ANUNCHAI ASSAWAMAKIN • *National Center for Genetic Engineering and Biotechnology (BIOTEC), Pathum Thani, Thailand*

KINMAN AU • *Division of Biostatistics, University of Massachusetts, Amherst, MA, USA*

SARA BALLOUZ • *Structural and Computational Biology Division, Victor Chang Cardiac Research Institute, Darlinghurst, NSW, Australia; School of Computer Science and Engineering, University of New South Wales, Kensington, NSW, Australia*

JENNIFER H. BARRETT • *Section of Epidemiology and Biostatistics, Leeds Institute of Molecular Medicine, University of Leeds, Leeds, UK*

HUGO P. BASTOS • *Department of Informatics, Faculty of Sciences, University of Lisbon, Lisbon, Portugal*

CHRISTOPHER G. BELL • *Medical Genomics, UCL Cancer Institute, University College London, London, UK*

ANDERS BERGKVIST • *Sigma-Aldrich Sweden AB, Stockholm, Sweden*

STEPHAN H. BERNHART • *Institute for Theoretical Chemistry, University of Vienna, Vienna, Austria*

STEPHEN BUSTIN • *Centre for Digestive Diseases, Barts and the London School of Medicine and Dentistry, Queen Mary University of London, The Royal London Hospital, London, UK*

FRANCISCO M. COUTO • *Department of Informatics, Faculty of Sciences, University of Lisbon, Lisbon, Portugal*

NORMAN DAVEY • *EMBL Structural and Computational Biology Unit, Heidelberg, Germany*

CHONGMEI DONG • *Plant Breeding Institute, The University of Sydney, Cobbitty, NSW, Australia*

C. GEORGE PRIYA DOSS • *School of BioSciences and Technology, Vellore Institute of Technology, Vellore, Tamil Nadu, India*

DANIEL FARIA • *Department of Informatics, Faculty of Sciences, University of Lisbon, Lisbon, Portugal*

ANDREA S. FOULKES • *Division of Biostatistics, University of Massachusetts, Amherst, MA, USA*

ANITA GRIGORIADIS • *Breakthrough Breast Cancer Research Unit, Guy's Hospital, King's Health Partners AHSC, London, UK*

PHILIP GROTH • *Research Laboratories, Bayer Schering Pharma AG, Berlin, Germany*

YIKE GUO • *Department of Computing, Imperial College London, London, UK; IDBS Limited, London, UK*

HERMAN VAN HAAGEN • *Department of Human Genetics, University Medical Center, Leiden, The Netherlands*

MARCUS HINCHCLIFFE • *Department of Molecular and Clinical Genetics, Royal Prince Alfred Hospital, The University of Sydney, Camperdown, NSW, Australia; Sydney Medical School (Central), The University of Sydney, Camperdown, NSW, Australia*

CLAUDE HOUDAYER • *Faculty of Pharmacy, Institut Curie, Paris Descartes University, Paris, France*
DIMITRIOS KALAITZOPOULOS • *IDBS Limited, London, UK*
ULF LESER • *Knowledge Management in Bioinformatics, Humboldt University of Berlin, Berlin, Germany*
VICTOR G. LEVITSKY • *Laboratory of Theoretical Genetics, Institute of Cytology and Genetics, Siberian Branch of the Russian Academy of Sciences, Novosibirsk, Russia*
HUI LI • *Department of Systems and Computer Science, Howard University, Washington, DC, USA*
CHUNMEI LIU • *Department of Systems and Computer Science, Howard University, Washington, DC, USA*
ALBERTO J.M. MARTIN • *Complex and Adaptive Systems Laboratory, University College Dublin, Belfield, Dublin 4, Ireland; Biocomputing UP, Department of Biology, University of Padua, Padova, Italy; School of Computer Science and Informatics, University College Dublin, Belfield, Dublin 4, Ireland*
BAREND MONS • *Netherlands Bioinformatics Centre (NBIC), Nijmegen, The Netherlands*
GRANT W. MONTGOMERY • *Queensland Institute of Medical Research, Brisbane, QLD, Australia*
CATHERINE MOONEY • *Complex and Adaptive Systems Laboratory, University College Dublin, Belfield, Dublin 4, Ireland; Conway Institute of Biomolecular and Biomedical Research, University College Dublin, Belfield, Dublin 4, Ireland; School of Medicine and Medical Science, University College Dublin, Belfield, Dublin 4, Ireland*
ROBIN E.J. MUNRO • *IDBS Limited, London, UK*
TANIA NOLAN • *Sigma-Aldrich, Haverhill, Suffolk, UK*
DALE R. NYHOLT • *Queensland Institute of Medical Research, Brisbane, QLD, Australia*
DMITRY Y. OSHCHEPKOV • *Laboratory of Theoretical Genetics, Institute of Cytology and Genetics, Siberian Branch of the Russian Academy of Sciences, Novosibirsk, Russia*
MARTIN OTI • *Structural and Computational Biology Division, Victor Chang Cardiac Research Institute, Darlinghurst, NSW, Australia*
JODIE N. PAINTER • *Queensland Institute of Medical Research, Brisbane, QLD, Australia*
CATIA PESQUITA • *Department of Informatics, Faculty of Sciences, University of Lisbon, Lisbon, Portugal*
JITTIMA PIRIYAPONGSA • *National Center for Genetic Engineering and Biotechnology (BIOTEC), Pathum Thani, Thailand*
GIANLUCA POLLASTRI • *Complex and Adaptive Systems Laboratory, University College Dublin, Belfield, Dublin 4, Ireland; School of Computer Science and Informatics, University College Dublin, Belfield, Dublin 4, Ireland*
R. RAJASEKARAN • *School of BioSciences and Technology, Vellore Institute of Technology, Vellore, Tamil Nadu, India*
RAO SETHUMADHAVAN • *School of BioSciences and Technology, Vellore Institute of Technology, Vellore, Tamil Nadu, India*
PHILIP J. SHAW • *National Center for Genetic Engineering and Biotechnology (BIOTEC), Pathum Thani, Thailand*
DENIS C. SHIELDS • *Complex and Adaptive Systems Laboratory, University College Dublin, Belfield, Dublin 4, Ireland; Conway Institute of Biomolecular and Biomedical*

Research, University College Dublin, Belfield, Dublin 4, Ireland; School of Medicine and Medical Science, University College Dublin, Belfield, Dublin 4, Ireland

BRUNO TAVARES • *Department of Informatics, Faculty of Sciences, University of Lisbon, Lisbon, Portugal*

M. DAWN TEARE • *Section of Epidemiology and Biostatistics, Leeds Institute of Molecular Medicine, University of Leeds, Leeds, UK*

NICKI TIFFIN • *The South African National Bioinformatics Institute, University of the Western Cape, Belville, Cape Town, South Africa*

SISSADES TONGSIMA • *National Center for Genetic Engineering and Biotechnology (BIOTEC), Pathum Thani, Thailand*

IAN WALSH • *Complex and Adaptive Systems Laboratory, University College Dublin, Belfield, Dublin 4, Ireland; Biocomputing UP, Department of Biology, University of Padua, Padova, Italy; School of Computer Science and Informatics, University College Dublin, Belfield, Dublin 4, Ireland*

PAUL WEBSTER • *Department of Molecular and Clinical Genetics, Royal Prince Alfred Hospital, The University of Sydney, Camperdown, NSW, Australia*

BERTRAM WEISS • *Research Laboratories, Bayer Schering Pharma AG, Berlin, Germany*

MERRIDEE A. WOUTERS • *School of Life & Environmental Sciences, Deakin University, Geelong, Victoria, Australia; School of Medical Sciences, University of New South Wales, Kensington, NSW, Australia; Structural and Computational Biology Division, Victor Chang Cardiac Research Institute, Darlinghurst, NSW, Australia*

BING YU • *Department of Molecular and Clinical Genetics, Royal Prince Alfred Hospital, Camperdown, NSW, Australia; Sydney Medical School (Central), The University of Sydney, Camperdown, NSW, Australia*

CHANGBIN ZHANG • *Prenatal Diagnostic Center, Guangdong Women and Children Hospital, Guangzhou, China*

Chapter 1

Accessing and Selecting Genetic Markers from Available Resources

Christopher G. Bell

Abstract

The history of genetic markers accurately partitions the progression of molecular genetics into three phases: the RFLP (restriction fragment length polymorphism), microsatellite and SNP (single nucleotide polymorphism) eras. This chapter focuses predominately on the current workhorse, the SNP, though briefly covers the former two and overviews current online databases and portals that act as central repositories as well as hubs to further detailed information. Central gene or disease-based searches are considered and then followed through systematically.

Key words: Restriction fragment length polymorphism (RFLP), microsatellite, single nucleotide polymorphism (SNP), HapMap.

1. Introduction

A genetic marker is any DNA sequence that can be assessed for variation. As technology has advanced, so have the variants used and their methods for measurement radically changed. Additionally, throughput has dramatically increased. Once a marker can be robustly determined, it can be used to enable differentiation or grouping by phenotype, trait or other category. A strong association with disease can enable these variants to be used as 'biomarkers' to infer on prognosis, drug choice or pharmacodynamics (1).

This chapter will discuss these variants with a *Homo sapiens* focus, but the principles are often universal, can be extrapolated, and many of the sites discussed include links to other data, such as the murine model organisms. After a brief overview of previously more widespread but now predominately historic markers,

B. Yu, M. Hinchcliffe (eds.), *In Silico Tools for Gene Discovery*, Methods in Molecular Biology 760,
DOI 10.1007/978-1-61779-176-5_1,

the majority of this chapter will discuss the currently widely used agent, the single nucleotide polymorphism (SNP).

2. Materials

2.1. Restriction Fragment Length Polymorphisms (RFLPs)

The discovery and application of restriction enzymes in the early 1970s by Danna, Nathans, Smith and Wilcox (2) enabled the initiation of the first detailed physical mapping of the genome. These enzymes digest DNA only at recognition sites, exact sequence motifs of generally 4–8 bps which are often palindromic. This leads to a double-strand break in DNA, which can either be blunt ended or sticky ended with base/s overhang. Their use to generate variable size lengths of DNA, dependent upon variation at the recognition site, produced RFLPs as the first generation of genetic markers. Initially visualised by Southern Blotting, these were later amplified by PCR around the recognition site, thereby enabling the identification of one whole or two cut fragments for each allele.

Whilst used extensively in the 1970s for mapping studies, although very restricted by their limited informativeness, today they are still, though decreasingly, used for some diagnostic assays. They are probably of most use as a quick supplementary means of confirmation of a critical mutation finding discovered by another method.

2.2. Microsatellites or Short Tandem Repeats (STRs)

Microsatellites were the primary tool of marker studies through the 1990s. They are defined as tandem repeats with simplistic motifs of one to six bases, though generally those of two (di-), three (tri-) or four (tetranucleotide) bases, usually less than 0.1 kb in length. These loci are widely dispersed throughout the genome with estimates that these variants account for 3% of the human genome, with numbers approximately around 1 million depending on the search criteria cutoffs used (3). However, the minimum number of bases or numbers of repeats and the amount of degeneracy in the repeat sequence allowed are not clearly defined, therefore these definitions are imprecise (4). Interestingly, the mouse genome appears to have a two- to threefold increase in number when compared with human (5) and this also appears to be the case of other rodent genomes (6).

Microsatellites can be classified by repeat motif and length, e.g. $(AT)_{12}$, and furthermore by three family classifications – i.e.

(i) Pure – ATATATATATATATATATATATAT

(ii) Compound – ATATATATGTGTGTGTGTGTGTGT – of two or more microsatellites

(iii) Interrupted – ATATATGGATATATATATATATAT

PCR amplification of these genomic regions from the end of the 1980s (7) and their use in the first detailed linkage mapping of the human genome (8) underlined their resourcefulness. This led to the considerable success in the identification of monogenic Mendelian diseases by linkage analysis (*see* **Chapter 2** for more discussion on 'Linkage Analysis') throughout the 1990s but less so when adapted for the study of complex traits (9, 10).

Mutation rate in microsatellites is high, with an estimate in humans of 10^{-4}–10^{-2} mutations per locus per generation, and this rate is additionally found to vary greatly between loci (4). A study by Kelkar et al. comparing microsatellite evolution in human and chimpanzee genomes managed to model and predict microsatellite mutability to <90% (11). This has obvious benefit for inclusion in probability calculations utilising microsatellites particularly in forensic analyses. The effectors of microsatellite mutagenesis are predominately found to be the inherent structure, including motif size, repeat number and length, which all affect the likelihood of replication slippage (11). Observations that mutability increases non-uniformly with microsatellite length suggest other processes, such as faulty repair, may also play a role. Furthermore, secondary structure differences and regional effects have a slight influence, although transcriptional status itself appears not to (11).

This predominate source of mutation, replication slippage, occurs due to dissociation after replication initiation and subsequent mismatched realignment, forward or reverse, of one strand to the other, leading to an increase or decrease in repeat number. Slippage may also occur during PCR amplification of loci leading to 'stutter' bands, usually of minor lower repeat numbers. Microsatellites are still used for 'DNA fingerprinting' in forensic identity analysis due to vastly increased informativeness compared with RFLPs and also SNPs, due to the multiple alleles per marker (e.g. AB AmpFℓSTR® Identifiler® PCR Amplification Kit).

Direct microsatellite pathogenicity is found in the trinucleotide or triplet repeat disorders that include Huntington disease, hereditary ataxias and spinobulbar muscular atrophy (12). Sizing of this subset of microsatellites enables diagnostic correlation with disease state.

2.3. SNPs (Single Nucleotide Polymorphisms)

The now ubiquitous SNP has facilitated the dramatic and detailed evaluation of common variation in the genome in large cohorts, thereby enabling estimates of population linkage disequilibrium and the subsequent explosion of genome-wide association (GWA) studies for a plethora of diseases and traits (*see* **Chapter 3** for more discussion on 'Association Mapping').

SNPS are simply due to a single base substitution, usually with only two possible alleles, a major and minor allele, although rarely triallelic SNP variants do exist. The replacement of a pyrimidine base for another pyrimidine (C↔T) or purine for a purine (A↔G) is termed a transition. Whereas the exchange between these two types of base is termed a transversion (A→C or T, C→A or G, G→T or C and T→A or G). SNPs are usually implied to have at least a minor allele frequency greater than 1% (13); however, this can obviously be population dependent. A single base insertion or deletion can also be referred to as a SNP, although the term single nucleotide variant (SNV) may be used inclusively to include these mutations together with substitution-only SNPs (14).

Base substitutions occur due to two major processes: replication errors or mutagenesis due to chemical or physical effects and agents. A major driver in SNP formation in the human genome is of the later means, the hypermutability of methylated cytosines in CpG dinucleotides, whereby the spontaneous deamination of these modified bases to thymine and consequent incorrect repair leads to the formation of TpG or CpA (15). This methylated cytosine mutational hotspot rate is 10–50 times that of non-CpG cytosines, although these bases have recently been identified to also have some lesser effect on the surrounding rate of non-CpG mutation as well (16).

3. Methods

3.1. Identification of Restriction Fragment Length Polymorphisms (RFLPs)

A comprehensive and fully referenced database of restriction enzymes can be found at Rebase from New England Biolabs (http://rebase.neb.com) (17). Recognition and cleavage sites, isoschizomers (those that recognise the same sequence), neoschizomers (recognise the same sequence, but cut at a differing position), plus extensive additional information on restriction-modification processes and other details such as methylation sensitivity is all readily presented here, together with commercial availability. This database is fully searchable and selected FTP download of datasets is also possible.

3.2. Searching for Microsatellites or Short Tandem Repeats (STRs)

Numerous bioinformatic methods of identifying microsatellites from raw sequence data are available and these include as follows:

(i) RepeatMasker (http://www.repeatmasker.org) identifies simple repeats less than 20 bp that do not diverge more than 10% from a perfect repeat.

(ii) Sputnik (http://espressosoftware.com/sputnik/index.html) utilises a recursive algorithm on FASTA formatted sequence files.

(iii) Tandem Repeats Finder (http://c3.biomath.mssm.edu/trf.html) (18) utilises statistically based recognition criteria with no requirement for specification of pattern or size.

(iv) BioPHP – Microsatellite Repeats Finder – http://www.biophp.org/minitools/microsatellite_repeats_finder/

The heterozygosity (the portion of individuals in a population that are heterozygous for a particular microsatellite) obviously greatly affects the usefulness of a microsatellite by increasing its informativeness. Information on this measure is available from CEPH (http://www.cephb.fr/en/cephdb/browser.php).

The GDB Human Genome Database (http://www.gdb.org/) was previously a large resource for human linkage map data; however, it is currently off-line, so its future is unclear.

The NCBI (National Center for Biotechnology Information) UniSTS database lists unique sequence-tagged sites (STSs) with a unique ID (http://www.ncbi.nlm.nih.gov/sites/entrez?db=unists) for multiple organisms, those that are polymorphic are utilised in map construction. The linkage maps available for humans include those listed in **Table 1.1** (*see* **Note 1**).

This database of STSs is defined by PCR primer pairs and associated information including genomic position, genes and sequences, including the UniSTS ID, locus, primer Information – forward and reverse, expected PCR range, GenBank Accession number and link for Sequence, cross reference to genes in region, mapping information to maps available, electronic PCR results on various available sequences and information for this marker in the *Pan troglodytes* sequence (*see* **Fig. 1.1**).

Table 1.1
Human linkage maps (listed on NCBI)

Map name	Map title	Total markers	Total UniSTS[a]
GeneMap99-G3	Human Transcript Map 99	7,056	7,040
GeneMap99-GB4	Human Transcript Map 99	45,138	44,277
Genethon	Genethon Human Linkage Map, 1995 release	5,264	5,264
Marshfield	Marshfield human genetic Map	7,698	7,694
NCBI	RH Computed integrated panel Map	23,727	23,699
NHGRI-7	NHGRI chr 7 Physical Map	2,117	2,117
Stanford-G3	Stanford G3 Map	7,198	7,149
TNG	Stanford TNG RH Map	36,634	35,608
WUSTL-X	WashU Chr. X STS Map	1,664	1,662
Whitehead-RH	Whitehead-RH Map, July 1997 release	14,658	14,627
Whitehead-YAC	Whitehead STS Map, July 1997 release	10,469	10,449
deCODE	deCODE high-resolution genetic Map	5,135	5,012

[a]Subset of markers mapped that are STS and available with primer sequence information in UniSTS (as 25 March 2010)

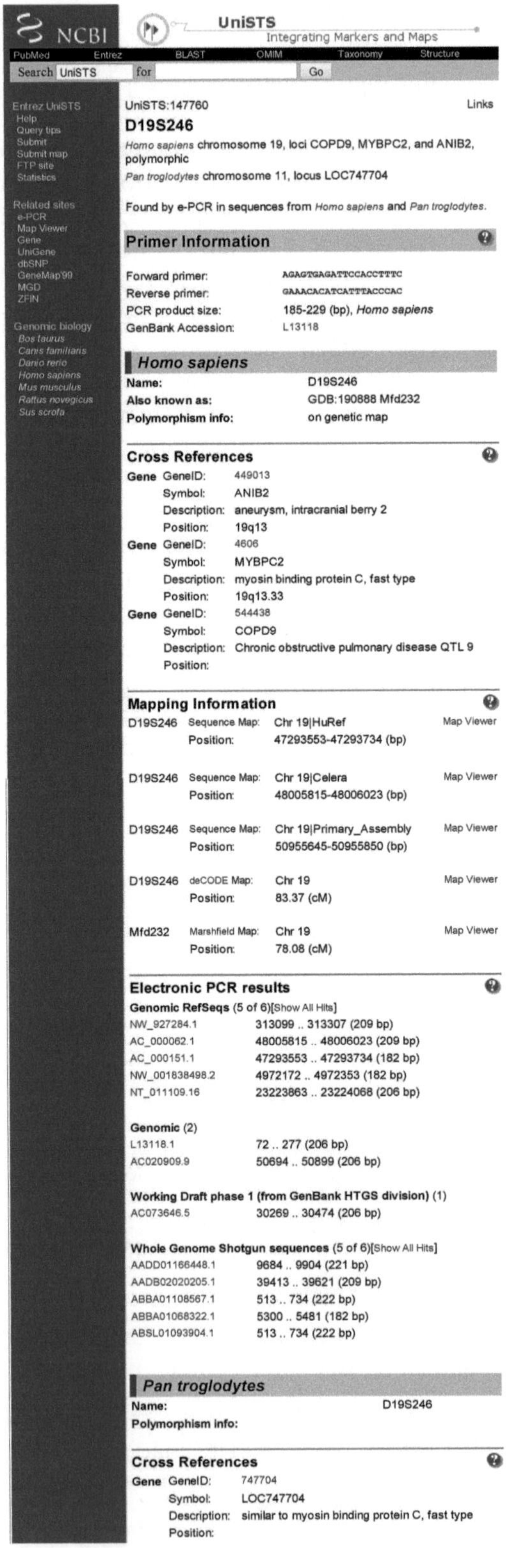

Fig. 1.1. The NCBI UniSTS database for D19S246.

Table 1.2
dbSNP query for Build 131

Organism	dbSNP build	Genome build	Number of submissions (ss #'s)	Number of RefSNP clusters (rs #'s) (# validated)	Number of (rs #'s) in gene	Number of (ss #'s) with frequency
Homo sapiens	131	37.1	105,098,087	23,652,081 (14,515,246)	10,372,495	10,679,869

3.3. Accessing and Selecting SNPs

3.3.1. dbSNP

The centre repository for SNP information is dbSNP, a SNP database from NCBI (http://www.ncbi.nlm.nih.gov/projects/SNP/) (19). All SNPs are assigned a RefSNP or rs number, and the database's current state is displayed in **Table 1.2**. Searching for a SNP by rs number reveals an identifier with 25 bp of flanking 5′ and 3′sequence, both variant alleles displayed in brackets, i.e. [A/T] and organism. Default tabs above include detail on this SNP in 1000 genomes data, cited in Pubmed links, clinical/locus-specific database (LSDB) submissions and human data. Clicking again on the SNP rs number will reveal this SNP's detailed individual dbSNP page with initial information detailed under categories of RefSNP (organism, molecular type, created/updated in build, map to genome build), allele (variation class, RefSNP alleles, ancestral allele (*see* **Note 2**), clinical association) and the HGVS (Human Genome Variation Society) official nomenclature for this variant (*see* **Note 3**). Then this page is divided into information on

(1) Maps – Integrated positions of this variant on various assemblies

(2) GeneView – Graph of position of SNP if within a genic region

(3) Submission – Details on submission history

(4) FASTA – FASTA formatted sequence 400 bp upstream and downstream of SNP with variant in single letter IUPAC format

(5) Resource – NCBI resource links to Genbank sequences

(6) Diversity – Information on assayed populations and their allele frequencies for this SNP

(7) Validation – Symbols to display level of validation and whether it is included in HapMap and 1000 genomes (*see* **Note 4**)

The complete database is also available for download (ftp://ftp.ncbi.nih.gov/snp).

Further SNP information is available from a number of sites including SNPedia (http://www.snpedia.com), which is a wiki style database with information including disease-related information and links related to these particular SNPs, and the HGVbaseG2P, which can be searched by SNP and other markers at http://www.hgvbaseg2p.org/markers. This site can also enable a multiple search input.

3.3.2. HapMap

The International HapMap Project (20) performed a vital role, building upon the success of the Human Genome Project (3), by enabling the identification of the most informative single nucleotide polymorphisms (SNPs) to assay in order to frugally capture human variation genome wide. This was possible because of the inherent redundancy that exists in the human genome, due to linkage disequilibrium. By dramatically reducing the genotyping requirements to capture common variants, this ushered in the era of high-throughput SNP chip or array genotyping, and due to this technological breakthrough true genome-wide SNP association studies (GWASs) were finally possible in large enough cohorts with enough resultant power (21) (*see* **Chapter 3** for more discussion on 'Association Mapping'). Since early 2007 this has led to a flurry of positive, and more importantly truly replicable, disease associations in complex traits. This notably included the Wellcome Trust Case Control Consortium (WTCCC) study, which investigated seven common diseases, in the UK Caucasian population, benefiting from the use of a collective control population (22). GWASs have radically increased our knowledge of definitive reproducible common genetic variants associated with common complex traits, such as type II diabetes, inflammatory bowel disease and breast cancer, which had been elusive up to this point. The potential benefits that will arise from these novel disease-associated genes and possible novel therapeutics pathways are only just beginning to be explored (23). The initial HapMap project detailed variation in a total of 270 people, comprising three groups: the Yoruba people of Ibadan, Nigeria (YRI), with 30 sets of parent–child trios, 45 unrelated Japanese from Tokyo and 45 unrelated Chinese from Beijing (ASN), and 30 US trios collected in 1980 from US residents with northern and western European ancestry by the CEPH – Centre d'Etude du Polymorphisme Humain (CEU) (*see* **Note 5**). The HapMap database has expanded from these initial three YRI, ASN and CEU, respectively, continental representative populations to Phase III, which now includes 10 ethnicities detailed in **Table 1.3**.

The site is accessible at http://hapmap.ncbi.nlm.nih.gov/index.html.en. The browser data is accessible here by clicking beneath project data for either Phases I and II (Only CEU, YRI, JPT and CHB) or Phase III for all ten ethnicity data. Browser information is split into

Table 1.3
HapMap Phase III populations and descriptors

ASW	African ancestry in Southwest USA
CEU	Utah residents with northern and western European ancestry from the CEPH collection
CHB	Han Chinese in Beijing, China
CHD	Chinese in Metropolitan Denver, Colorado
GIH	Gujarati Indians in Houston, Texas
JPT	Japanese in Tokyo, Japan
LWK	Luhya in Webuye, Kenya
MEX	Mexican ancestry in Los Angeles, California
MKK	Maasai in Kinyawa, Kenya
TSI	Toscans in Italy
YRI	Yoruban in Ibadan, Nigeria

(1) Search – where the Landmark or Region to be viewed is entered, also where Reports & Analysis can be configured and downloaded.

(2) Overview – entire chromosome position and ideogram, contigs, number of genotyped SNPs represented graphically/500 kb, location of any OMIM disease associations and locations of any GWA studies SNPs (from the Catalog of Published genome-wide association studies, http://www.genome.gov/gwastudies/) (24).

(3) Region – close up chromosome position, number of genotyped SNPs represented graphically/20 kb, location of copy number variants (CNVs).

(4) Detail – position, genotyped SNPs – with pie graphs representing allele frequencies, gene Location – entrez number ID and link, GWA study loci and reactome pathway links.

These default tracks can all be toggled at the click boxes below and additional information such as LD graphics can be accessed, as well as enabling custom tracks to be imported.

However, this information and downloaded genotype data from HapMap is best viewed utilising the HaploView software for detailed analysis (25). This is accessible from http://www.broadinstitute.org/haploview/haploview (*see* **Fig. 1.2** and **Note 6**).

Genotype information is downloaded from HapMap by utilising the Reports & Analysis Files dropdown option and selecting Download SNP Genotype Data, then clicking on the Configure button to its right. This leads to a new Configure SNP Genotype Data screen. Here population (CEU, YRI, JPT+CHB, JPT

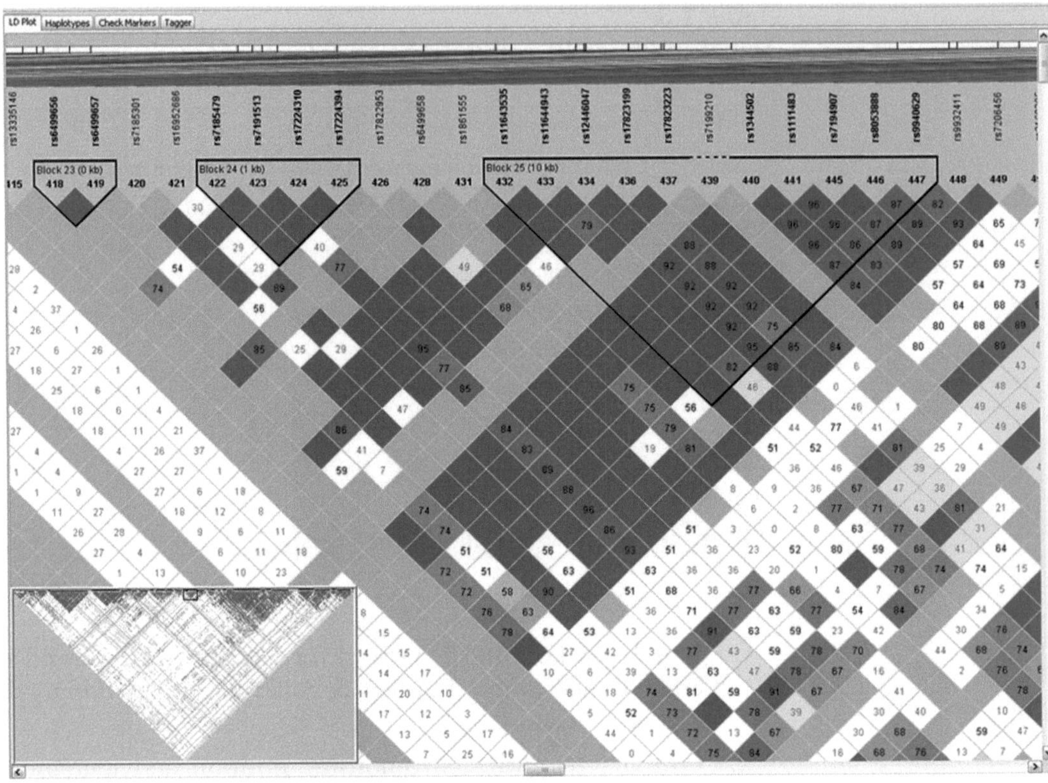

Fig. 1.2. Linkage disequilibrium visualisation from Haploview (25).

or CHB), strand (fwd, rev or rs (*see* **Note 7**)) and Output format as text or Save to Disk or Open directly in HaploView (*see* **Note 8**) functions are available. HaploView enables detailed visualisation of linkage disequilibrium (LD) Blocks (*see* **Note 9**), haplotypes, markers which can be manually selected and TAGGER software can be run (26). This program can be used to not only remove those SNPs which are captured by pairwise comparison with a specified r^2 value or above but aslo remove those made redundant by the use of two or three SNP haplotypes of genotyped SNPs.

These HapMap SNPs have been analysed for evidence of positive selection in the human genome and this data can be accessed from Haplotter (27) (http://hg-wen.uchicago.edu/selection/haplotter.htm). Additional information on SNPs population diversity for 53 populations can be found in HGDP Selection Browser (28, 29) (http://hgdp.uchicago.edu/).

3.3.3. 1000 Genomes Project

The 1000 genomes project (http://www.1000genomes.org/), by use of second-generation sequencing technologies, plans to extend on the catalogue of human diversity begun with the HapMap database (30). After an initial pilot phase comprising low coverage sequencing of the original 180 HapMap Phases I and II unrelated individuals, deep sequencing of two trios and exome only sequencing in 900 individuals will be followed by full genome sequencing of approximately 2000 genomes at 4x depth coverage, depending on pilot information adjustments. This later group will consist of 22 different populations and all these data will be publicly available and incorporated into databases such as dbSNP.

3.4. Copy Number Variants

The extent of copy number variant (CNV) polymorphism in the human genome has gradually become apparent over the last few years (31), although with less success with common disease association (32). Information on population copy number variation is available in browser format from the Database of Genomic Variants (33) at http://projects.tcag.ca/variation/.

3.5. Investigating an Individual Gene or Disease

Initial assessment for genetic markers will usually either be for (1) a particular gene of interest or for (2) the disease being investigated. An excellent first stop from a gene angle is the HUGO Gene Nomenclature Committee search page (http://www.genenames.org) to confirm the gene's Approved Gene Symbol and check that a colloquial or historical name is not being used. Once this is identified, clicking on the Gene Symbol produces the Symbol Report page. This central hub then enables connection to many relevant databases categorised by Core Data, Database Links, Gene Symbol Links and any Locus or Specialist-Specific Databases for this gene (*see* **Fig. 1.3** with an example for *MLH1*). Definitions for all of these links can be found at http://www.genenames.org/data/gdlw_columndef.html.

The online version of the well-known Mendelian Inheritance in Man (OMIM) is linked from here and contains direct disease-related information, association between polymorphisms and disease with comprehensive references of associated papers (http://www.ncbi.nlm.nih.gov/omim). With respect to genetic markers the locus-specific databases will give links to curated disease-related variation. A full list of these databases is given at www.hgvs.org/dblist/glsdb.html. Additionally, to explore known polymorphisms within the gene, links are given to the major Genome Browsers: Ensembl and UCSC. Furthermore the European Bioinformatics Institute now includes a very comprehensive data portal (http://www.ebi.ac.uk/).

NCBIs homepage http://www.ncbi.nlm.nih.gov/ enables a search performed across all of the extensive NCBI databases at once, or a selected one, with the Entrez Lifesciences Search Engine. The example result is given for *MLH1* in **Fig. 1.4**.

3.6. Biomarkers

Any genetic marker may be useful as a biomarker. The NIH Biomarker Working Group definition is 'A characteristic that is

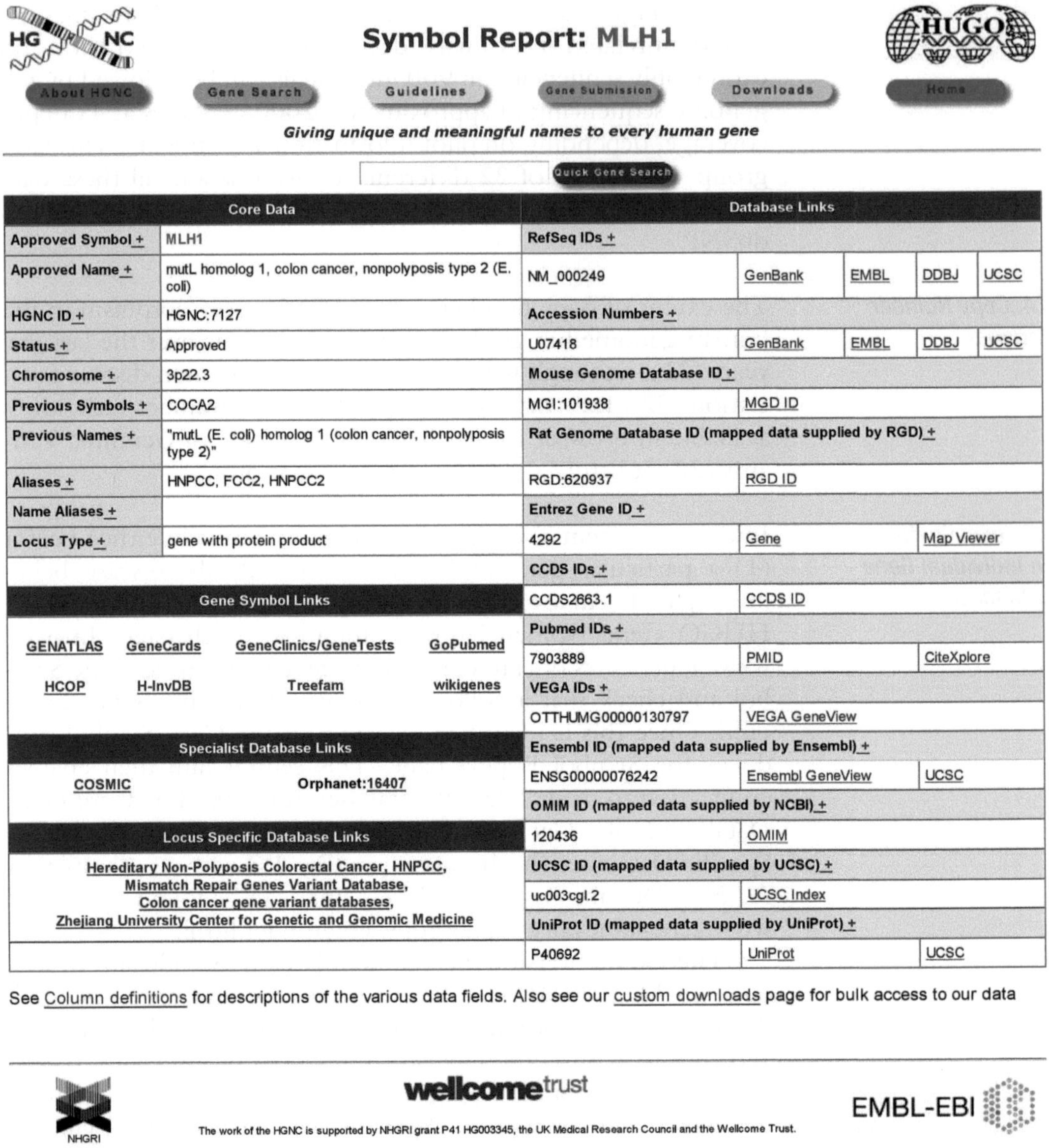

Fig. 1.3. HUGO Gene Symbol Report.

objectively measured and evaluated as an indicator of normal biologic processes, pathogenic processes or pharmacologic response to a therapeutic intervention.' Biomarkers validated by genetic methods can be classified into three types (1).

(1) Type 0 – Natural history of disease

(2) Type 1 – Drug activity markers

(3) Type 2 – Surrogate markers – substitute for a clinical endpoint

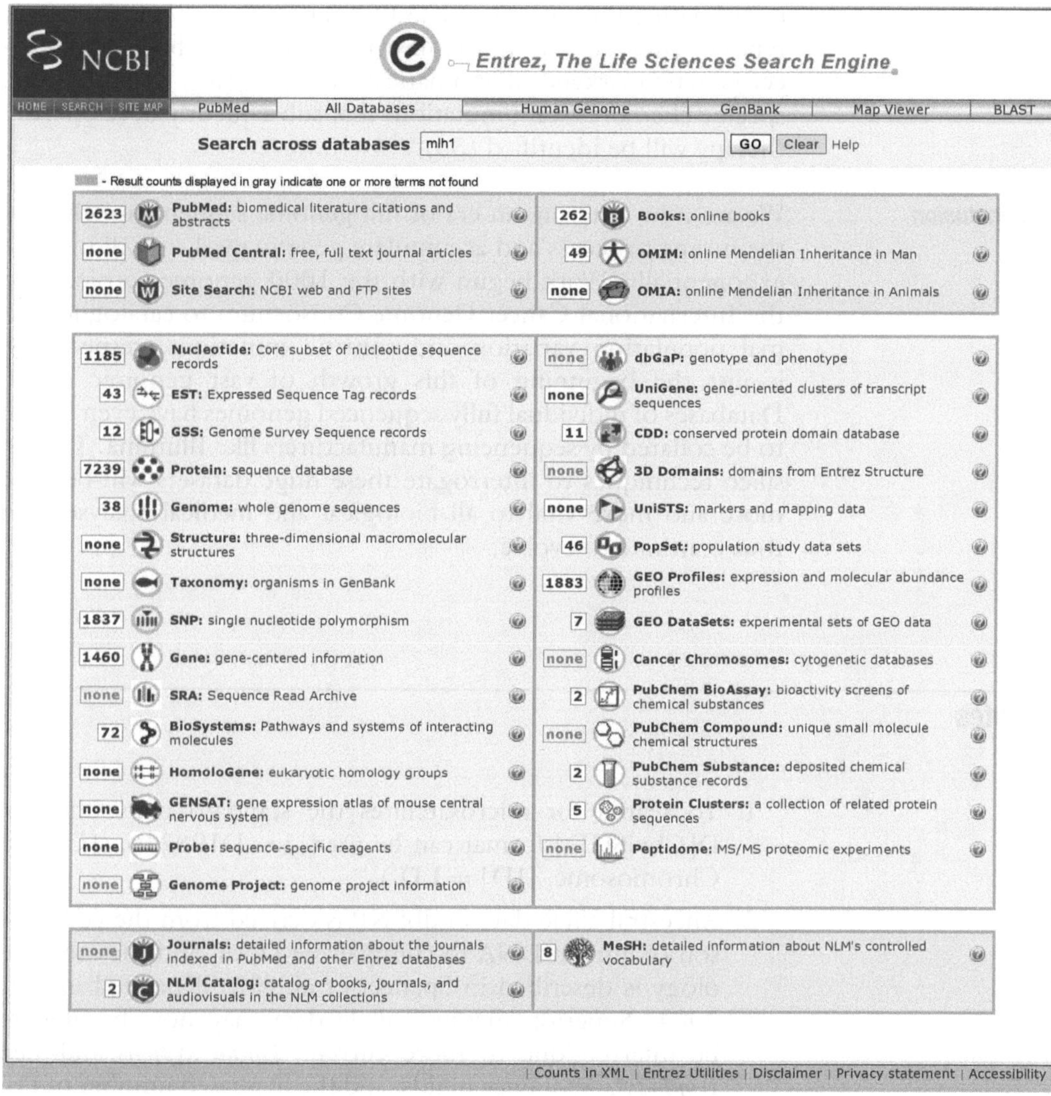

Fig. 1.4. NCBI Entrez search.

Cancer biomarkers may, for example, infer on the natural course of the tumour, good or poor outcome, who to treat or how aggressively to treat. The Cancer Genetic Markers of Susceptibility (CGEMS) project is at http://cgems.cancer.gov/ and Catalogue of Somatic Mutations in Cancer (COSMIC) is at http://www.sanger.ac.uk/genetics/CGP/cosmic/. With the large-scale cancer sequencing projects currently underway, including the Cancer Genome Project in the United Kingdom (http://www.sanger.ac.uk/genetics/CGP/) and the Cancer Genome Atlas (http://cancergenome.nih.gov/) in the United States, brought together under the umbrella of the International Cancer Genome Consortium (ICGC) (http://www.icgc.org/)

coordinating the analysis of >25,000 cancer genomes in 50 cancer types or subtypes within the next few years (34) the level of cancer genetic markers will dramatically increase (35). Furthermore, specific chemoresistant mutations that subsequently develop from therapy will be identified (36).

3.7. Conclusion

We are now entering an era of full genome sequencing whereby the means to access and accumulate genetic markers will increase exponentially. Work begun with the 1000 genomes project and the International Cancer Genome Consortium to catalogue normal population variation and somatic mutations, respectively, is just the beginning of this growth of vast genomic detail. Databases of individual fully sequenced genomes have even begun to be collated by sequencing manufacturers like Illumina. Thus in silico techniques to interrogate these huge datasets will become more and more vital to all biological and medical analyses and thus continue to evolve.

4. Notes

1. To search for microsatellites the standard convention of D[Chr]S[ID] format can be used, i.e. D19S246, ([Chr] = Chromosome, [ID] = I.D.).
2. Ancestral allele data in dbSNP is derived from the comparison of human DNA to chimpanzee DNA, and the methodology is described in Spencer et al. (37) deposited in May 2004. Superior ancestral allele data may now be able to be inferred due to more current *Homo sapiens* and *Pan troglodytes* sequence builds, and the increased number of Primate sequences available.
3. This recent addition will facilitate consistent cataloging of pathogenic variants and should be used in describing all clinically significant mutations.
4. The incorporation of 1000 genomes data will help in quality control assessment of SNPs in dbSNP. Sequencing artefacts leading to SNP inclusion in this database due to paralogous or duplicated genes have been recently estimated to be as high as 8.32% (38). Abnormal Hardy–Weinberg Equilibrium (HWE) test calculations may be indicative of this (http://www.oege.org/software/hwe-mr-calc.shtml) (13).
5. Therefore in some analyses of these data that require non-relatedness, only 210 individuals are included, i.e. the offspring of the CEU and YRI trios are excluded.

6. The Phase II populations (CEU, YRI and ASN combined or as separate CHB and JPT groups) genotype data download from HapMap is only presently viewable with HaploView, although all Phase III populations should be able to be correctly read by HaploView with the next software update.
7. Strand assignment of SNPs so that SNP alleles are given for either forward (fwd), reverse (rev) or rs which gives SNP variation displayed in dbSNP for the rs number that may be either forward or reverse.
8. It is stated that this option to directly open the file in HaploView will not work on all OS platforms or browsers; however, in fact it has not been found to work on any Windows or Linux-based systems attempted currently.
9. Linkage Disequilibrium can be defined by Gabriel et al. (39), four gamete rule, solid spline of LD or custom methods.

URLS

1000 genomes project (http://www.1000genomes.org/)

BioPHP – Microsatellite Repeats Finder (http://www.biophp.org/minitools/microsatellite_repeats_finder/)

Cancer Genetic Markers of Susceptibility (CGEMS) Project (http://cgems.cancer.gov/)

Cancer Genome Project (http://www.sanger.ac.uk/genetics/CGP/)

Catalog of Published Genome-Wide Association Studies (http://www.genome.gov/gwastudies/)

Catalogue Of Somatic Mutations In Cancer (COSMIC) (http://www.sanger.ac.uk/genetics/CGP/cosmic/)

CEPH (http://www.cephb.fr/en/cephdb/browser.php)

Database of Genomic Variants (http://projects.tcag.ca/variation)

dbSNP (http://www.ncbi.nlm.nih.gov/projects/SNP/)

Ensembl (http://www.ensembl.org/index.html)

GDB Human Genome Database (http://www.gdb.org/)

Haplotter (http://hg-wen.uchicago.edu/selection/haplotter.htm)

Haploview (http://www.broadinstitute.org/haploview/haploview)

Hgdp Browser (http://hgdp.uchicago.edu/)

HGDP Selection Browser (http://hgdp.uchicago.edu)

HGVbaseG2P (http://www.hgvbaseg2p.org/markers)

HUGO Gene Nomenclature Committee search page (http://www.genenames.org)

International Cancer Genome Consortium (http://www.icgc.org/)

International HapMap Project (http://hapmap.ncbi.nlm.nih.gov/index.html.en)

Locus-Specific Databases (http://www.hgvs.org/dblist/glsdb.html)

Minisatellites (http://minisatellites.u-psud.fr/GPMS/human_minisat.htm)

NCBI (http://www.ncbi.nlm.nih.gov/)

NCBI UniSTS (http://www.ncbi.nlm.nih.gov/sites/entrez?db=unists)

OMIM (http://www.ncbi.nlm.nih.gov/omim)

Rebase from New England Biolabs (http://rebase.neb.com)

RepeatMasker (http://www.repeatmasker.org)

SNPedia (http://www.snpedia.com)

Sputnik (http://espressosoftware.com/sputnik/index.html)

Tandem Repeats Finder (http://c3.biomath.mssm.edu/trf.html)

The Cancer Genome Atlas (http://cancergenome.nih.gov/)

UCSC Browser (http://genome.ucsc.edu/)

European Bioinformatics Institute (http://www.ebi.ac.uk/)

References

1. Frank, R., Hargreaves, R. (2003) Clinical biomarkers in drug discovery and development. *Nat Rev Drug Discov* 2, 566–580.
2. Roberts, R. J. (2005) How restriction enzymes became the workhorses of molecular biology. *Proc Natl Acad Sci USA* 102, 5905–5908; Danna, K., Nathans, D. (1971) *Proc Natl Acad Sci USA* 68, 2913–2917; Smith, H. O., Wilcox, K. W. (1970) *J Mol Biol* 51, 379–391.
3. Lander, E. S., Linton, L. M., Birren, B., et al. (2001) Initial sequencing and analysis of the human genome. *Nature* 409, 860–921.
4. Ellegren, H. (2004) Microsatellites: simple sequences with complex evolution. *Nat Rev Genet* 5, 435–445.
5. Waterston, R. H., Lindblad-Toh, K., Birney, E., et al. (2002) Initial sequencing and comparative analysis of the mouse genome. *Nature* 420, 520–562.
6. Gibbs, R. A., Weinstock, G. M., Metzker, M. L., et al. (2004) Genome sequence of the Brown Norway rat yields insights into mammalian evolution. *Nature* 428, 493–521.
7. Litt, M., Luty, J. A. (1989) A hypervariable microsatellite revealed by in vitro amplification of a dinucleotide repeat within the cardiac muscle actin gene. *Am J Hum Genet* 44, 397–401.
8. Weissenbach, J., Gyapay, G., Dib, C., et al. (1992) A second-generation linkage map of the human genome. *Nature* 359, 794–801.
9. Davies, J. L., Kawaguchi, Y., Bennett, S. T., et al. (1994) A genome-wide search for human type 1 diabetes susceptibility genes. *Nature* 371, 130–136.

10. Ogura, Y., Bonen, D. K., Inohara, N., et al (2001) A frameshift mutation in NOD2 associated with susceptibility to Crohn's disease. *Nature* 411, 603–606.
11. Kelkar, Y. D., Tyekucheva, S., Chiaromonte, F., Makova, K. D. (2008) The genome-wide determinants of human and chimpanzee microsatellite evolution. *Genome Res* 18, 30–38.
12. Molla, M., Delcher, A., Sunyaev, S., et al. (2009) Triplet repeat length bias and variation in the human transcriptome. *Proc Natl Acad Sci USA* 106, 17095–17100.
13. Day, I. N. (2010) dbSNP in the detail and copy number complexities. *Hum Mutat* 31, 2–4.
14. Hawkins, R. D., Hon, G. C., Ren, B. (2010) Next-generation genomics: an integrative approach. *Nat Rev Genet* 11, 476–486.
15. Duret, L. (2009) Mutation patterns in the human genome: more variable than expected. *PLoS Biol* 7, e1000028.
16. Walser, J. C., Furano, A. V. (2010) The mutational spectrum of non-CpG DNA varies with CpG content. *Genome Res*20, 875–882.
17. Roberts, R. J., Vincze, T., Posfai, J., Macelis, D. (2010) REBASE – a database for DNA restriction and modification: enzymes, genes and genomes. *Nucleic Acids Res* 38, D234–236.
18. Benson, G. (1999) Tandem repeats finder: a program to analyze DNA sequences. *Nucleic Acids Res* 27, 573–580.
19. Sherry, S. T., Ward, M. H., Kholodov, M., et al. (2001) dbSNP: the NCBI database of genetic variation. *Nucleic Acids Res* 29, 308–311.
20. Altshuler, D., Brooks, L. D., Chakravarti, A., et al. (2005) A haplotype map of the human genome. *Nature* 437, 1299–1320.
21. Zeggini, E., Rayner, W., Morris, A. P., et al. (2005) An evaluation of HapMap sample size and tagging SNP performance in large-scale empirical and simulated data sets. *Nat Genet* 37, 1320–1322.
22. The Wellcome Trust Case Control Consortium (2007) Genome-wide association study of 14,000 cases of seven common diseases and 3,000 shared controls. *Nature* 447, 661–678.
23. McCarthy, M. I., Abecasis, G. R., Cardon, L. R., et al. (2008) Genome-wide association studies for complex traits: consensus, uncertainty and challenges. *Nat Rev Genet* 9, 356–369.
24. Hindorff, L. A., Sethupathy, P., Junkins, H. A., et al. (2009) Potential etiologic and functional implications of genome-wide association loci for human diseases and traits. *Proc Natl Acad Sci USA* 106, 9362–9367.
25. Barrett, J. C., Fry, B., Maller, J., Daly, M. J. (2005) Haploview: analysis and visualization of LD and haplotype maps. *Bioinformatics* 21, 263–265.
26. de Bakker, P. I., Yelensky, R., Pe'er, I., et al. (2005) Efficiency and power in genetic association studies. *Nat Genet* 37, 1217–1223.
27. Voight, B. F., Kudaravalli, S., Wen, X., Pritchard, J. K. (2006) A map of recent positive selection in the human genome. *PLoS Biol* 4, e72.
28. Pickrell, J. K., Coop, G., Novembre, J., et al. (2009) Signals of recent positive selection in a worldwide sample of human populations. *Genome Res* 19, 826–837.
29. Coop, G., Pickrell, J. K., Novembre, J., et al. (2009) The role of geography in human adaptation. *PLoS Genet* 5, e1000500.
30. Via, M., Gignoux, C., Burchard, E. G. (2010) The 1000 Genomes Project: new opportunities for research and social challenges. *Genome Med* 2, 3.
31. Redon, R., Ishikawa, S., Fitch, K. R., et al. (2006) Global variation in copy number in the human genome. *Nature* 444, 444–454.
32. Conrad, D. F., Pinto, D., Redon, R., et al. (2010) Origins and functional impact of copy number variation in the human genome. *Nature* 464, 704–712.
33. Iafrate, A. J., Feuk, L., Rivera, M. N., et al. (2004) Detection of large-scale variation in the human genome. *Nat Genet* 36, 949–951.
34. The International Cancer Genome Consortium (2010) International network of cancer genome projects. *Nature* 464, 993–998.
35. Golub, T. (2010) Counterpoint: Data first. *Nature* 464, 679.
36. Stratton, M. R., Campbell, P. J., Futreal, P. A. (2009) The cancer genome. *Nature* 458, 719–724.
37. Spencer, C. C., Deloukas, P., Hunt, S., et al. (2006) The influence of recombination on human genetic diversity. *PLoS Genet* 2, e148.
38. Musumeci, L., Arthur, J. W., Cheung, F. S., et al. (2010) Single nucleotide differences (SNDs) in the dbSNP database may lead to errors in genotyping and haplotyping studies. *Hum Mutat* 31, 67–73.
39. Gabriel, S. B., Schaffner, S. F., Nguyen, H., et al. (2002) The structure of haplotype blocks in the human genome. *Science* 296, 2225–2229.

Chapter 2

Linkage Analysis

Jennifer H. Barrett and M. Dawn Teare

Abstract

Linkage analysis is used to map genetic loci using observations on relatives. It can be applied to both major gene disorders (parametric linkage) and complex diseases (model-free or non-parametric linkage), and it can be based on either a relatively small number of microsatellite markers or a denser map of single nucleotide polymorphisms (SNPs). We describe the methods commonly used to map loci influencing disease susceptibility or a quantitative trait. Application of these methods to simulated but realistic datasets is illustrated in some detail using the program Merlin. We provide some guidance on the best methods to use in different situations and on the interpretation of output.

Key words: Linkage analysis, genetic mapping, parametric, non-parametric, Merlin, quantitative traits.

1. Introduction

Genetic linkage analysis observes the segregation of alleles at meiosis to infer the distances between genetic loci. In the context of disease or trait gene mapping, a panel of established genetic markers (i.e. ones where the chromosomal location is known) are used to effectively label the participants' genomes so that the segregation of genetic material can be observed or followed (*see* **Chapter 1** for more discussion on genetic markers). In the genetic analysis of quantitative traits, the families may be a random population sample. However, in most disease mapping studies, the families have been selected due to the presence of the trait of interest occurring in at least one of the family members. The linkage analysis consists of studying the pattern of co-inheritance of marker alleles and the presence/absence or quantitative measure of a phenotype. The evidence against the null hypothesis (that the risk locus is unlinked to this position) is then reported at

B. Yu, M. Hinchcliffe (eds.), *In Silico Tools for Gene Discovery*, Methods in Molecular Biology 760,
DOI 10.1007/978-1-61779-176-5_2, © Springer Science+Business Media, LLC 2011

each examined position in the genome. In the context of linkage analysis the term genome does not include mitochondrial DNA.

In this chapter, two forms of linkage analysis are presented: parametric (or model based) and non-parametric (model-free). Parametric linkage analysis requires the investigator to specify the genetic model in advance of mapping the locus. For simple fully penetrant Mendelian traits (such as recessive or dominant traits), there is frequent evidence from clinical experience to support the assumed mode of inheritance. In more common diseases where only a component of the disease risk is attributable to genetic causes, the genetic model can be estimated through segregation analyses or familial aggregation studies. Before its characterisation it is usual to assume that the genetic risk locus will have only two alleles: the common normal form or wild type (denoted by **d**) and the mutant risk-associated form (**D**). There are four model parameters which must be specified. These are the population allele frequency of the **D** allele, and the probabilities of being affected (penetrances) for each of the three genotypes: **dd**, **Dd**, and **DD**. For a simple dominant fully penetrant disorder the respective penetrances would be 0, 1, and 1. A dominant disorder with incomplete penetrance of 80% would have penetrances specified by 0, 0.8, and 0.8. The allele frequency parameter can be estimated from population incidence. In complex disease it is common to allow for a sporadic rate of disease, which means that there is risk of disease in the **dd** genotype, so the corresponding penetrance is greater than zero. In addition, the risk for the **Dd** and **DD** genotypes is generally relatively low, and the penetrance of the **DD** genotype is often higher than that of the **Dd** genotype.

In parametric linkage, the alleles present in an individual at the disease locus are not observed directly but can be inferred through the individual's observed phenotype, the genetic risk model, and the pattern of inheritance of phenotypes in the family. In its simplest form, genetic linkage analysis or mapping attempts to estimate the genetic distance between a pair of loci by studying informative meioses and counting recombinations. An informative meiosis requires heterozygous genotypes at both marker and disease locus. The recombination fraction represents the probability of a gametic recombination of alleles occurring between a pair of loci during meiosis. If the recombination fraction equals $^1/_2$, then recombinants and non-recombinants are equally likely and the two loci are said to be unlinked. The smaller the recombination fraction the closer two loci are located along the same chromosome.

When considering several loci along the same chromosome, it is more common to see genetic distance reported than the recombination fraction. The recombination fractions between each pair of loci can be transformed to the additive genetic distance (and vice versa) by an appropriate mapping function such as Haldane or

Kosambi (2). Genetic distance is reported in centiMorgans (cM), where a recombination fraction of 0.01 is equivalent to 1 cM.

The statistical evidence for linkage is traditionally reported as a maximum LOD (logarithm of the odds) score. The LOD score function summarises the statistical evidence resulting from the joint analysis of all of the families. It compares the evidence that the disease risk locus resides at a specific location with the evidence that it resides at an unlinked part of the genome (i.e. on a different chromosome or a very distant part of the same chromosome). Parametric linkage analysis is very powerful for mapping rare risk loci with strong effects (3). It can also be successful in detecting linkage when there is locus heterogeneity, i.e. when distinct genes can independently give rise to the same phenotype. To allow for heterogeneity in the parametric framework, an additional parameter is estimated, which is the proportion of families linked (α). The evidence for linkage is assessed by computation of a heterogeneity LOD score (or HLOD). The value of the LOD score captures the evidence of linkage: a high positive score is evidence for linkage and a large negative score is evidence against. For the early years when genetic markers were not so numerous, the threshold of '+3' was required to be reached to declare evidence of linkage. Since the availability of high-density genomic markers, several authors reviewed the thresholds for a variety of study designs (4, 5). Empirical p values associated with a peak LOD score can now be calculated post-linkage analysis by simulation.

Though a parametric heterogeneity LOD score analysis can detect linkage if a small proportion of families are unlinked to the candidate region, a dramatic loss in power is seen as the unlinked proportion increases. Once substantial genetic heterogeneity is suspected (generally after parametric linkage analysis has been unsuccessful), a non-parametric or model-free approach is favoured. In this context non-parametric means that a genetic model is not specified. The model-free approach studies the pattern of alleles shared identical by descent (IBD) between pairs or groups of relatives. Relatives may carry copies of alleles that are descended from recent common ancestors, and such alleles are said to be IBD. Assuming neutral alleles and random mating, the expected IBD sharing probabilities for any pair (or group) of relatives can be calculated (6). Non-parametric linkage requires at least two affected relatives per family, the hypothesis being that, if there is an inherited genetic component to the disease, increased IBD sharing between affected relatives will be seen in the genomic location of the risk loci. In the model-free context, the evidence to support linkage can also be reported with LOD scores, but often a Z-score is reported. It is important to be clear as to whether one is reporting a LOD score or a Z-score, as the thresholds corresponding to the same p values are different.

2. Materials

There are many available software packages for linkage analysis, most of which are freely available. These include Linkage (7), one of the earliest linkage analysis programs, with a faster adaptation in Fastlink (8), Genehunter (9), which is widely used for non-parametric linkage analysis, and Allegro (10) (a faster and modified version of this), Morgan (11), which uses Monte Carlo Markov Chain methods and is suited to handle large complex pedigrees, Solar (12) for quantitative trait linkage analysis and Merlin (1), which can cope with very large numbers of marker loci. A more comprehensive list can be found on the Web site http://www.nslij-genetics.org/soft/. We have chosen to use Merlin to illustrate the methods outlined in this chapter, since Merlin is simple to use, has good documentation, can be used in a variety of computing environments, is very fast, and can be used to carry out a wide range of different analyses. The principles we discuss are general, and many of the methods can be implemented similarly in other software; although each program has its own particular features, there is also a degree of consistency in file formats used.

The methods behind Merlin are described in detail elsewhere (1) but the program uses a fast algorithm based on sparse trees to represent the flow of genes through pedigrees. The methodology enables Merlin to handle large numbers of markers such as are found in more recent linkage analyses based on single nucleotide polymorphisms (SNPs) (*see* **Section 3.3**). Besides parametric and non-parametric linkage analysis of binary traits (**Sections 3.4** and **3.1**, respectively), Merlin can be used for quantitative trait linkage analysis (**Section 3.2**) and for simulation and has additional capabilities not discussed here such as error detection and haplotype estimation.

The methods described here are illustrated by applying them to a simulated dataset derived from a large affected sibling pair study of cardiovascular disease (13). The study design was to collect pairs of siblings both of whom were affected by cardiovascular disease before age 66 years. Altogether over 4000 individuals were collected in 1933 families; parents were not genotyped. Some families had three or more affected siblings, some siblings were found to be half-siblings and recoded as such, and a small number of multi-generational families were identified. For the purposes of this analysis, data were used from chromosome 10, including the marker map and independently ascertained allele frequencies for the 20 microsatellite markers used in the original study. Using the simulation facility in Merlin, a disease locus was simulated at position 120 cM, between markers 13 and 14, with a genetic relative risk of 2 (penetrances assumed to be 0.001, 0.002 and 0.004 for the three genotypes) and allele frequency of 0.1. Genotypes were simulated conditional on the observed affection status of individuals in the family, preserving the family structures and pattern of missing genotype data in the original study. For the analysis described in **Section 3.2**, Merlin was again used to simulate a quantitative trait using the same family structures and patterns of missing data. We assumed that 20% of the variance of the trait was accounted for by a SNP, with minor allele frequency 0.3, again at position 120 cM, with polygenic effects explaining in total 30% of the variance (The locus-specific effect is actually much stronger than we might expect to find, but quantitative trait linkage analysis based on this study design would have low power to detect

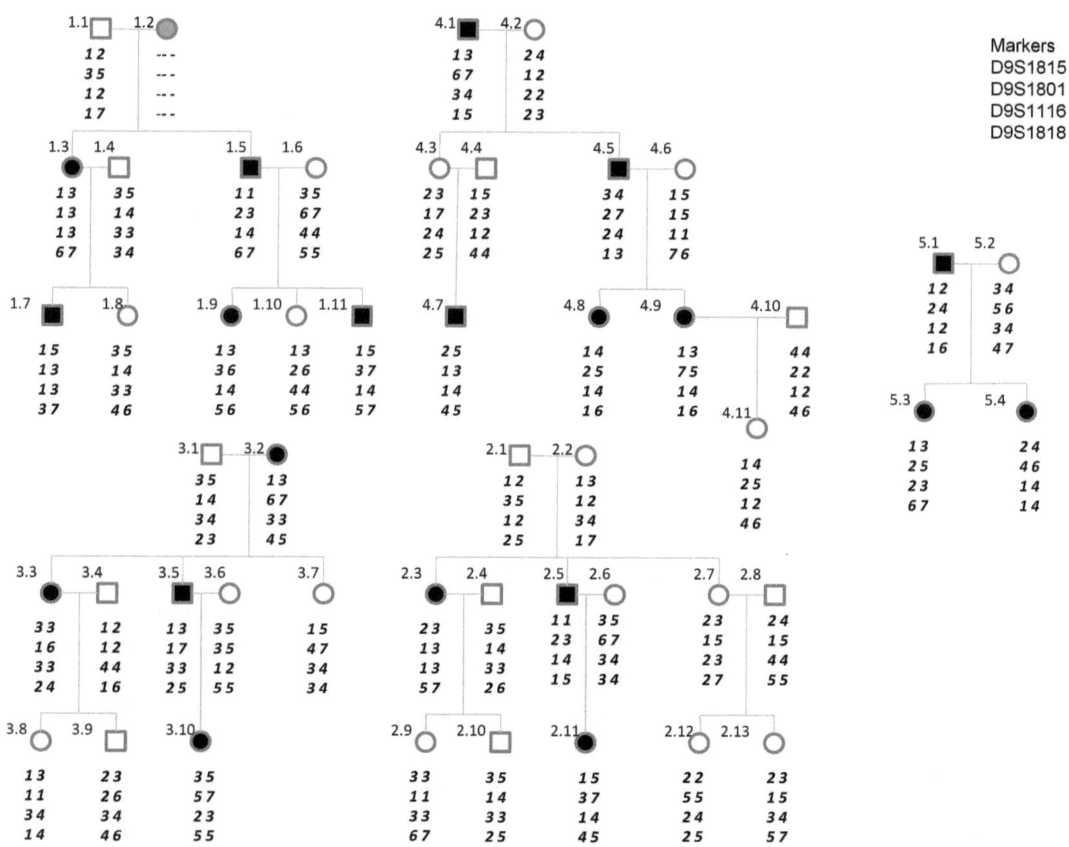

Fig. 2.1. The figure displays five families segregating a rare dominant disorder labelled ACC. *Squares* represent males and *circles* represent females. *Black-filled shapes* indicate the person is affected with the disorder. *Non-filled shapes* indicate the person is not affected, and grey shading indicates the status with respect to the phenotype is unknown. Below each person is a column of genotypes for the chromosome 9 markers D9S1815, D9S1901, D9S1116 and D9S1818. Information about these and other microsatellite markers can be found at http://research.marshfieldclinic.org/genetics. The index number to the *top left* of each individual is of the form 'x.y', where 'x' is the family ID and 'y' is the individual ID within the pedigree. The person labelled 1.2 is of unknown phenotype and unknown genotype. She is still required to be entered into the analysis so that 1.3 and 1.5 are correctly analysed as full siblings.

a weaker effect.). The simulated datasets are available for download (details can be found at http://limm.leeds.ac.uk/research_sections/epidemiology_and_biostatistics/groups/barrett.htm).

The dataset simulated for the parametric example (**Fig. 2.1**) consists of five pedigrees segregating a rare autosomal dominant trait. Members of the families have been genotyped at four microsatellite markers on chromosome 9. The column of numbers below each person lists the genotype observed at each marker.

3. Methods

3.1. Non-parametric Linkage Analysis

Non-parametric or *model-free* linkage analysis refers to the investigation of linkage without specification of a disease model. As explained earlier, regardless of the mode of inheritance, pairs of relatives affected by the disease are expected to show greater sharing of haplotypes that are IBD in the region of the disease gene. Various methods test whether IBD sharing at a locus is greater than expected under the null hypothesis of no linkage. Non-parametric linkage analysis requires family data where more than one individual in the family is affected, but it does not require large pedigrees. It is suitable for complex diseases where risk is influenced by a number of genes, usually in addition to environmental factors.

The simplest approach is to study sibling pairs, both of whom are affected. At any locus, according to the null hypothesis of no linkage, the number of alleles shared IBD by a pair of siblings is 0, 1 or 2, with probabilities 0.25, 0.5 and 0.25, respectively. If IBD sharing in the families is known, evidence for excess sharing at any locus can be tested by comparing the observed proportions with these expectations. In practice, IBD sharing usually has to be estimated, either because parental genotypes are unknown or because the markers are not sufficiently polymorphic.

There are several steps to carrying out linkage analysis:

1. Create files for analysis

   The key information is contained in a pedigree file, which includes the pedigree structure and all individual genotypes. The file contains one row for every individual in the pedigrees, including those with no genotype information but whose offspring are included. The format of the file is common to most linkage analysis software and contains the following fields: *Pedigree, Individual, Father, Mother, Sex*, followed by affection status and genotype information.

   The first four columns contain identifiers for the family, the individual, their father and their mother. For founders (first generation in the pedigree), the parental codes are set to 0. The following field by convention contains the individual's sex (1 for male, 2 for female and 0 for unknown), generally followed by a field for affection status (1 for unaffected, 2 for affected and 0 for unknown). The genotype information follows, recording the two alleles for each marker, either in two separate columns or concatenated (e.g. "1/3"). An example of such a file can be found in *chr10-grr2.ped*.

Merlin also requires a file containing information about the structure of the pedigree file. This allows for more flexibility so that, for example, quantitative phenotypes can be included as well as or instead of affection status and the order of the fields can be specified (*see* **Section 3.2**). This basic data file contains descriptions of the fields in the pedigree file; the first five columns up to and including sex are taken as read. Each line begins either "A" (for affection), "T" (for quantitative trait) or "M" (for marker) and is followed by the name of the disease, trait or marker respectively. An example of such a file is *chr10-grr2.dat*, which describes a file such as *chr10-grr2.ped*, with 20 markers and affection status (named "disease").

Information may also be required about the markers genotyped, in the form of a genetic map and allele frequencies. In Merlin the marker map can consist of three columns listing for each marker the chromosome, the marker name and the position (in cM), headed "CHR," "MARKER" and "POS" (*see chr10-replicate.map*).

2. Check data integrity
   Prior to running analyses it is advisable to check that the data are as expected. This can be done using the pedstats program (14) (available with Merlin):

   >pedstats -d chr10-grr2.dat -p chr10-grr2.ped

   The program output confirms that there are 8352 individuals, consisting of 4071 founders and 4281 non-founders, in 1983 pedigrees, mainly (99.7%) of 2 generations (the remainder with 3 generations), and with family size ranging from 3 to 9. Most pedigrees (81.4%) are of size 4, and 4223 individuals (50.6%) are affected, reflecting the affected sibling pair ascertainment scheme. For each marker the proportion of subjects genotyped is given, together with the proportion of founders genotyped. Finally heterozygosity is calculated, which reflects the degree of polymorphism and hence informativeness of the marker.

3. Analysis options
   Before carrying out the linkage analysis various choices are to be made regarding method of analysis:

a. Single-point or multipoint analysis
In single-point analysis each marker is analysed separately. It is generally preferable to use multipoint analysis, which makes use of the marker map and the information from all markers in the region to estimate IBD sharing, potentially more accurately (*see* **Note 1**). For multipoint analysis the points along the chromosome at which IBD sharing is estimated can be specified either as the number of points between markers (--steps n) or as equally spaced points (--grid n for every n cM).
b. Allele frequency estimation
Allele frequencies can either be obtained from an independent source and supplied in a file or be estimated from the dataset (*see* **Note 2**). The allele frequency file contains two rows for each marker: one giving the marker name preceded by "M" and one listing the frequencies in order preceded by "F" (*see chrom10.freq*). An alternative format, which may be preferable for highly polymorphic markers, is illustrated for the same markers in *chr10-grr2.freq*. If this information is not provided then estimates are obtained by counting across all individuals (the default), across all founders (-ff option) or by maximum likelihood (-fm).
c. Statistical analysis
The original idea behind non-parametric linkage analysis is to take pairs of related affected individuals and compare their (estimated) IBD sharing with the expected distribution under the null hypothesis. Each pedigree is assigned a score that measures IBD sharing, and the test for linkage is based on comparing this score with the expected score according to the null hypothesis (combining over pedigrees) (*see* **Note 3**). If IBD information is complete, then, under the null hypothesis, the resulting non-parametric-linkage test statistic is normally distributed with mean of 0 and variance of 1, for large enough samples sizes. In the absence of complete information, the test as initially proposed is conservative. In response to this, the approach has been modified to provide accurate likelihood-based tests which are implemented in Merlin (*see* **Note 4**).

4. Running the analysis
Once the input files have been correctly constructed, carrying out the analysis is simple and fast. The command below, for example, carries out a multipoint non-parametric linkage analysis based on the IBD sharing among all affected individuals in each family, using allele frequencies specified in *chr10-grr2.freq*:

merlin -d chr10-grr2.dat -p chr10-grr2.ped -m chr10-grr2.map -f chr10-grr2.freq --npl --steps 3 --tabulate --pdf --prefix grr2

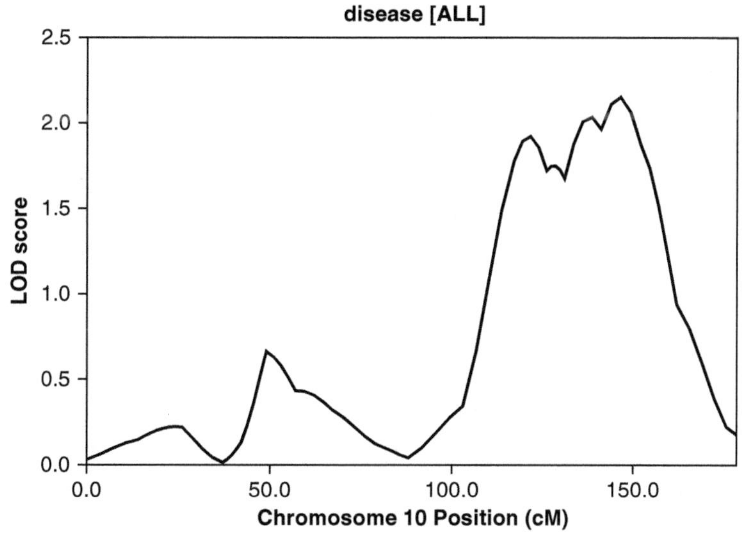

Fig. 2.2. Output from Merlin showing LOD score along the chromosome from non-parametric linkage analysis of a binary disease trait.

The main output from the program is now available in a file named *grr2-nonparametric.tbl* and the graphical representation in **Fig. 2.2** is saved to file *grr2.pdf*.

5. Interpretation of output

   At each point along the chromosome at which analysis has been requested (e.g. in the above example at each marker and 3 points between them, as specified by the **step 3** option), four measures are given: the *Z*-score, delta, LOD score, and *p* value. The *Z*-score is based on the non-parametric linkage statistic as proposed by Whittemore and Halpern (15) which should follow a standard normal distribution under the null hypothesis of no linkage. Delta is the parameter of interest in the allele-sharing model proposed by Kong and Cox (16) (*see* **Note 4**), taking the value 0 under the null hypothesis; and the LOD score and *p* value refer to tests of this hypothesis.

   For the example above, **Fig. 2.2** shows that the linkage peak is quite broad. The maximum LOD score of 2.15 ($p = 0.0008$) is attained at position 146.5 cM, between markers D10S1693 and D10S587 (*see* **Note 5**). This is simulated data, and in fact the true location of the marker is at 120 cM, where the evidence for linkage is slightly weaker (LOD score $\sim = 1.9$, $p \sim = 0.002$). It is common to find in linkage analysis that the highest signal occurs some distance from the disease locus (17).

The conclusion of this analysis would be that there is some suggestive evidence of linkage in the broad region covered by the peak in **Fig. 2.2**, although the evidence is not significant at the genome-wide level (*see* **Note 6**).

3.2. Quantitative Traits

Analysis of a quantitative trait can also be carried out without assuming a genetic model, and various different approaches to this have been proposed and are implemented in Merlin. The variance components approach is applicable to general pedigrees; the trait covariance matrix between relatives in the pedigree is modelled as a component due to a specific chromosomal region (on the basis of estimated IBD sharing at the locus) and a component due to other unlinked genes (on the basis of degree of kinship, see for example Almasy and Blangero (12)).

For sibling pairs, the classical Haseman–Elston method was based on regression of the squared difference in trait values between the two siblings on the estimated proportion of alleles they share IBD at a locus (18); numerous extensions and variations of this method have been proposed, and Merlin includes a separate regression program (Merlin-Regress) that implements one of these (19). In this approach, multivariate regression is used to regress the estimated IBD sharing among all pairs of relatives in the pedigree on the squared difference and the squared sum of trait values of the relative pairs.

To carry out linkage analysis of a quantitative trait, most of the steps are similar to those described above for binary traits. The pedigree file will now contain the following fields: *Pedigree, Individual, Father, Mother, Sex, Trait,* in addition to genotype information and possibly affection status. As before another file must also be constructed describing the pedigree file; the file *chr10-qtl.dat* for example describes the structure of *chr10-qtl.ped.* Data integrity can be checked as before using pedstats, which now also reports the minimum, maximum, mean and variance of the trait values in the pedigree file and an estimate of correlation between siblings.

For the statistical analysis, variance components analysis can be selected using the --vc option:

merlin -d chr10-qtl.dat -p chr10-qtl.ped -m chr10-qtl.map -f chr10-qtl.freq --vc --steps 3 --tabulate --pdf --prefix traitvc

The on-screen output reports that overall heritability of the trait is estimated to be 33.1% (true value in simulation 30%). At each analysis point four measures are estimated: H2, which is an estimate of locus-specific heritability, the chi-squared statistic, corresponding LOD score and associated p value (for a one-sided test of heritability greater than zero). From **Fig. 2.3** it can be seen that the linkage peak is at 117 cM, quite close to the true locus at 120 cM; the estimated locus-specific heritability here is 15.7% (true value 20%), $p = 0.004$.

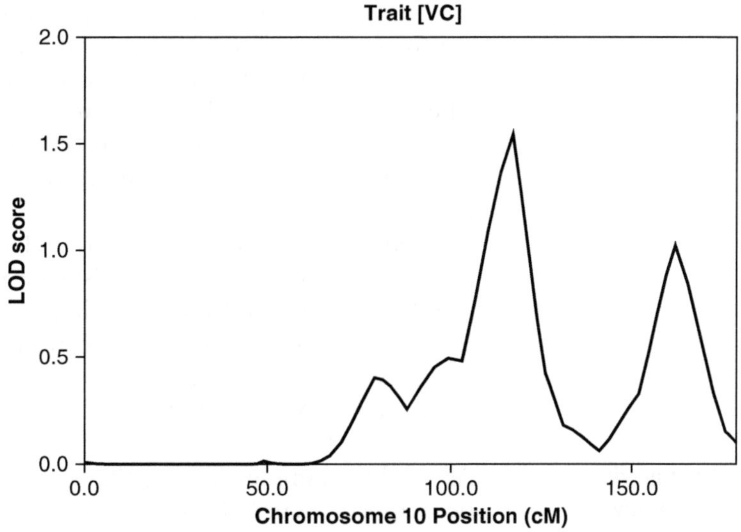

Fig. 2.3. Output from Merlin showing LOD score from quantitative trait linkage analysis.

A disadvantage of the variance components approach is that the method is inappropriate for samples selected on the basis of their phenotype; the method implemented in Merlin-regress by contrast is robust to sample selection. Using the same data files, the analysis can be run using the following command:

merlin-regress -d chr10-qtl.dat -p chr10-qtl.ped -m chr10-qtl.map -f chr10-qtl.freq --steps 3 --randomSample --tabulate --pdf --prefix traitregress

For this dataset of unselected samples and sibling pairs, the methods give almost identical results, but the regression analysis has the advantage of being many times faster.

For a sample selected on phenotype, "--randomSample" would be replaced by estimates of the mean, variance and heritability of the trait in the population, e.g.:

merlin-regress -d chr10-qtl.dat -p chr10-qtl.ped -m chr10-qtl.map -f chr10-qtl.freq --steps 3 --mean0.0 --var1.0 --her 0.3 --tabulate --pdf --prefix traitregress

The choice of appropriate method may also be influenced by the distribution of the trait (*see* **Note 7**).

3.3. Linkage Analysis Using Single Nucleotide Polymorphisms

Linkage analysis is now often carried out using a dense set of SNPs instead of a smaller number of microsatellite markers (20). Although the basic methods are no different, one complication that arises is that the SNP markers are likely to be in linkage disequilibrium (LD). It has been shown that ignoring the LD between SNPs can lead to false positive linkage signals (21).

In Merlin, this problem is approached by creating clusters of contiguous correlated markers and then assuming that there is no recombination within the clusters and no LD between clusters. These assumptions will only be approximately correct; data which violate the assumptions, such as obligatory recombination events within the clusters, can be analysed by setting such genotypes to missing.

Clusters can be created either based on distance (i.e. any markers within a very small distance of each other are formed into one cluster, and the map file is adjusted so that these markers are mapped to the same location) or on the r^2 measure of LD between them. The clusters can be defined independently or generated from the data by Merlin.

3.4. Parametric Linkage Analysis

As in the examples above, the genetic markers are assumed to be mapped accurately, so the order and distances between each locus are specified in the '.map' file and the evidence for linkage is computed at many locations within the range of the genetic markers. The format of the pedigree (.ped) file is the same as before. The individuals are coded as affected (2), unaffected (1) and unknown (0). Here it is assumed that the marker allele frequencies have been independently estimated, but in this example estimating the alleles from the data will make very little difference as only one person is not directly genotyped. The parametric model is assumed to be rare dominant (labelled 'ACC' in .model file) with allele frequency 0.005. There is no sporadic rate, and carriers have incomplete penetrance of 90%. The analysis is performed with the command below:

merlin --d rd5.dat --p rd5.ped --m rd5.map --f rd5.freq --model rd5.model --step 3

The output is listed on the screen. The default is to list both LODs and HLODs. The '**Step 3**' option delivers 3 evenly spaced Scores per marker. The -perFamily option prints the LOD scores by family to a file.

```
Parametric Analysis, Model rare-dom
```

Position	LOD	Alpha	HLOD
99.400	-11.483	0.150	0.243
103.718	-3.177	0.299	0.523
108.035	-2.206	0.386	0.819
112.353	-2.061	0.429	1.082
116.670	-3.642	0.448	1.316
120.133	1.414	0.726	1.967

123.595	2.238	0.789	2.632
127.058	2.622	0.796	3.071
130.520	2.478	0.780	3.393
135.620	2.945	0.832	3.178
140.720	2.644	0.848	2.807
145.820	1.851	0.816	2.105
150.920	-3.713	0.174	0.111

The maximum LOD score of 2.945 is reported at position 135.620. When allowing for heterogeneity, the maximum HLOD is reported one step away at 130.520. Allowing for heterogeneity, there appears to be marginally significant evidence of linkage to this region. The maximum likelihood estimate of the proportion linked is 78%, and the strongest evidence is coincident with marker D9S1116. The true location of the risk locus in the simulations was between the two markers D9S1801and D9S1116 (position 125.00), and two of the five families were unlinked to this locus. Examining the individual by family LOD scores at this position, it can be seen which families provide the evidence for and against linkage. Examining the LOD scores, post analysis, by family is useful for identifying those who are currently not very informative and may benefit from more genotyping at intervening markers. In this dataset, family 5 shows strong evidence against linkage as the two affected offspring do not share any alleles IBD (**Fig. 2.1**).

4. Notes

1. In the Introduction linkage analysis is described with respect to two loci, but it is now usually performed in multipoint form (multiple markers per chromosomal region) as this provides much better information on the origin of each chromosomal segment segregating through a family, and much better estimates of IBD sharing. Multipoint linkage analysis is quite sensitive to the correctness of the map on which it is based, so if there are doubts about the accuracy of the map it may be wise to compare results from multipoint and single-point analyses.
2. If good estimates of allele frequencies, applicable to the population from which the families are drawn, can be obtained independently, then these should be used. In the absence of such estimates, frequencies can be estimated from the dataset itself, especially if the sample size is large. However this can

lead to a conservative test for linkage, since the frequencies of any alleles associated with disease will tend to be overestimated.

3. When larger numbers of affected relatives are included within a family, a more powerful alternative to pairwise analysis has been proposed, which considers the sharing of alleles among all affected relatives in the family. This is based on a score that increases more sharply as the number of affected members sharing the same allele IBD increases (15).
4. Kong and Cox (16) proposed an alternative approach to overcome the conservative nature of the "NPL" scores in the presence of incomplete genotype data. For any of the proposed scores, a one-parameter model can be constructed, the free parameter (δ) of which is chosen such that $\delta = 0$ under the null hypothesis of no linkage and $\delta > 0$ in the presence of linkage. The test of $\delta = 0$ is carried out by a likelihood ratio test, and can be converted to a traditional $\log_{10}$ LOD score, for comparability with parametric methods. Two versions of the model are proposed, known as the linear and the exponential models. In most situations very similar results are obtained from the two approaches and the linear model would be used; the exponential model allows δ to take large values, and may be preferable given a small number of pedigrees with extreme IBD sharing.
5. Slightly different results are obtained from the *Z*-score, where the peak is at 140 cM with a *Z*-score of 2.51 (*p* value 0.006). In general, the LOD score analysis is to be preferred.
6. As mentioned in the Introduction, evidence for linkage can now be evaluated by calculating empirical *p* values, which avoids the need to agree LOD score thresholds for declaring significant evidence of linkage. Data are simulated under the null hypothesis of no linkage preserving the original data structure, and the LOD score is compared with the distribution of LOD scores obtained from the analysis of many such simulated datasets to obtain an empirical *p* value.
7. Although both the above methods assume normality of the trait, the regression method is more robust than variance components methods to departures from normality. An alternative approach also available in Merlin is an extension of the non-parametric methods for binary data and is based on comparing the IBD sharing among individuals at the tails of the trait distribution (*see* the --qtl option). This method is less commonly used and has the disadvantage of relatively low power but the advantage of avoiding distributional assumptions. When applied to the example dataset this method provides very little evidence for linkage.

References

1. Abecasis, G. R., Cherny, S. S., Cookson, W. O., and Cardon, L. R. (2002) Merlin-rapid analysis of dense genetic maps using sparse gene flow trees. *Nature Genetics* 30, 97–101.
2. Ott, J. (1999) *Analysis of Human Genetic Linkage*, Second ed. The Johns Hopkins University Press, Baltimore, MD.
3. Teare, M. D., and Barrett, J. H. (2005) Genetic epidemiology 2 – Genetic linkage studies. *Lancet* 366, 1036–1044.
4. Chiano, M. N., and Yates, J. R. W. (1995) Linkage detection under heterogeneity and the mixture problem. *Annals of Human Genetics* 59, 83–95.
5. Lander, E., and Kruglyak, L. (1995) Genetic dissection of complex traits – guidelines for interpreting and reporting linkage results. *Nature Genetics* 11, 241–247.
6. Cannings, C., and Thompson, E. A. (1981) *Genealogical and Genetic Structure*. Cambridge University Press, Cambridge.
7. Lathrop, G. M., and Lalouel, J. M. (1984) Easy calculations of lod scores and genetic risks on small computers. *American Journal of Human Genetics* 36, 460–465.
8. Cottingham, R. W., Idury, R. M., and Schaffer, A. A. (1993) Faster sequential genetic-linkage computations. *American Journal of Human Genetics* 53, 252–263.
9. Kruglyak, L., Daly, M. J., ReeveDaly, M. P., and Lander, E. S. (1996) Parametric and nonparametric linkage analysis: a unified multipoint approach. *American Journal of Human Genetics* 58, 1347–1363.
10. Gudbjartsson, D. F., Jonasson, K., Frigge, M. L., and Kong, A. (2000) Allegro, a new computer program for multipoint linkage analysis. *Nature Genetics* 25, 12–13.
11. Wijsman, E. M., Rothstein, J. H., and Thompson, E. A. (2006) Multipoint linkage analysis with many multiallelic or dense diallelic markers: Markov chain-Monte Carlo provides practical approaches for genome scans on general pedigrees. *American Journal of Human Genetics* 79, 846–858.
12. Almasy, L., and Blangero, J. (1998) Multipoint quantitative-trait linkage analysis in general pedigrees. *American Journal of Human Genetics* 62, 1198–1211.
13. The BHF Family Heart Study Research Group (2005) A genomewide linkage study of 1933 families affected by premature coronary artery disease: The British Heart Foundation (BHF) family heart study. *American Journal of Human Genetics* 77, 1011–1020.
14. Wigginton, J. E., and Abecasis, G. R. (2005) PEDSTATS: descriptive statistics, graphics and quality assessment for gene mapping data. *Bioinformatics* 21, 3445–3447.
15. Whittemore, A. S., and Halpern, J. (1994) A class of tests for linkage using affected pedigree members. *Biometrics* 50, 118–127.
16. Kong, A., and Cox, N. J. (1997) Allele-sharing models: LOD scores and accurate linkage tests. *American Journal of Human Genetics* 61, 1179–1188.
17. Roberts, S. B., MacLean, C. J., Neale, M. C., Eaves, L. J., and Kendler, K. S. (1999) Replication of linkage studies of complex traits: an examination of variation in location estimates. *American Journal of Human Genetics* 65, 876–884.
18. Haseman, J. K., and Elston, R. C. (1972) Investigation of linkage between a quantitative trait and a marker locus. *Behavior Genetics* 2, 3–19.
19. Sham, P. C., Purcell, S., Cherny, S. S., and Abecasis, G. R. (2002) Powerful regression-based quantitative-trait linkage analysis of general pedigrees. *American Journal of Human Genetics* 71, 238–253.
20. Schaid, D. J., Guenther, J. C., Christensen, G. B. et al (2004) Comparison of microsatellites versus single-nucleotide polymorphisms in a genome linkage screen for prostate cancer-susceptibility loci. *American Journal of Human Genetics* 75, 948–965.
21. Huang, Q., Shete, S., and Amos, C. I (2004) Ignoring linkage disequilibrium among tight linked markers induces false-positive evidence of linkage for affected sib pair analysis. *American Journal of Human Genetics* 75, 1106–1112.

Chapter 3

Association Mapping

Jodie N. Painter, Dale R. Nyholt, and Grant W. Montgomery

Abstract

Association mapping seeks to identify marker alleles present at significantly different frequencies in cases carrying a particular disease or trait compared with controls. Genome-wide association studies are increasingly replacing candidate gene-based association studies for complex diseases, where a number of loci are likely to contribute to disease risk and the effect size of each particular risk allele is typically modest or low. Good study design is essential to the success of an association study, and factors such as the heritability of the disease under investigation, the choice of controls, statistical power, multiple testing and whether the association can be replicated need to be considered before beginning. Likewise, thorough quality control of the genotype data needs to be undertaken prior to running any association analyses. Finally, it should be kept in mind that a significant genetic association is not proof positive that a particular genetic locus causes a disease, but rather an important first step in discovering the genetic variants underlying a complex disease.

Key words: Genetic association, allele, single nucleotide polymorphism (SNP), genotype, genome-wide association (GWA), genetic power.

1. Introduction

Association mapping seeks to identify marker alleles present at significantly different frequencies in cases carrying a particular phenotype (a disease or trait) compared with controls. This contrasts with linkage mapping (covered in **Chapter 2**) which searches for chromosomal regions shared by family members who are affected by the disease under study. Association mapping relies on linkage disequilibrium (LD), where some combinations of alleles at loci close together in the genome occur more often than by chance because of previous population history. A genetic marker close to and in LD with a causal variant will show significantly different allele frequencies in cases compared with appropriate control

B. Yu, M. Hinchcliffe (eds.), *In Silico Tools for Gene Discovery*, Methods in Molecular Biology 760,
DOI 10.1007/978-1-61779-176-5_3, © Springer Science+Business Media, LLC 2011

individuals. One consequence is that in a successful association mapping study the marker associated with a disease is unlikely to be the casual variant. The marker locus will likely be located close to the variant or variants contributing to disease risk, but further studies will be required to locate and characterise these casual variants.

Association studies can include family-based designs (1, 2). In general, case–control studies have greater power than family-based designs when genotyping equivalent numbers of individuals and for simplicity in this chapter we have restricted the discussion and examples to case–control studies. Association mapping designs range from genotyping a single marker in a 'candidate' gene through to genome-wide association (GWA) studies. Current GWA studies genotype 300,000–2,500,000 single nucleotide polymorphisms (SNPs) per individual, and this number will soon reach 5,000,000 SNPs per individual. Prior to the development of genotyping methods using high-density SNP 'chips', studies concentrated on genotyping markers in candidate genes chosen from an understanding of the biological mechanisms thought to contribute to the disease under study. Most studies genotyped small numbers of selected variants within the target gene and sample sizes were often low.

Genome-wide association strategies developed from advances in genotyping technology, greater understanding of the structure of common variation in the human genome and continued advances in computing power and software tools. The discoveries from many association studies in complex diseases clearly demonstrate that the effect size for common risk variants for most diseases is low with odds ratio's for the risk allele in the range of 1.1–1.5 (3–5). Large studies with several thousand cases and equivalent numbers of controls are required to have sufficient power to detect these small effects. For some traits, large international collaborations have developed to conduct association studies with samples sizes around 100,000 cases.

There are a number of different options for the analysis of association studies. However, as noted above, recent studies demonstrate that large sample sizes are necessary to have sufficient power to detect 'true' associations for most diseases. We have therefore discussed association mapping and provide examples using software that can be applied to both small and large studies.

2. Materials

The basic requirements for an association study are DNA genotypes and a computer with an Internet connection (in fact, many genetic data analysts work exclusively with electronic data!). First,

DNA samples must be extracted and genotyped to a high quality, and the methodology and techniques used to do both will depend on the scale of the project. While most laboratories are equipped to extract DNA and perform basic genotyping, a growing number of laboratories offer extraction and genotyping as a commercial service. This can be efficient for large-scale projects (*see* **Note 1**).

For association analyses there are a growing number of software programs being developed by commercial companies; however, all quality control and analysis stages can be either conducted using programs with a worldwide web interface or downloadable onto a personal computer directly from a Web site. Specialist software and the Web sites from which these are available will be presented in the relevant sections below (*see* **Note 2**).

3. Methods

3.1. Planning Your Study

Aspects that should be considered during the project planning phase are outlined briefly below, and the overall order of steps to perform an association study is shown in **Fig. 3.1**. There are now increasing numbers of reviews in the genetic literature dealing with specific aspects of association study design that should be referred to for more detail (*see* **Note 3**). These include reviews on issues to consider while planning association studies (6–9), data quality control (10), data analysis (11) and interpretation (4, 12) and replication analyses (13).

3.1.1. Selection of Cases and Controls

The first aspects to consider when designing an association study are that the trait or disease under investigation is heritable, and that all of your case subjects have the same phenotype. These seem obvious; however, complex diseases may have low levels of heritability and many are likely to be genetically heterogeneous and influenced by environmental risk factors. As a result, studies of complex diseases typically require extremely large sample sizes (e.g. 1000s of cases and controls) (10) in order to detect an association, particularly if the effect size is expected to be low. Careful phenotyping during case recruitment should reduce the risk of collecting a heterogeneous case sample, although the sample size attainable may need to be balanced with the cost of obtaining phenotypic information (e.g. clinical assessment versus detailed questionnaires).

Control subjects should ideally come from the same population as the cases to avoid issues of sample stratification (*see* **Section 3.1.2**). Controls can be ‘selected’, where each individual has been screened for the disease under investigation, or ‘unselected’, where individuals are taken from a general population

Study design stage:
- Collect well-phenotyped cases and appropriate controls
  1. Consider potential stratification issues
- Calculate the genetic power of the study
- Plan analyses considering significance levels and issues of multiple testing
- Chose SNPs
- Plan for replication testing of significant associations

↓

Genotyping quality control stage:
1. Perform lab-based quality control measures
- SNP genotypes clearly distinguishable?
1. Format data files according to the program to be used for analyses
2. Determine missing data rates for individuals
3. Determine missing data rates for markers
4. Perform Hardy-Weinberg tests in controls

Additional tests for GWA studies:
- Check missing data rates between cases and controls
- Remove individuals with excess homozygosity or heterozygosity rates
- Remove individuals mismatched for sex
- Remove ancestry outliers
- Remove related samples
- Remove SNPs with extremely low minor allele frequencies

↓

Association testing stage:
1. Perform appropriate test for association
   1. Case-control analyses
   2. Family-based tests (e.g. TDT tests)
   3. Haplotype-based tests
2. Perform meta-analyses for combined data sets taking population stratification into account

↓

Replication stage:
- Test significantly associated SNPs in an independent case-control group

↓

Plan future studies:
- Bioinformatic analyses to explore the genetic architecture of the associated region
- Further genotyping to search for the causal SNP
- Functional analyses to confirm causality

Fig. 3.1. Association study flow from initial planning to investigate a significant, replicated, association signal.

and for whom there is typically no information on disease status. Depending on the population prevalence a non-negligible proportion of unselected controls may carry the disease under investigation, hence a higher number of unselected controls is typically required than if controls are selected. The number of controls should equal or exceed the number of cases.

3.1.2. Stratification

Stratification refers to differences in allele frequencies of genetic variants between cases and controls due to the underlying sampling scheme, which may lead to false-positive signals of association. To avoid technical stratification resulting from systematic differences in the way samples are handled, the collection of biological samples, DNA extraction and subsequent storage and genotyping should be performed in the same manner (and where possible in the same laboratories) for both cases and controls. Where case and control datasets have been collected and processed separately, for example GWA studies using large publically available control datasets (14), the quality of the genotyping should be compared prior to conducting association analyses.

Cases and controls should also be matched for ancestry to avoid population stratification due to genetic admixture (15). The inclusion of subgroups of genetically distinct individuals may lead to false-positive signals of association particularly if one ancestral population is over-represented amongst either the case or the control groups. Apparent association signals may then be due to differences in frequencies at ancestry-informative alleles, which have systematic differences in frequencies amongst populations. Ancestry should be determined at the subject recruitment stage by including questions on the birthplace of the subject and/or the subject's parents and grand parents in questionnaires, although ancestry outliers can now easily be detected with GWA data (**Section 3.3.4**, QC measure 7).

3.1.3. Statistical Power

The power of a study is the probability of rejecting your null hypothesis (*Ho*: that there are *no* differences in allele frequencies between cases and controls) when it is false (i.e. when association between a gene or locus and a disease actually exists). Power calculations allow estimation of the power of the study given the sample size, frequency of the disease-associated allele and the effect size associated with the risk allele.

Power calculations should be performed over a range of allele frequencies and effect sizes, as these are typically unknown for complex diseases (*see* **Note 4**). The web-based Genetic Power Calculator (16) (http://pngu.mgh.harvard.edu/~purcell/gpc/) allows power to be estimated for a number of study types (e.g. case–control studies for discrete or quantitative traits and family-based studies), while the program Power for Association with Error (17) (http://linkage.rockefeller.edu/pawe/) calculates power in the presence of a small proportion of genotyping errors. Power for studies using a two-stage design, where a large number of SNPs are first genotyped in a case–control group (stage 1) and only the most promising SNPs subsequently genotyped in a larger, independent case–control group (stage 2), and under different genetic models can be calculated using the CaTS program (18) (http://www.sph.umich.edu/csg/abecasis/cats/). The program Quanto (http://hydra.usc.edu/GxE/)

allows power to be calculated in the presence of gene × environment or gene × gene interactions.

3.1.4. Significance and Multiple Testing

Multiple testing refers to the increasing number of hypotheses that can be tested in a genetic association study, such as testing for association with over 500,000 markers in a GWA study or testing multiple SNPs per gene or multiple subgroups for a particular disease. As multiple testing increases the chance of obtaining a false-positive result the significance threshold should take the number of tests performed into account (19). The simplest method is the 'Bonferroni' correction, where the pre-determined threshold for significance is divided by the number of tests performed. For example, the significance threshold for a study that genotyped 30 'tagging' SNPs (*see* **Section 3.1.5**) would require a p value lower than $0.05/30 = 0.00167$ to claim association with a type I error (false-positive) rate of 5%. However, this method can be overly conservative and result in stringent thresholds for evidence of association (19). More specifically, performing such a correction assumes that each test is completely ***independent*** of all others, which is typically not the case due to LD between SNPs located within the same genomic region. The web-based program SNPSpD (20) (http://gump.qimr.edu.au/general/daleN/SNPSpD/) allows p value correction in the presence of LD by estimating an 'effective' number of independent SNPs. However, this method may also result in overly conservative p values, hence permutation and/or simulation procedures are considered the 'gold standard', although these are generally computationally intensive. Significance thresholds for GWA studies can also be determined on a per-project basis using permutation, although values $<5\text{–}10 \times 10^{-8}$ (i.e. 0.05/500,000–1,000,000 independent tests) are often taken as evidence of significant association (21, 22).

The goal of such Bonferroni-type corrections and adjusted significance thresholds is to guard against any single false positive occurring. However, in the high-dimensional setting of GWA studies one may also aim to identify as many true positive findings as possible while incurring a relatively low number of false positives. The false discovery rate (FDR) (23, 24) is designed to quantify this type of trade-off, making this particularly useful to identify loci worth further investigation.

3.1.5. Choosing SNPs

Nowadays, association studies are typically performed using SNPs as the genetic marker (*see* **Chapter 1** for more discussion on genetic markers). Candidate gene/region studies may include SNPs chosen as biologically plausible candidates for which positive associations have previously been reported (usually as an attempt to replicate such a finding) and, increasingly, 'tagging' SNPs to comprehensively account for common genetic variation across a gene. Tagging relies on LD, the correlation between alleles at SNPs located in the same chromosomal region, and effectively reduces the numbers of SNPs that need to be typed as the genotype at one locus is highly correlated with loci in high LD, thus testing these loci too. Tagging can be performed through the HapMap database (http://www.hapmap.org) and using programs such as Haploview (25) (http://www.broadinstitute.org/haploview/haploview) or Goldsurfer2 (26) (http://www.well.ox.ac.uk/gs2/) (9). SNPs for GWA studies are provided on commercially produced genotyping chips designed to tag >90% of the common variation present in the human genome.

3.1.6. Replication

The gold standard for accepting that an association between a marker and a disease potentially exists and is worthy of further investigation is replication, where significant association to the same allele is detected in a completely independent case–control group. Many candidate gene associations fall down at this stage, as subsequent studies fail to replicate the initial findings. This may be due in part to the 'winner's curse', where the first report of an association is typically the most significant (27), or underlying risk alleles differing between populations. However, a careful review of associations that subsequently fail to replicate typically reveals that initial associations were either weak (with p values close to the significance threshold or where multiple testing was not taken into account) or underpowered due to low sample size. Replication studies should therefore be interpreted with respect to their level of power and whether there is strong statistical or biological evidence underpinning the original association.

3.2. Programs for Association Mapping Analyses

Association analyses test for differences in genotype or allele frequencies between cases and controls using for instance Chi-squared (χ^2) tests. For small numbers of SNPs, association tests can be performed by hand or using a pocket calculator by constructing a 2 × 2 table of allele counts. For the larger numbers of SNPs typically included in a candidate gene SNP tagging or GWA study, specialist analysis software is more practical. Any program that performs χ^2 tests can be used to test association, including SAS or SPSS. There are also a growing number of programs written specifically for the analysis of genetic association data, including plugins for the R package of statistical programs (e.g. GenABEL (28), http://mga.bionet.nsc.ru/~yurii/ABEL/GenABEL/) and SNPTEST (10, 29) (http://www.stats.ox.ac.uk/~marchini/software/gwas/snptest.html) for the analysis of GWA data or the web-based SNPStats (30) (http://bioinfo.iconcologia.net/snpstats/start.htm) for smaller association studies. In the sections below we provide the options for performing quality control and association analyses using the program PLINK

(31) (http://pngu.mgh.harvard.edu/~purcell/plink/). While PLINK requires the user to be familiar with MS-DOS or Unix/Linux environments, it is a user-friendly program for the analysis of GWA data that allows rapid and flexible analyses to be performed on 1 to more than 1 million SNPs for 1000s of individuals, with an upper limit to the size of datasets determined only by computing power (*see* **Note 5**).

3.3. Data Quality Control

3.3.1. Laboratory-Based Quality Control

Genotyping studies should include appropriate controls to test for correct orientation of DNA sample tubes or plates and repeatability of genotype results across the study. Initial quality control (QC) is typically performed in the laboratory in which the genotypes were generated. Laboratory-based QC measures should focus on ensuring that all individuals and SNPs have genotyped accurately. For each SNP, homozygotes for the alternative alleles and heterozygotes for both alleles should be clearly distinguishable. For large-scale projects conducted using genotyping chips, this can be visualised as genotype 'clusters' (**Fig. 3.2**) (4).

3.3.2. Analysis File Preparation

The minimum requirement for an association study is individual genotype data assigned to case and control individuals and knowledge of the order and position of SNPs along a chromosome. File formats will depend on the analysis program that is utilised. Depending on the amount of data, files can be created and edited in a spreadsheet program such as Microsoft Excel or a text editor, and association analysis programs can then produce correctly formatted files. PLINK requires two files: a pedigree file containing individual information including disease status and genotype data and a map file containing the chromosomal positions of SNPs (*see* **Note 6**).

3.3.3. Running PLINK

PLINK can be driven by a graphical user interface (GUI) in Windows, command-line instructions typed directly into a MS-DOS or Unix command window or via a –script option, where the options are read from a text file. To save disk space and reduce analysis time, particularly for large GWA data files, PLINK can covert pedigree and map files to 'binary' files, which will have the endings *.bed* (containing genotype information), *.fam* (containing pedigree information) and *.bim* (containing map information). In the following sections we assume that data files have been converted to binary format. Note also that by default all output files will be named *plink.xxx* unless an outfile name (using the '--out' option) is specified.

The command line for a basic PLINK run has the format:

plink --bfile *mydatafile* --assoc --out *mydatafile*

This will call PLINK to perform an association analysis using information included in the *mydatafile.bed*, *mydatafile.fam*

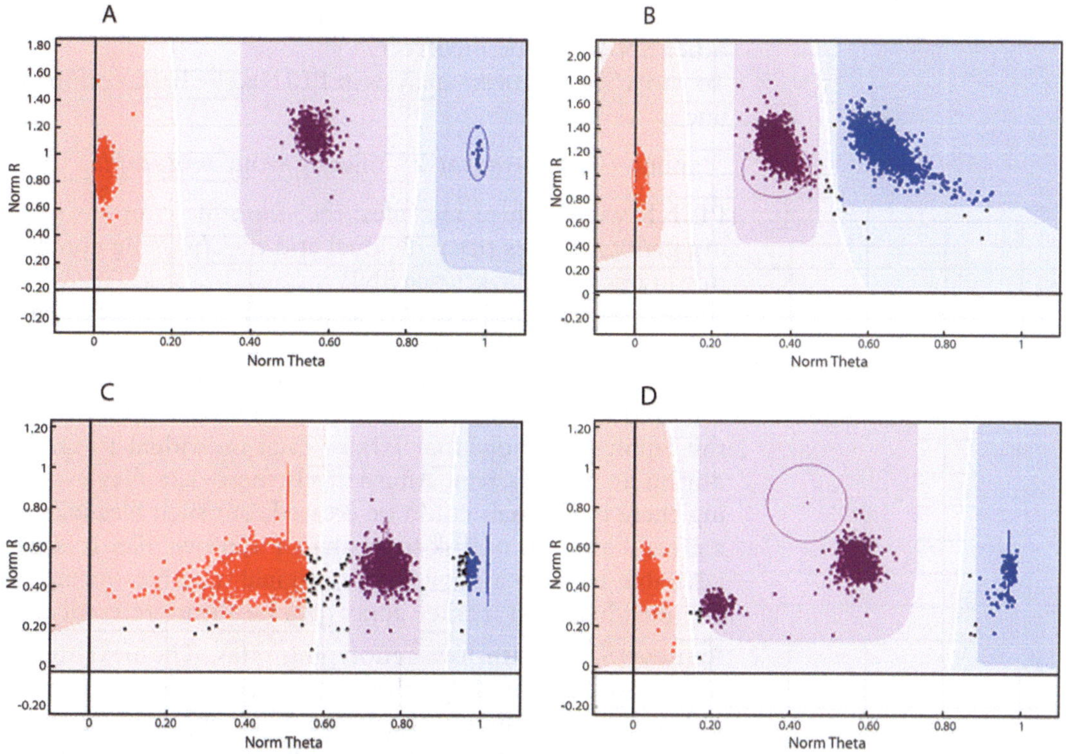

Fig. 3.2. SNP genotyping cluster plot examples. (**a**) SNP genotypes cluster well and homozygotes for either allele as well as heterozygotes carrying both alleles can be clearly distinguished from each other even though few samples are homozygous for one of the alleles. (**b**) Homozygotes for one allele cluster well but the range of values seen for heterozygotes and the homozygotes for the alternative allele cluster reasonably loosely. *Black dots* indicate samples with values outside of which genotypes can be confidently called. Such a SNP may fail quality control. (**c**) Although the clusters appear reasonably tight a number of samples carrying all three genotypes fall outside of the values for which genotypes can be confidently called. Data for SNPs clustering as in b and c could be rescued following visual inspection of the cluster plots. (**d**) Heterozygous genotypes for this SNP appear in two clusters, indicating the presence of a so-called null or non-amplifying allele (typically due to the presence of a SNP in the PCR primer site, preventing amplification in any DNA sample carrying such a variant). Such a SNP would likely *pass* quality control, but should in fact be removed from the dataset. Cluster plots of at least all significantly associated SNPs should be inspected before data analyses are taken further. This is particularly important for GWA studies that include 100,000 s of SNPs.

and *mydatafile.bim* files and produce a result file named *mydatafile.assoc* (or by default *plink.assoc* if no output file name was specified). Output files can be viewed and manipulated in a text editor or spreadsheet program (*see* **Note 7**).

3.3.4. In Silico Quality Control

In silico QC measures can be performed either in PLINK, other genetic analysis software or a spreadsheet program.

1. Remove individuals with low genotyping rates. The threshold for the removal of individuals due to missing data is dependent on the number of SNPs genotyped but is often set at 5%. Low individual genotyping rates are generally due to low concentration or poor quality DNA, and such

individuals should be removed as the genotypes obtained for other SNPs may be incorrect.

To run a 'missingness' analysis in PLINK the basic command line is

plink --bfile *mydatafile* --missing --out *mydatafile*

PLINK will produce two files: the *.imiss* file contains missing genotype rates per individual and the *.lmiss* file contains missing genotype rates per SNP.

Individuals with an excess of missing data (e.g. missing genotypes for >5% of the total number of SNPs genotyped) should be omitted from the next round of QC. This can be achieved in PLINK by including a 'remove' file containing the family and individual IDs of each individual to ignore during an analysis run. Alternatively, new data files excluding these individuals could be created, but such files take up a greater amount of disk space than a 'remove' file. It is also advisable to keep a copy of the original data files including all individuals and marker genotypes for future reference.

2. Remove SNPs with low genotyping rates. The next step is to remove SNPs with high rates of missing genotypes in the individuals remaining in the dataset following the first round of QC. Typically, SNPs missing more than 1–5% of data are excluded from further analyses.

   Re-run the PLINK '--missing' option. Note that the *.imiss* file will be overwritten if a new outfile name is not provided.

   plink --bfile *mydatafile* --missing --remove *removeindividualslist.txt* --out *mydatafileQCII*

   SNPs with an excess of missing data should be excluded from the next round of analysis by including the names of the SNPs in a separate file using the '--exclude' option or by creating new data files.

3. Investigate SNPs for evidence of Hardy–Weinberg disequilibrium (HWD). Under a neutral genetic model the frequencies of homozygote and heterozygote genotypes for a particular SNP are expected to equal the products of the allele frequencies: if the frequency of an allele 'A' = p and the frequency of the alternative allele 'G' = q, then the frequencies of AA, AG and GG genotypes should equal p^2, $2pq$ and q^2, respectively. Departures from Hardy–Weinberg equilibrium (HWE) may occur due to true association, where certain genotypes are over-represented in the case group. In GWA studies, HWE tests are generally performed only in controls where such departures are often due to poor genotyping. Departures from HWE in cases should be checked for any SNPs showing association to ensure the

departure is in the expected direction of the genotype over-representation/association. SNPs with extremely low HW *p* values ($<10^{-6}$) should be excluded.
To perform HWE tests in PLINK:

plink --bfile *mydatafile* --remove *removeindividualslist.txt* --exclude *excludeSNPlist.txt* --hardy --out *mydatafile*

PLINK will output a *.hardy* file. Any SNP markers that are not in HWE and have clear clustering issues should be added to the list of SNPs to exclude in further analyses (*see* **Note 8**).

The following additional QC measures are undertaken in GWA studies where the numbers of SNPs and individuals are large enough to provide accurate estimates. Typically, exclusion thresholds are determined on a per-project basis.

4. Check missing data rates between cases and controls and across all genotyping chips. To avoid stratification due to technical issues SNP missing data rates should be equivalent in the case and control groups, and across all genotyping chips included in an association analysis. In PLINK the test for differences in missing rates between cases and controls is performed using the '--test-missing' option. More complex group comparisons, such as chip effects (where genotyping success rates differ per chip), can be performed using the '--loop-assoc' option which automatically tests each group (defined by a categorical factor) versus all other individuals for a variety of statistics.
5. Remove individuals showing excessive homozygosity or heterozygosity. Excessive levels of either homozygosity or heterozygosity can indicate poor genotyping, typically due to low-quality DNA. 'Normal' individual heterozygosity levels using GWA data are typically of the order of ~0.3. Heterozygosity is measured as an inbreeding coefficient (denoted as *F*, the observed versus expected number of homozygous genotypes). The PLINK option to calculate heterozygosity is '--het'.
6. Remove individuals mismatched for sex. Large-scale genotyping chips include markers for both the X and the Y chromosomes. Males should be homozygous for X chromosome markers, while females should show a degree of X chromosome heterozygosity and have no genotypes for Y chromosome markers. The PLINK option to calculate F for the X chromosome is '--check-sex'.
7. Remove ancestry outliers. Many SNPs have systematic differences in allele frequencies between populations. On a genome-wide scale such SNPs can be used to determine

genetic ancestry. Programs such as Eigenstrat (32) (http://genepath.med.harvard.edu/~reich/Software.htm) are used to perform multidimensional scaling of pairwise 'identity by state' (IBS) values in comparison to reference populations from, e.g. the HapMap (*see* **Note 9**). The first two principle components of the IBS values for each individual are then plotted to reveal ancestry. In PLINK, outlying individuals can either be excluded from further analysis or the principal components be included as covariates ('--covar') in a logistic regression ('--logistic') test for association.

8. Remove related samples. Cryptic (unknown) relatedness between samples can produce erroneous association results due to increased allele sharing amongst relatives. Relatedness is generally estimated by calculating measures of IBS and/or 'identity by descent' (IBD). In PLINK the option '--genome' will generate a *.genome* file containing estimated IBD values for each pair of individuals in the dataset.

9. Exclude SNPs with very low minor allele frequencies (MAFs). While rare SNPs (MAFs <1%) of large effect are likely to be important in at least some complex diseases, SNPs with very rare minor allele frequencies may cause spurious association signals if present in one group (e.g. cases) but not the other (e.g. controls). Very rare alleles are more likely to differ in frequency due to chance, and due to their rarity any truly disease-associated variant must be of particularly large effect for a real association signal to be detected. Unless the effect is large (odds ratio >2) most case–control samples (those with <10,000 individuals) have minimal power to detect association to less common alleles (e.g. MAFs <5%).
   Allele frequencies can be calculated in PLINK using the '--freq' option, and SNPs with MAFs less than the threshold for inclusion can then be added to the 'exclude' file. Alternatively, PLINK can filter SNPs based on allele frequencies using the option '--maf 0.01' (for example), which will exclude SNPs with MAFs <0.01 from the analysis.

3.4. Association Analyses

1. Running a basic association analysis. Once all QC steps have been completed the next step is to perform the association analysis on the clean dataset.
   In PLINK the '--assoc' option will perform χ^2 tests of association on each SNP in the data file, producing an *.assoc* output file containing *p* values and odds ratios for each marker. PLINK allows for the use of separate phenotype files that over-ride the phenotypes in the main .fam or .ped files. This

option is particularly useful if the trait under investigation has distinct, well-characterised sub-phenotypes that could be run in alternative analyses without the need for multiple pedigree files to be produced. Individuals failing QC could also be removed from the analysis by setting their phenotype to '0' in the phenotype file to avoid the need to include a '--remove' file.

--bfile *mydatafile* --pheno *phenotypefilename.txt* --remove *removeindividualslist.txt* --exclude *excludeSNPlist.txt* --assoc

2. Running an association analysis in the presence of population stratification. Due to the extremely large sample sizes required to find variants of even moderate effect, it is becoming increasingly common for researchers from different centres to combine their data sets prior to running GWA analyses to maximise the power to detect association. Analyses should then be run taking potential population stratification into account. This can be done in two ways depending on the data files at hand.
   If genotype data are available the Cochran–Mantel–Haenszel (CMH) test can be used to test for association in the presence of different population groups, while possible heterogeneity in disease-marker associations between the different groups can be estimated using Breslow-Day (BD) tests. An additional 'within' file is required to indicate the group (or 'cluster') to which each individual belongs:

   plink --bfile *mydatafile* --pheno *phenotypefilename.txt* --remove *removeindividualsfile.txt* --exclude *excludeSNPs-file.txt* --within *individualclusterinfo.txt* --mh --bd --out *mydatafile*

   PLINK will produce two files, *.cmh* and *.bd*. Confidence intervals for odds ratios can be calculated using the option '--ci 0.95'.

   PLINK can also run 'meta-analyses' using files containing only the results (p values, etc.,) for different projects. The options here are

   plink --meta-analysis *project1.assoc project2.assoc* --out *meta-analysisresults*

3.5. Visualising and Interpreting Your Results

The results generated in small-scale studies can be easily accessed from the output of the program used to perform the association testing. The interpretation of GWA studies, where 100,000 s of tests have been performed, is simpler if the results are visualised as plotted figures. The first plot that should be made is a diagnostic quartile–quartile (q–q) plot (**Fig. 3.3**), produced by plotting

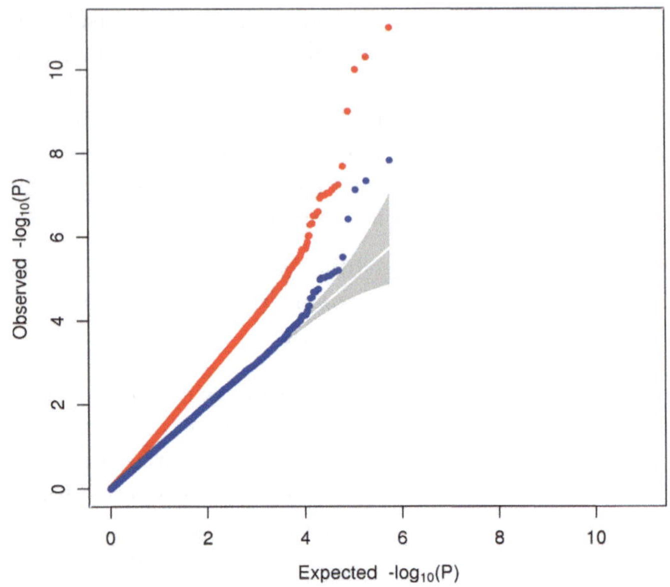

Fig. 3.3. Quartile–quartile (q–q) plot of hypothetical GWA results. The solid *white line* represents the expected (reference) distribution under the null hypothesis of no association and the *grey shaded region* indicates the point-wise 95% confidence interval envelope based on the standard errors of order statistics. The *red points* indicate population stratification and/or cryptic relatedness (substructure), while the blue points show no evidence for substructure, but convincing evidence for an excess of disease associations.

the observed values of the association statistics (e.g. the χ^2 or *p* values) ranked in order from smallest to largest against those expected under a null distribution. Deviations from the diagonal line give an indication of the quality of the data, in terms of controlling for population stratification and the strength of the associations detected (4, 12).

The second plot is a display of the association results themselves, termed a Manhattan plot (**Fig. 3.4**). Here the $-\log_{10}$ of the *p* values generated by the association analysis are plotted against chromosomal location, allowing interesting association signals to be clearly seen against background signals. Two user-friendly programs that can generate both q–q plots and Manhattan plots directly from PLINK output files are Haploview and WGAViewer (33) (http://people.genome.duke.edu/~dg48/WGAViewer/). These and other programs (e.g. SNAP, http://www.broadinstitute.org/mpg/snap/ldplot.phpcan – change the 'plot type' drop-down window to 'regional association plot' – and LocusZoom, http://csg.sph.umich.edu/locuszoom/) can then be used to focus on the areas harbouring interesting association signals, for example displaying the genes and features such as microRNAs present in the region and providing links to genetic databases that can serve as the starting point for in silico investigation of the area surrounding significant association signals.

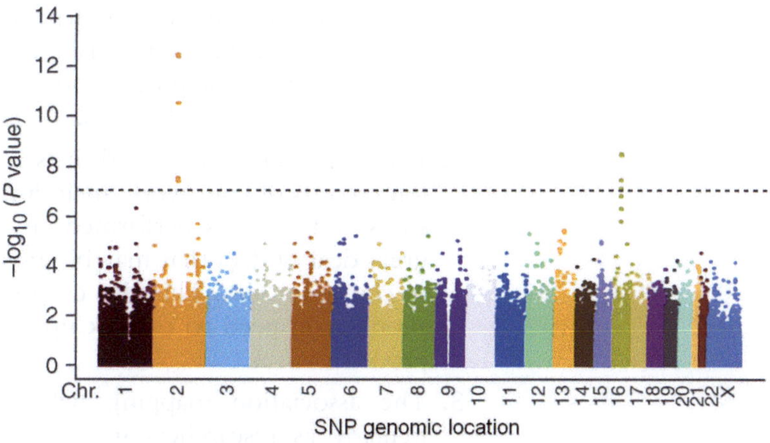

Fig. 3.4. Manhattan plot of hypothetical GWA results. *P* values for each SNP analysed in the GWA study are shown as their $-\log_{10}$ values. Each chromosome is represented by a different colour. The *dashed line* shows the threshold for genome-wide significance (accounting for the number of independent tests performed). Two regions in this example have reached genome-wide significance and should be targeted for replication.

3.6. Additional Considerations

It is increasingly clear that very large samples of well-phenotyped individuals are required to detect the typically modest effect sizes for risk alleles underlying susceptibility to complex genetic diseases or traits. The association analysis field is changing rapidly to adapt to the increasing complexities involved in mapping human disease genes. In addition to careful planning and QC, once at the analysis phase there are a growing number of methods that can be employed to increase the likelihood of detecting an association. For example, genotypes for untyped SNPs can be generated by imputation (34) in reference to individuals taken from HapMap or the 1000 Genomes project (http://www.1000genomes.org), increasing the total number of loci that can be analysed. Haplotype associations can be examined to determine the genetic background on which a causal variant may lie. Potential interactions between loci can also be investigated. While it should be remembered that even a highly significant association signal replicated in an independent case–control group is not absolute proof that a marker or gene is associated with the phenotype under investigation, such results are extremely encouraging and indicate that further in silico and genetic analyses and subsequent functional investigations should be carried out.

4. Notes

1. There is no substitute for high-quality DNA with carefully measured concentrations. The tissue type (e.g. blood), collection method, storage and transport of samples, DNA

extraction and subsequent storage of the DNA itself need to be carefully planned well in advance. Poor quality DNA will result in genotyping errors or failure, wasting considerable time and research funds.

2. Just as for laboratory work it is a good idea to keep written records of your work, including all quality control measures and analyses performed, as you will quickly amass a great deal of data that may be spread across a large number of computer files. This also ensures you can repeat analyses should you need to or pick up any errors in the analytical process.
3. The association mapping field is rapidly evolving, particularly as researchers gain more experience with GWA data. Literature searches (using a site such as the NCBI PubMed http://www.ncbi.nlm.nih.gov/pubmed/) should be undertaken regularly to keep up with new methodologies as they are published.
4. If risk allele frequencies and effect sizes are unknown, power calculations should be run over a realistic range, for example allele frequencies from 0.05 to 0.4 and odds ratios of 1.1–2.0 (although odds ratios for complex disease are typically in the range of 1.1–1.5). These can then be plotted on a graph to visualise the power expected over the range of values.
5. Another advantage of using PLINK is that the Web site has extensive, easy to read, documentation on all aspects of file preparation, quality control and analysis and is therefore an extremely useful resource even for those using other analysis programs.
6. The most common input file format used is the so-called linkage format, following that initially required by the original 'Linkage' program (*see* http://linkage.rockefeller.edu/soft/list2.html#l under 'L'). PLINK is reasonably flexible with regards to input file formats, consult the Web site to determine what is most appropriate for your study.
7. PLINK will also output a *.log* file containing all details of the analysis that has just run (input files and commands, etc.,) that should be kept for future reference. This *.log* file will have the default name *plink.log* and will be overwritten with each new analysis if an output file name is not specified via the '--out' option.
8. Various QC steps, including the 'missing' and 'hardy' steps, can also be performed during an association analysis by providing pre-determined thresholds for each measure in a single command line (*see* the 'filter' section of the PLINK

documentation). However, it is highly recommended that all QC steps are performed individually as this ensures a greater understanding of the quality of the dataset and allows decisions of what data should be excluded to be made based on actual missing data and HWD rates.

9. The HapMap (at http://www.hapmap.org) is an invaluable resource for association mapping projects providing genotyping data for millions of SNPs in a genomic context. Other easy to use databases that the reader should become familiar with as a starting point for genetic research are the UCSC Genome Browser (http://genome.ucsc.edu/), ENSEMBL (http://www.ensembl.org/index.html) and NCBI (http://www.ncbi.nlm.nih.gov/) databases.

References

1. Laird, N. M., and Lange, C. (2006) Family-based designs in the age of large-scale gene-association studies. *Nat Rev Genet* 7, 385–394.
2. Benyamin, B., Visscher, P. M., and McRae A. F. (2009) Family-based genome-wide association studies. *Pharmacogenomics* 10, 181–190.
3. Hindorff, L. A., Sethupathy, P., Junkins, H. A., Ramos, E. M., Mehta, J. P., Collins, F. S., and Manolio, T. A. (2009) Potential etiologic and functional implications of genome-wide association loci for human diseases and traits. *Proc Natl Acad Sci USA* 106, 9362–9367.
4. McCarthy, M. I., Abecasis, G. R., Cardon, L. R., Goldstein, D. B., Little, J., Ioannidis, J. P., and Hirschhorn, J. N. (2008) Genome-wide association studies for complex traits: consensus, uncertainty and challenges. *Nat Rev Genet* 9, 356–369.
5. Visscher, P. M., and Montgomery, G. W. (2009) Genome-wide association studies and human disease: from trickle to flood. *JAMA* 302, 2028–2029.
6. Zondervan, K. T., Cardon L. R., and Kennedy, S. H. (2002) What makes a good case-control study? Design issues for complex traits such as endometriosis. *Hum Reprod* 17, 1415–1423.
7. Hirschhorn, J. N., and Daly, M. J. (2005) Genome-wide association studies for common diseases and complex traits. *Nat Rev Genet* 6, 95–108.
8. Wang, W. Y., Barratt, B. J., Clayton, D. G., and Todd, J. A. (2005) Genome-wide association studies: theoretical and practical concerns. *Nat Rev Genet* 6, 109–118.
9. Pettersson, F. H., Anderson, C. A., Clarke, G. M., Barrett, J. C., Cardon, L. R., Morris, A. P., and Zondervan, K. T. (2009) Marker selection for genetic case-control association studies. *Nat Protoc* 4, 743–752.
10. Wellcome Trust Case Control Consortium (2007) Genome-wide association study of 14,000 cases of seven common diseases and 3,000 shared controls. *Nature* 447, 661–678.
11. Balding, D. J. (2006) A tutorial on statistical methods for population association studies. *Nat Rev Genet* 7, 781–791.
12. Pearson, T. A., and Manolio, T. A. (2008) How to interpret a genome-wide association study. *JAMA* 299, 1335–1344.
13. Kraft, P., Zeggini, E., and Ioannidis, J. P. (2009) Replication in genome-wide association studies. *Stat Sci* 24, 561–573.
14. Zhuang, J. J., Zondervan, K., Nyberg, F., Harbron, C., Jawaid, A., Cardon, L. R., Barratt, B. J., and Morris, A. P. (2010) Optimizing the power of genome-wide association studies by using publicly available reference samples to expand the control group. *Genet Epidemiol* 34, 319–326.
15. Cardon, L. R., and Palmer, L. J. (2003) Population stratification and spurious allelic association. *Lancet* 361, 598–604.
16. Purcell, S., Cherny, S. S., and Sham, P. C. (2003) Genetic Power Calculator: design of linkage and association genetic mapping studies of complex traits. *Bioinformatics* 19, 149–150.
17. Gordon, D., Haynes, C., Blumenfeld, J., and Finch, S. J. (2005) PAWE-3D: visualizing power for association with error in case-control genetic studies of complex traits. *Bioinformatics* 21, 3935–3937.

18. Skol, A. D., Scott, L. J., Abecasis, G. R., and Boehnke, M. (2007) Optimal designs for two-stage genome-wide association studies. *Genet Epidemiol* 31, 776–788.
19. Cardon, L. R., and Bell, J. I. (2001) Association study designs for complex diseases. *Nat Rev Genet* 2, 91–99.
20. Nyholt, D. R. (2004) A simple correction for multiple testing for single-nucleotide polymorphisms in linkage disequilibrium with each other. *Am J Hum Genet* 74, 765–769.
21. Dudbridge, F., and Gusnanto, A. (2008) Estimation of significance thresholds for genomewide association scans. *Genet Epidemiol* 32, 227–234.
22. Pe'er, I., Yelensky, R., Altshuler, D., and Daly, M. J. (2008) Estimation of the multiple testing burden for genomewide association studies of nearly all common variants. *Genet Epidemiol* 32, 381–385.
23. Benjamini, Y., Drai, D., Elmer, G., Kafkafi, N., and Golani, I. (2001) Controlling the false discovery rate in behavior genetics research. *Behav Brain Res* 125, 279–284.
24. Storey, J. D., and Tibshirani, R. (2003) Statistical significance for genomewide studies. *Proc Natl Acad Sci USA* 100, 9440–9445.
25. Barrett, J.C., Fry, B., Maller, J., and Daly, M. J. (2005) Haploview: analysis and visualization of LD and haplotype maps. *Bioinformatics* 21, 263–265.
26. Pettersson, F., Morris, A. P., Barnes, M. R., and Cardon, L. R. (2008) Goldsurfer2 (Gs2): a comprehensive tool for the analysis and visualization of genome wide association studies. *BMC Bioinformatics* 9, 138.
27. Kraft, P. (2008) Curses—winner's and otherwise – in genetic epidemiology. *Epidemiology* 19, 649–651.
28. Aulchenko, Y. S., Ripke, S., Isaacs, A., and van Duijn, C. M. (2007) GenABEL: an R library for genome-wide association analysis. *Bioinformatics* 23, 1294–1296.
29. Marchini, J., Howie, B., Myers, S., McVean, G., and Donnelly, P. (2007) A new multipoint method for genome-wide association studies by imputation of genotypes. *Nat Genet* 39, 906–913.
30. Sole, X., Guino, E., Valls, J., Iniesta, R., and Moreno, V. (2006) SNPStats: a web tool for the analysis of association studies. *Bioinformatics* 22, 1928–1929.
31. Purcell, S., Neale, B., Todd-Brown, K., et al. (2007) PLINK: a tool set for whole-genome association and population-based linkage analyses. *Am J Hum Genet* 81, 559–575.
32. Price, A. L., Patterson, N. J., Plenge, R. M., et al. (2006) Principal components analysis corrects for stratification in genome-wide association studies. *Nat Genet* 38, 904–909.
33. Ge, D., Zhang, K., Need, A. C., et al. (2008) WGAViewer: software for genomic annotation of whole genome association studies. *Genome Res* 18, 640–643.
34. Li, Y., Willer, C. J., Sanna, S. and Abecasis, G. R. (2009) Genotype Imputation. *Ann Rev Genomics Hum Genet* 10, 387–406.

Chapter 4

The ForeSee (4C) Approach for Integrative Analysis in Gene Discovery

Yike Guo, Robin E.J. Munro, Dimitrios Kalaitzopoulos, and Anita Grigoriadis

Abstract

The development of high-throughput experimental techniques has made measurements for virtually all kinds of cellular components possible. Effective integration and analysis of this diverged information to produce insightful knowledge is central to biological study today. In this chapter, we present a methodology for building integrative analytical workbenches using the workflow technology. We focus on the field of gene discovery through the combined study of transcriptomics, genomics and epigenomics, although the methodology is generally applicable to any *omics*-data analysis for biomarker discovery. We illustrate the application of the methodology by presenting our study on the identification of aberrant genomic regions, genes and/or their regulatory elements with their implications for breast cancer research. We also discuss the challenges and opportunities brought by the latest development of the next generation sequencing technology.

Key words: *Omics*, genomics, gene discovery, integrative analysis, workflow, data flow, process-driven, ForeSee approach, breast cancer, next generation sequencing.

1. Introduction

Over the last 15 years, various technologies have emerged that produce genome-wide or *omics*-datasets, providing measurements for virtually all kinds of cellular components. The development of these high-throughput experimental techniques has transformed biological research into a data-rich discipline where informatics plays a key role. An important challenge that is faced by investigators today lies not only in the interpretation of these large datasets but also in tackling the problem of the fragmented nature of biological research and thus the need to integrate several sources

B. Yu, M. Hinchcliffe (eds.), *In Silico Tools for Gene Discovery*, Methods in Molecular Biology 760,
DOI 10.1007/978-1-61779-176-5_4, © Springer Science+Business Media, LLC 2011

of heterogeneous information to produce insightful knowledge. Effective information integration for knowledge production is a non-trivial task. To maximise the extraction of biological knowledge, while recognising and accommodating the specific statistical and computational requirements of each platform in its correct biological context, a consistent and reproducible approach is the essential basis for working with *omics*-data. In this post-genomic era, the integration of disparate data sources with different modalities and the bridging of phenotypic data with *omics* knowledge will be the key to analyse research data for modelling the molecular basis of diseases. In this chapter we briefly introduce representative *omics* technologies for genomic biomarker discovery (or gene discovery) including transcriptomics, genomics and epigenomics. Naturally, the combination and integration of *omics*-data goes far beyond these three *omics* areas and could also include proteomics, metabolomics, glycomics and lipidomics, to mention but a few, and undoubtedly also contribute to the cellular phenotype. We then discuss several challenges unique to the integrative analysis of data from these different platforms. Based on workflow technology, we present a methodology applicable in generic biomarker and gene discovery contexts for efficiently achieving an integrative analytics task. We call this methodology the 'Fore-See approach (4C)'. We illustrate the application of our Fore-See approach with the identification of aberrant genomic regions, genes and/or their regulatory elements, and their implications for breast cancer research using information at several different levels of biological and clinical research. Finally, the chapter will conclude with a discussion of the challenges and opportunities that face this field with the advent of the latest high-throughput technology, namely next generation sequencing (NGS).

2. Integrative Analysis for Gene Discovery

In the mid-1990s the functional genomics era started with serial analysis of gene expression (SAGE) using DNA sequencing (1). This was soon followed by several different technological innovations, providing genome-wide measurements for all kinds of molecular species within the cell. Nowadays, many routinely used analytical platforms are microarray-based for which a huge variety of different microarray systems have been developed. The basic principle is very similar across all platforms: a two-dimensional substrate (e.g. membrane, glass slides, silicon beads (Illumina) or nanoparticles) is spotted with thousands of molecules of known sequence and location across the genome (also known as microarray features), these are then hybridised with the biological sample of interest, and after sequential chemical reactions, the raw data is obtained by laser scanning or autoradiographic imaging. These images are then analysed using a variety of statistical methods. The most familiar microarray-based *omics* technology is, without a doubt, transcriptomics: the study of gene expression profiles, measuring both the presence and the relative abundance of RNA transcripts. Recently, due to advances in microarray technologies in conjunction with the completion of the sequencing of the human genome, expression profiling has been expanded by the ability to examine the abundance of all known exons, as well as of post-transcriptional regulators such as microRNAs (miRNAs). The latter is a class of short non-coding RNAs which regulate gene expression of several transcripts by binding to the complementary sequences in target mRNAs and thereby block their selective translation and/or degradation. Because of their redundancy (exon skipping and the 'one to many corresponding relations' between a miRNA and a set of mRNAs), both new areas provide an extra dimension of complexity to the integration with other analytical platforms.

Genomics, which refers to the study of the whole genome sequence and the information (including variations) contained therein, can be interrogated by analytical platforms such as array genomic comparative hybridisation (aCGH) (2) and single nucleotide polymorphism (SNP) microarrays (3). While aCGH combines the conventional CGH with DNA microarray for the detection of DNA copy number variation (CNV) of larger genomic regions (e.g. entire chromosomal or interstitial DNA losses or gains), SNP microarrays have the advantage of providing high-resolution information with regard to allelic copy number changes, loss of heterozygosity (LOH) and genotypes within a single experiment.

In contrast, epigenomics is the study of heritable changes across the entire genome in the regulation of gene activity and expression that are not coded in the DNA sequence (epigenetics) (4). In general, epigenetic mechanisms such as DNA methylation and modification to histone proteins differ from genetic events mainly in that they are reversible and typically happen with a higher frequency. A number of microarray platforms have been developed on a medium- to high-throughput scale, while methylation arrays interrogate the DNA hypermethylation of CpG islands within the promoter of genes; ChIP-chip technologies (5) combine chromatin immunoprecipitation (ChIP) and microarray technology (chip) to directly identify protein–DNA interaction.

All of these different genomic variations as well as the epigenetic modifications have an impact on the expression state of the active component within the cell (**Fig. 4.1**). Several integrated meta-analysis methods have already been developed and applied to different types of *omics*-data, using simple non-parametric rank

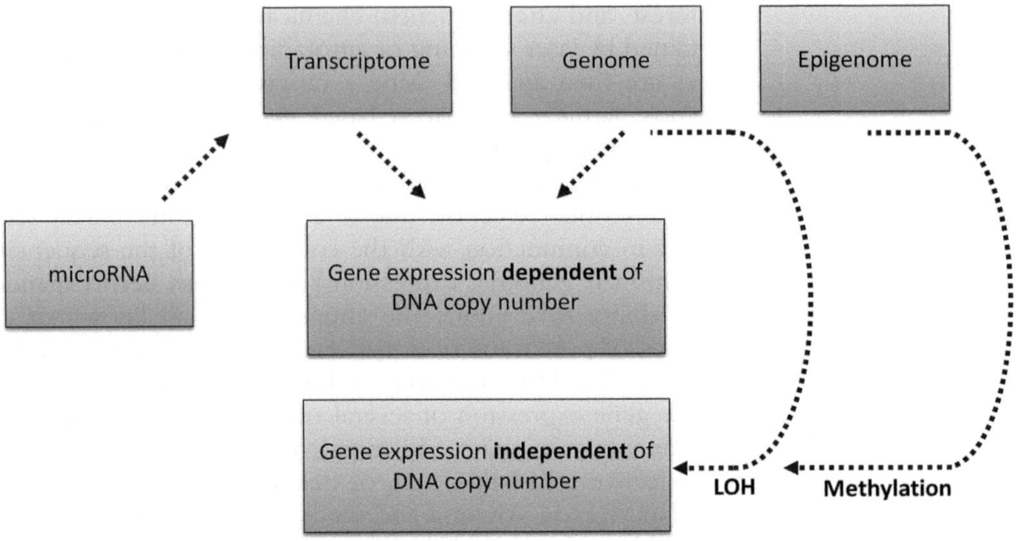

Fig. 4.1. Schematic representation of the correlation between different omics-data. Expression levels of certain genes can be dependent on DNA copy number, under the influence of the methylation state of their regulator features, or post-transcriptionally controlled by microRNAs. Genomic aberrations such as LOH can alter the levels of gene expression independent of DNA copy number changes.

statistics to Bayesian methods (6). Interestingly, while current meta-analyses have so far provided an unprecedented capability to model cellular processes on two levels (most commonly the integration of gene dosage and gene expression), integrative analysis and visualisation, using multi-modality *omics*-datasets are still in their infancies.

Due to the fast growing platform technology, the continuing development of our understanding on the molecular mechanism and the ad hoc nature of gene discovery make a standard data model equipped with a well-defined processing and analysis tools impossible. More flexible and systematic ways of integrating and analysing *omics*-data are therefore needed.

3. Methods

3.1. The ForeSee (4C) Approach for Integrative Analysis for Gene Discovery

In this section we describe a systematic approach for integrative analysis of multi-modality genomics information based on our experiences in using commercial workflow platforms (e.g. InforSense Suite (http://www.idbs.com/) or the open source platform Taverna (http://www.taverna.org.uk/)). Workflow technology is based on the principle that by providing commonly used functions as components software can be built by orchestrating these components together using a graphical language (*see*

Note 1). By applying such a component-based approach for integrative analysis of *omics*-data, several analytical tasks can be constructed with different workflows (*see* **Notes 2 and 3**). The key concept underlying this component-based approach is that an ad hoc integration mechanism, in addition to traditional rigid integration approaches (such as data warehousing), is crucial to provide the capability to form subject-oriented integrative analysis workbenches (*see* **Note 4**).

Most of the integrative analysis is composed of four levels, namely, data integration, processing and analysis, correlating different discovery results and knowledge management by integrating putative genes with more information from the literature and other contextual information.

3.2. Methodology

Here we present the methodology in workflow building for the four levels by emphasising the key focus at each level, namely:

(1) Building a data integration workflow by joining data using a common reference key (**C**RK).

(2) Building an analysis workbench by composing common analytical components (**C**AC).

(3) Correlating discovery results by examining the collective patterns (**C**P).

(4) Using a context mapping (**C**M) concept to annotate the discovery results with literature, curated databases and other information.

We refer to it as the 'ForeSee approach (4C)' for integrative analytics, which is also illustrated in **Fig. 4.2**.

3.2.1. The 1st 'C' – Information Integration Based on a Common Reference Key (CRK)

For an integrative analytics task with *omics*-data, the complexity of data integration is introduced not only by the multi-modality of the information generated by multiple platforms with different focuses but also by the different data models where the information is managed. For example, the query: 'How many patients have HER2-positive breast cancer, responded to treatment, have a chromosome 17q21 amplification and have blood and epithelium samples in the our biobank?' relates to at least three different data management systems: patient diagnosis information management (HER2-positive breast cancer patients response to treatment), genomics study information system (chromosome information) and biobank which stores all the tissue samples. This query may be followed by another one such as 'for all those patients, which pathways have more than 10 genes co-expressed in the gene expression profiles studied and for all these pathways, which one is correlated most closely to the methylation studies conducted so far'. While the first query can still be handled by the traditional data federation system, the second query is much harder to handle since it cannot be strictly formalised as

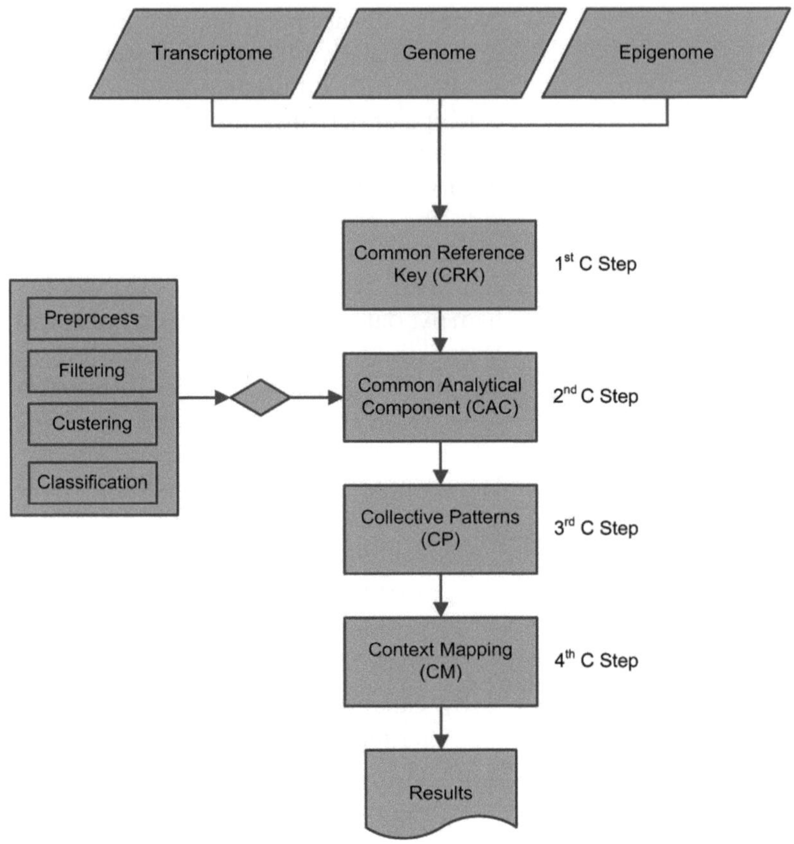

Fig. 4.2. The ForeSee (4C) approach.

a relational one. Querying conditions such as 'most closely correlated' require analytical computation with a non-conventional strategy. Thus, to deal with those problems efficiently, which are very common in research, flexible mechanisms such as workflow approaches to build an integration structure can be employed.

A workflow-based integration mechanism is based on the simple approach of using a common reference key (CRK) to join the different data sources. That is, data from different platforms can be retrieved and then put together into a single table based on a given common identifier (CRK) from the different platforms. Based on this single table, queries can be mapped to a set of workflows. This approach shares the similar principle as that of the multi-tenant data model where different data users from different organisations (tenants) share the same database and the same schema (7). Instead of multiple data users from different organisations as in the multi-tenant data model, in our cases, multiple users of the same project write different type of queries against a simple data table. The CRK approach is based on the observation that for a specific research project, users always have a common conceptual data model in mind (*see* **Note 5**). This

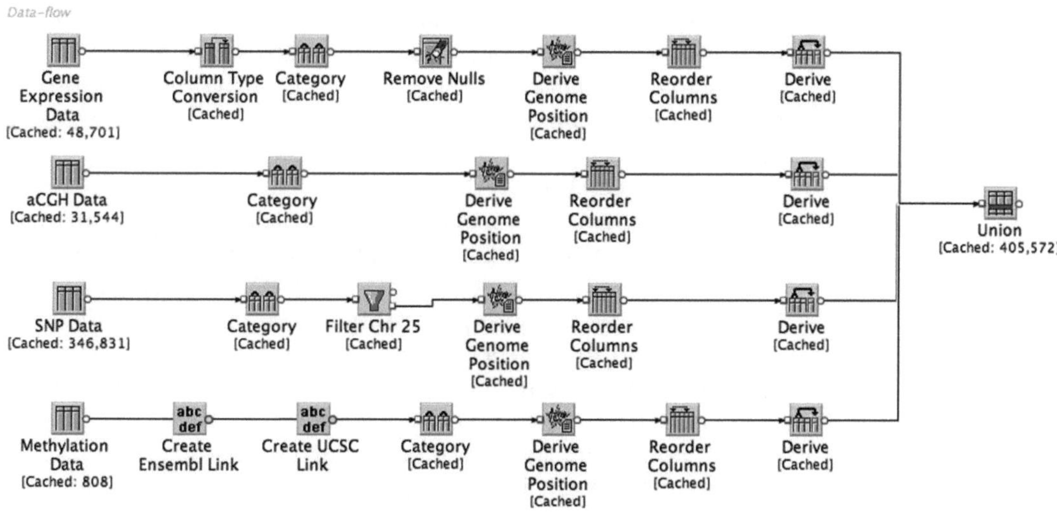

Fig. 4.3. Representation of a workflow unifying different omics-data. Each of these datasets has been pre-processed in separate workflows (not shown) and is mapped to human genome build 18 (CRK) using a 'Derive Genome Position' service, which in turn is based on a component-based workflow (not shown). The 'Union' is a table containing 405,572 keys. Using Categories allows reuse of this workflow so that other metadata types can be mapped together to generate the CRK.

data model should be built to have the generality to support various forms of ad hoc queries and should be simple as it is usually short lived and only deals with a small subpart of the information space for a particular project. Workflows can be used to build a CRK-based table, as illustrated in **Fig. 4.3**, where relevant data from different sources are retrieved through the workflow and using the CRK they are joined together to form a single table. For a successful integration mechanism, the mapping of proper identifiers from different data sources into a single CRK is essential. This can be achieved by simple mechanisms ranging from using dictionaries, lookup tables of existing annotations or employing an ontology through to more complex methods that employ computational searches for mapping sequence fragments to a common reference version of the human genome using tools like BLASTX and/or BLAT searches. These latter mapping techniques are strongly suggested when analytical platforms such as transcriptomics, genomics and epigenomics are used, to achieve a rigorous, consistent and traceable comparison based on a CRK, i.e. one version of a genome assembly.

3.2.2. The 2nd 'C' – Using a Common Analytical Component (CAC) for Building a Consistent Analytical Process

For *omics*-data analysis, although data modality may be different, an analytical process in gene discovery studies will have some similarities. Defining and using a set of well-defined components is not only important for reducing variances introduced by the diversity of analytical methods but also makes the validation as well as the cross comparisons of results easier. Here we are focusing on the analytical components for microarray-based data;

however, the principles are also applicable for other data types such as short read sequences or mass spectroscopy data.

We have categorised these common analytical components (CACs) into pre-processing, filtering, clustering and classification methods:

1. **Pre-processing Methods**

   Data pre-processing plays a crucial role in *omics*-data analysis. Data pre-processing can be applied at two different levels: at the raw data level and at the derived measurement level. The goal of raw data pre-processing is to transform the detected signals from an experiment platform into biologically meaningful measurements. Significant efforts have been devoted in the past 10 years to develop various methods (8).

   For all the array-based data analysis (for expression, SNP or methylation profiling), pre-processing of raw data usually includes the task of background correction, normalisation and summarisation. While background correction (e.g. RMA (Robust multi-array analysis) and MLE (maximum likelihood estimation) aim to removing non-specific signal from total signal, normalisation and summarisation methods, such as median polish median (per-array summarisation) and FARMS (factor analysis for Robust microarray summarisation are used to remove non-biological variance and aggregate probe signals into the measurement. Most importantly, pre-processing of raw data is platform specific. Thus, for any analysis, when raw data is provided, applying proper validated pre-processing methods is the critical first step. When measurements are derived from the raw data, pre-processing analyses of the derived can be performed using operators of relational algebra, including table-level operators such as join or projection, and column/row-level operators for data transformations (*see* **Note 6**). **Figure 4.4** illustrates a typical workflow for data pre-processing.

2. **Filtering Methods**

   After pre-processing, one of the important analytical tasks in gene discovery studies is to identify genes that can differentiate sample groups (disease versus control or different disease types). From an analytical point of view, this task can be viewed as a filtering or feature selection problem whereby genes are features (variables) and sample types are classes. The task is to identify a set of features (genes), which can characterise a disease group, or to remove all features which do not contribute to the differentiation. Apart from directly using the intensity and/or variance to select differentiated genes, commonly used methods include hypothesis test-based filtering, correlation-based filtering and the combined correlation-adjusted t scores (CAT scores) approach and many more. Hypothesis test-based filtering is based on

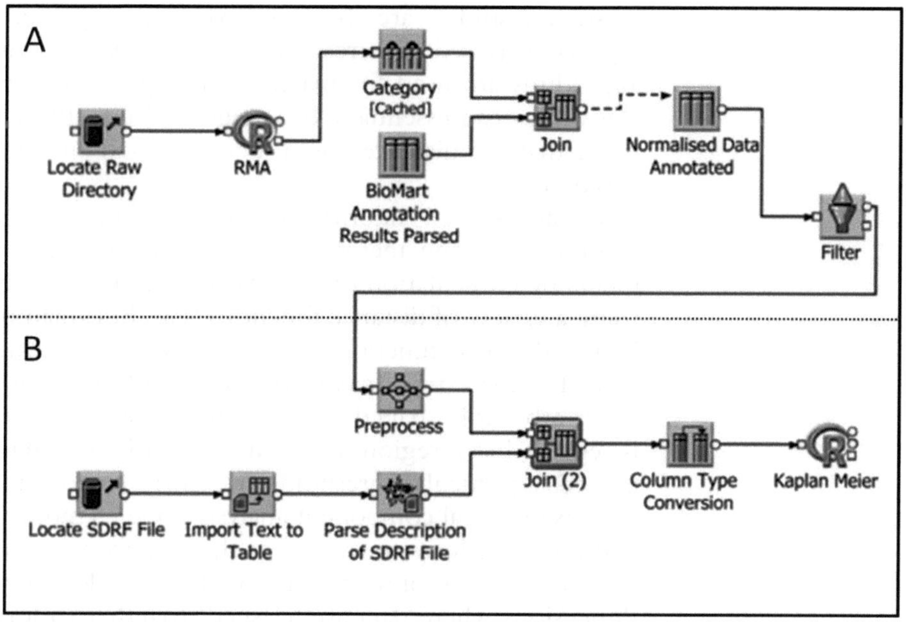

Fig. 4.4. A workflow representing an analytical path from pre-processing (**a**) to survival analysis (**b**). 'Locate Raw Directory' provides a file pointer to the raw expression data, which is pre-processed with a workflow component using a statistical method (RMA) from R environment. Followed by table-level operators such as join and filter, the expression measurement matrix is annotated with sequence (Biomart Annotation) and sample information (SDRF File) to be used for Kaplan–Meier analysis (9).

the traditional statistical testing framework, whereby features are identified if their differences among the groups are unlikely to have occurred by chance. Methods include *t* tests, when the comparison is made between two groups; ANOVA (10) when the comparison is made among more than two groups; and Wilcoxon rank sum tests (11) when no assumption of the distribution of the mean values of the groups can be made. In contrast to filtering by hypothesis testing, correlation-based filtering evaluates the importance of individual features for predicting the group membership along with the level of intercorrelation among them by employing heuristics such as mutual information. The CAT scores filtering method combines both of the above approaches by extending the *t* test method to incorporate not only information of the mean difference and its variance but also feature–feature (i.e. gene–gene) correlation, thereby improving the quality of feature selection (12). For gene discovery studies, CACs like these are essential filtering methods for gene ranking and other differentiation studies.

3. **Clustering Methods**

Clustering studies in gene discovery group genes based on similar behaviour. In the case of functional genomics, clustering studies are the standard technology for revealing co-expressed features. For studying SNPs, clustering algorithms are used for making genotype calls. Clustering algorithms can essentially be categorised into three classes, those that are distance based, density based and transform based (13).

Distance-based algorithms, such as K-means and hierarchical clustering methods, model similarity between elements by a calculation of how close they are to each other, using a variety of distance functions (e.g. Euclidian or Manhattan distance functions). Density-based clustering, such as EM (expectation maximisation algorithm), aims to discover arbitrarily shaped clusters. In this approach, a cluster is regarded as a region in which the density of data objects exceeds a particular threshold. Transform-based algorithms, such as principal component analysis (PCA), employ mathematical procedures to transform the data from a space with high dimensions into a space with a smaller number of dimensions where data are 'clashed' together to form clusters. In PCA, the reduced dimensions are called principal components or Eigen vectors. The first principal component (the vector which has the highest Eigen value) accounts for as much of the variability in the data as possible, and each successive component accounts for as much of the remaining variability as possible. All three clustering methods are widely used in gene discovery studies providing possible options as CACs.

4. **Classification Methods**

To establish predictive patterns of gene signatures (biomarkers), classification methods are another CAC used in gene discovery and in combination with filtering methods provide more complete patterns in predicting a phenotype or diagnostic outcome. Classification, which is also called supervised learning, uses a training set consisting of pairs of input data (e.g. abundance measurement of certain gene behaviour) and desired outputs (phenotypes) to then learn a predictive function. The output of the function can be a continuous value (called regression) or can predict a class label of the input object (called classification). The task of the classification (or learning) is to form such a function, called a model, which can compute the predictive value for any valid input object after learning from the training set. The commonly used learning methods include support vector machine, decision trees, k-nearest neighbours, linear discriminant analysis, logistic regression, partial least squares and naïve Bayes (14). An example of a decision tree-based workflow for building a predictive model for classification of tumour types is shown in **Fig. 4.5**. In addition to

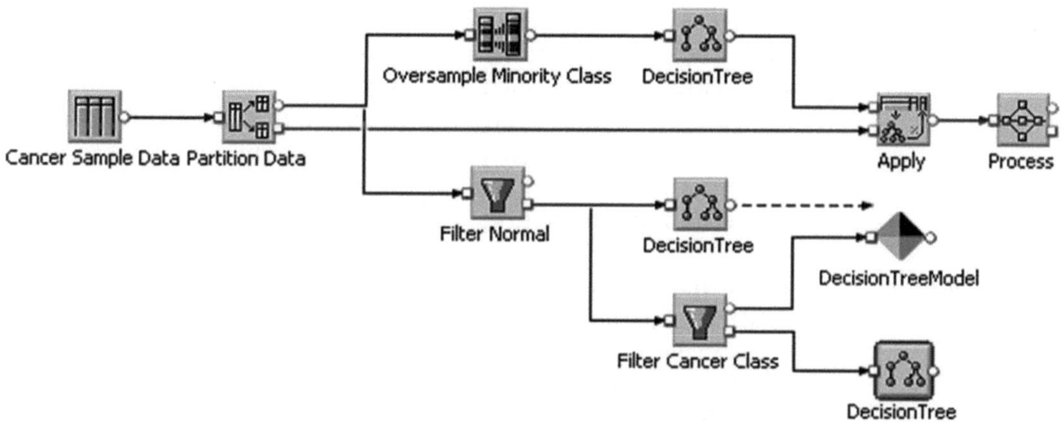

Fig. 4.5. Workflow illustrating the building and the application of a predictive model, using a decision tree classifier, image data of cancer tumours is used to classify different tissue samples into normal or two different classes of malignancy.

providing these algorithms as CACs for building models, a set of methods for model evaluation should also be adopted to support the selection of high-quality models. These methods are used to assess various quality measurements for a predictive model such as predictive accuracy, sensitivity and specificity, area under curve, receiver operating characteristic, positive prediction value, negative prediction value and lift. Together, these methods can be used within a model evaluation process, i.e. cross-validation, to score the models and can then be used for predictive analysis in diagnosis and outcome (*see* **Note 7**).

3.2.3. The 3rd 'C' – Correlating Discovery Results by Comparing Collective Patterns (CP)

The fast development of platform technologies made different biological measurements in gene discovery easier. Transcriptomics, genomics and epigenomics datasets for a given set of genes or a given set of samples can be quickly acquired and analysed. One of the key tasks in integrative analysis is to correlate across the different discovery results in a study to provide a complete biological picture of genes and their interactions. Such correlation can be studied through correlation statistical analysis. For example, transcriptomics and GWAS (genome-wide association studies) can be used for a given sample set for cancer study (or other disease) (15). Using filtering and classification, gene expression studies can identify candidate genes associated with cancer development and progression. With GWAS, a difference in allelic or genotype frequencies between cases and controls can suggest an association between cancer risk and the SNP, a linked gene or its regulatory region. Thus, it is natural to study the correlation of the two studies based on the assumption that the resulting gene sets from the two separate studies should be closely related. Such relationships can be revealed via a functional annotation of the top genes identified in both transcriptomics and GWAS along with the related pathway information. Statistical approaches of correlation analysis, such as Mann–Whitney U test (6), can also be used to directly study the different measurements to reveal the correlation. In a later section, we present a working example of breast cancer *omics* analysis where various discovery results are correlated for an integrated study.

3.2.4. The 4th 'C' – Applying Context Mapping (CM)

After having processed through the three 'Cs' and identified collective patterns in the *omics*-data, a key feature in integrative analysis is to understand or map the functional context of these common patterns (so-called context mapping (CM)). Several approaches are commonly used to create pathway networks, originally based on metabolic pathways, but more recently also protein, drug interactions, regulatory processes and disease maps are used. Pathway information is made publicly available by systems like KEGG (http://www.genome.jp/kegg/) and on commercial platforms from GeneGo (http://www.genego.com), Ingenuity (http://www.ingenuity.com/) and Ariadne Genomics (http://www.ariadnegenomics.com/) and can be integrated into workflow-based approaches. Given the growing number of excellent resources that are currently being made available as web services by many research organisations, CM can be easily integrated into workflow-based approaches enabling access to the latest information on demand.

An additional very useful source of CM is always biomedical literature. There are over 19 million citations within the MEDLINE database that are made available in abstract form by PubMed (http://www.ncbi.nlm.nih.gov/pubmed/). Current literature mining tools and the application of controlled vocabularies and ontologies allow fast context-based searching of these comprehensive databases. An example for such a tool is GoPubMed (http://www.gopubmed.org/) which allows enhanced structured browsing across the MEDLINE database based on Gene Ontology and MeSH terms. In addition, an ever growing wealth of data has become available in full text articles and companies like Thomson Reuters and Elsevier provide highly curated information, particularly in the areas of chemistry and biomarkers (*see* **Note 8**).

Last but not least is the visualisation of the obtained results, starting from the integration of the different *omics*-data to the functional mapping of biological context. Given the large amounts of data produced across the different platforms, we need a flexible way to interrogate, browse and add value to our *omics*-data. Thus visualisation tools are key features of organising context and contribute significantly in making sense of the data generated (*see* **Note 9**). Publicly available genome browsers such as UCSC (http://www.genome.ucsc.edu/) and Ensembl (http://www.ensembl.org/) have started to provide the facility to display *omics*-data together in its genomic context. Systems like Cytoscape (http://www.cytoscape.org) offer network analysis, and software such as InforSense Suite and Tibco Spotfire (http://www.spotfire.tibco.com/) make integration and visualisation of different clinical and research data possible.

3.3. Breast Cancer Omics as a Working Example of the ForeSee Approach

Basic breast cancer research tries to understand the molecular mechanisms of the origin and progression of cancer, as well as its invasion leading to metastatic disease. Over the years many studies have searched for prognostic and diagnostic biomarkers with the ultimate aim of developing therapeutic interventions to disturb the workings of genes and their involved pathways perturbed by their associated disease. All of the previously mentioned *omics* technologies have not only dramatically changed how breast cancer research has been conducted but also significantly contributed to the discovery of key genes and pathways, altered in some way and thereby defining specific molecular phenotypes and breast cancer types. Model systems such as breast cancer cell lines have played a significant role in our current understanding of breast cancer and were among the first to be extensively analysed by several different analytical platforms (16).

By using the InforSense Suite and by applying the ForeSee approach, we have combined *omics*-data from gene expression, DNA copy number and DNA methylation profiles together to systematically characterise, identify and verify possible new biomarkers or therapeutic targets for breast cancer research. For a panel of breast cancer cell lines, transcriptomic data was derived from Illumina human WG6 version 2 expression arrays; the genomic profiles were interrogated by two different platforms, namely a 32k tiling path bacterial artificial chromosome aCGH and the Human CNV370 Genotyping BeadChips (http://www.illumina.com/); and the epigenome was determined using the Illumina Golden Gate methylation array, providing methylation levels of ~1500 CpG islands.

Applying the first 'C' and thereby ensuring comprehensive coverage and achieving maximal information retrieval of each analytical platform and as well as the ability to perform cross-platform analyses, microarray features from each platform were sequence matched to the human genome build 18 of the UCSC genome assembly using BLAT (**Fig. 4.3**). Since all datasets were mapped to a CRK, it was possible to scale all data points to one scatter or overlay plot (as shown in **Fig. 4.6a**) and to visually interrogate millions of data points across the genome across different technologies, as well as gradually add more context to the data being viewed. In concordance with the second 'C', each platform was separately pre-processed, normalised and filtered, using in-house R scripts in combination with several Bioconductor packages (e.g.

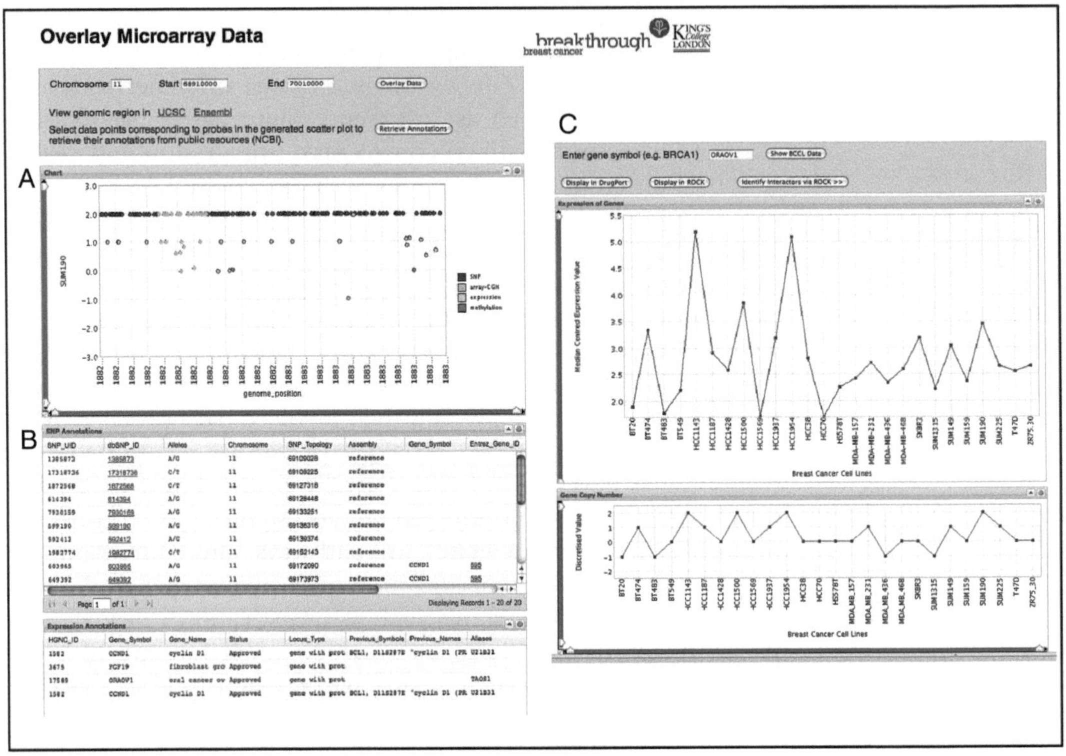

Fig. 4.6. Screenshots of different perspectives to visually interrogate integrative analytical platforms. (**a**) Overlay plot of microarray data, showing data points from SNPs, aCGH, expression and methylation omics-data across the chromosome 11: 68.91–70.01 MB for one case (e.g. breast cancer cell line SUM190). Annotations of selected features (**b**) as well as data across sample set (**c**) or external data can be retrieved and displayed.

lumi, *multitest*) of the R environment. CACs were wrapped up in workflows, providing a reusable service and self-documenting record of the analysis processes. The relationship between the expression matrix of robustly detected transcripts with defined levels of DNA copy number variation, genotype calls and loss of heterozygosity, as well as methylation measurements for each loci were combined, using the third 'C' approach. Transcriptomics, genomics and epigenomics datasets were merged by overlaying data at fixed genomic positions, and if necessary an average of measurements within genomic intervals was taken. Using correlation analysis as well as Mann–Whitney U tests for comparing the three datasets, genes whose expression was dependent on DNA copy number levels or those genes under DNA methylation influence, in addition to region of DNA hypomethylation and LOH were identified (**Fig. 4.1**). In concordance with the fourth 'C', gene sets with common patterns, e.g. co-expression of genes in certain breast cancer cell lines, genes whose expression was DNA copy number dependent or commonly hypermethylated, were subjected to pathway analysis to identify the biological context of their concurrences. Finally, as part of our ForeSee approach, we

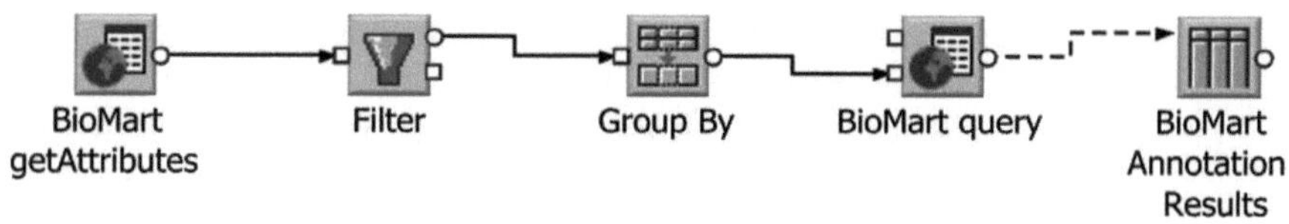

Fig. 4.7. Retrieval of BioMart annotations using a series of BioMart WebService queries.

also combined web service queries from ArrayExpress (http://www.ebi.ac.uk/microarray-as/ae/) and BioMart (http://www.biomart.org/) to access external transcriptomics data and annotated it to the same human genome build as our *omics*-data, so that we can integrate and cross-validate our results (**Fig. 4.7**).

3.4. The Impact of Next Generation Sequencing to Integrative Gene Discovery

The developments in new massively parallel sequencing technologies have made available a next generation of sequencing platforms. These NGS machines produce large numbers of short sequence reads which are used in 're-sequencing' applications where the availability of a reference sequence identical, or highly similar, to the investigating genetic material is assumed. This feature makes it fit well as the uniform technology for various gene discovery tasks. While SNP discovery can be regarded a typical re-sequencing application, the high throughput of short sequence reads enables the technology to be efficiently applied to a wide range of other functional genomics applications. Depending on the objective of a study, one can directly focus on selecting small fractions of a genome that appear as mRNA, as methylated or unmethylated fragments, as DNA or RNA bound by specific proteins or DNA regions that are hypersensitive to nucleases. These fragments can then be sequenced, mapped and then counted to provide a measurement of their abundance.

In general, NGS technology enables the, so-called, sequence census method: where the content of a complex nucleic acid sample can be measured by sequencing the sample directly, with the goal of getting just enough sequence to assign the site of origin in the genome for each read (17). A small snippet of 25–35 base pairs is enough to enable informatics to identify the location of each fragment on the reference genome. Once mapped, the abundance can be estimated by counting the hits and analysing their distribution throughout the genome.

As an example to illustrate this, by aligning 'reads' of cDNA to a reference genome, we can estimate the abundance of transcripts (digital expression profile) by counting the reads in the mapped exon region. Such a mapping can help to identify novel transcripts as well as splice variants. Thus, although there are technical challenges in making a correct expression estimation, such an RNA-seq technology, which produces expression profiles with digital counts, has a clear advantage over the microarray-based analogue expression profiles derived from decoding signal intensity.

With NGS technology, all the experiment platforms we have described above could be systematically replaced with the Seq-methods:

- Targeted discovery of mutations or polymorphisms and mapping of structural rearrangements, such as copy number variation, can both be done via resequencing.
- Transcriptomics studies can be run using the RNA-Seq consensus approach, analogous to the SAGE.
- Large-scale analysis of DNA methylation can be studied by deep sequencing of bisulphite-treated DNA.
- Genome-wide mapping of DNA–protein interactions by deep sequencing of DNA fragments pulled down by chromatin immunoprecipitation (called ChIP-Seq method).

Having many different kinds of functional genomics measurements made possible by these new sequencing-based methods, NGS provides a new paradigm for integrative analysis in gene discovery (18).

With regard to gene discovery based on integrative analysis, as proposed in our ForeSee approach, data modality would significantly be reduced by using a single sequence-based technology. In theory, a tuple of <gene-name, mapping-position, value>, where value can be counts or variants, will give most of the information needed for a gene discovery study. Such a simple data model will make the CRK-based integration easier. Also, the sequence-based methods would moderate data pre-processing since many variances introduced by signal detection and conversion are all removed. Single modality of data facilitates the identification of a well-defined set of common analytical components and also diminishes significantly the complexity of cross-modality comparison of different discovery results. In conclusion, using NGS will make the study of integrative genomics a uniform data science and the proposed ForeSee approach can be applied for building analytical workbenches.

In summary, our workflow-based ForeSee approach provides a reusable representation of the analysis process, the opportunity to build the individual components from several different angles and can be easily adjusted to accommodate new technologies such as NGS.

4. Notes

1. Workflows, sometimes also called pipeline or dataflow programming, are now widely adopted in life science informatics. The key concept of a workflow is to build up applications by linking computational components together. Since each

component performs a specific function which can be reused in any particular order, its application is ideal for the integrative analysis of ***omics***-data (*see* **Chapter** 7 for an exome data workflow). Each component in a workflow (representing either a data source or an analytical tool) is represented as a node in a graph. This graph provides a description of the input and output ports of the component, the type of data that can be passed to the component and parameters of the node that a user might want to change. Each node descriptor contains information, or metadata, covering three aspects: the tool's parameters, the node history within the context of the workflow (changes to parameter settings, user information, etc.) and user-added comments. Using the metadata information the user is guided in building the visual graphs as only nodes with corresponding inputs and outputs may be connected together.

2. InforSense workflows are represented and stored using DPML (Discovery Process Markup Language) which is an XML-based file format. The language supports both a dataflow model of computation for analytical workflows and control flow operations for linking and orchestrating multiple workflows together. Workflows can be therefore stored and distributed as a new means of conveying the knowledge about analysis processes. Thus, workflow is a good way to support collaborative and reproducible research.
3. In workflow systems, third party algorithms can be embedded into a workflow by making them new nodes. A new node can be made either using the APIs provided or using the web service interface. Thus, a workflow system is an open system in the sense that its functionality can be extended by adding new nodes.
4. Ad hoc integration is a technology which is complementary to the systematic integration technologies such as data warehousing and federation structures of integration are defined through building new data models. Ad hoc integration brings data together via an in-memory data management engine and is useful when the integration is specific to a particular subject or query. In life science, since most of queries have the exploratory nature, ad hoc integration is quite adequate.
5. To address the scientific questions in mind appropriately and still provide the flexibility for future research, an ideal common reference key for integrating data of several different sources and formats should be identified. When defining the common reference key, data dictionary and ontology can be used to map syntactic different names with the same semantics into a unique key.

6. Before progressing with the integration of *omics*-data, significant attention should be paid to data quality as well as the individual statistical models used in each step of analysis. An analytical workflow system is usually equipped with components to assess data quality.
7. For predictive modelling, -it is important to evaluate the quality of the derived models. Cross-validation is a commonly used technology. One round of cross-validation divides dates into two subsets: performing the analysis on one subset (*training set*) and validating the analysis on the other subset (*testing set*). To reduce variability, multiple rounds of cross-validation are performed using different partitions, and the validation results are averaged over the rounds.
8. Due to the vast size of *omics*-data, biological interpretation of integrative data analysis is the ultimate challenge. As a starting point for the validity of the result, it is advised to look for known biological characteristics (e.g. known copy number variation in specific genomic locations, higher expression levels of specific gene).
9. Each step in the process of data integration and analysis – such as data quality control, predictive modelling, overlaying of different datasets, biological interpretation – is best evaluated by good graphical displays. Thus a strong emphasis should be given to the visualisation of the data and the results.

Acknowledgements

The authors would like to acknowledge Andrew J. Tutt for his contribution to the breast cancer study presented in **Section 3.3**.

References

1. Velculescu, V. E., Zhang, L., Vogelstein, B., and Kinzler, K. W. (1995) Serial analysis of gene expression. *Science 270*, 484–487.
2. Shinawi, M., and Cheung, S. W. (2008) The array CGH and its clinical applications. *Drug Discov Today 13*, 760–770.
3. Yue, P., and Moult, J. (2006) Identification and analysis of deleterious human SNPs. *J Mol Biol 356*, 1263–1274.
4. Bird, A. (2007) Perceptions of epigenetics. *Nature 447*, 396–398.
5. Aparicio, O., and Geisberg, J. V. (2004) Chromatin immunoprecipitation for determining the association of proteins with specific genomic sequences in vivo. In, Chapter 17, Unit 17.7 *Current Protocols in Cell Biology*. Juan S. Bonifacino, Mary Dasso, Joe B. Harford, Jennifer Lippincott-

Schwartz, and Kenneth M. Yamada (Eds.) Wiley, Los Angeles, CA.

6. Conover, W. J. (1980) *Practical Nonparametric Statistics*, 3rd ed. Wiley, New York, NY.
7. Chong, F., Carraro, G., Wolter, R. (2009) Multi-Tenant Data Architecture. http://msdn.microsoft.com/en-us/library/aa479086.aspx
8. Stafford, P. (2008) *Methods In Microarray Normalization*. CRC Press, New York, NY.
9. Kaplan, E. L., and Meier, P. (1958) *Nonparametric Estimation from Incomplete Observations. J Am Stat Assoc* ***53***(282), 457–481.
10. Freedman, D. A. (2007) *Statistics*. W.W. Norton & Company, New York, NY.
11. Corder, G. W., and Foreman, D. I. (2009) *Nonparametric Statistics for Non-Statisticians: A Step-by-Step Approach*. Wiley, River Street Hoboken, NJ.
12. Zuber, V., and Strimmer, K. (2009) Gene ranking and biomarker discovery. *Bioinformatics* 25, 2700–2707.
13. Tan, P., Steinbach, M., and Kumar, V. (2002) Clustering analysis: basic concepts and algorithms. In *Introduction to Data Mining*, Chapter 8, 487–559. Addison-Wesley, Boston, MA.
14. Klosgen, W., and Zytkow, J. M. (2002) *Handbook of Data Mining and Knowledge Discovery*. Oxford University Press, Oxford.
15. Gorlov, I. P., Gallick, G. E., Gorlova, O. Y., Amos, C., and Logothetis, C. J. (2009) GWAS meets microarray: are the results of genome-wide association studies and gene-expression profiling consistent? Prostate cancer as an example. *PLoS One* ***4***, e6511.
16. Neve, R. M., Chin, K., Fridlyand, J., Yeh, J., Baehner, F. L., Fevr, T., Clark, L., Bayani, N., Coppe, J. P., Tong, F., Speed, T., Spellman, P. T., DeVries, S., Lapuk, A., Wang, N. J., Kuo, W. L., Stilwell, J. L., Pinkel, D., Albertson, D. G., Waldman, F. M., McCormick, F., Dickson, R. B., Johnson, M. D., Lippman, M., Ethier, S., Gazdar, A., and Gray, J. W. (2006) A collection of breast cancer cell lines for the study of functionally distinct cancer subtypes. *Cancer Cell* ***10***, 515–527.
17. Wold, B., and Myers, R. M. (2008) Sequence census methods for functional genomics. *Nat Methods* ***5***, 19–21.
18. Mardis, E. R. (2008) The impact of next-generation sequencing technology on genetics. *Trends Genet* ***24***, 133–141.

Chapter 5

R Statistical Tools for Gene Discovery

Andrea S. Foulkes and Kinman Au

Abstract

A wide assortment of R tools are available for exploratory data analysis in high-dimensional settings and are easily applicable to data arising from population-based genetic association studies. In this chapter we illustrate the application of three such approaches, namely conditional inference trees, random forests, and logic regression. Through applications to simulated data, we explore the relative utility of each approach for uncovering underlying association between genetic polymorphisms and a quantitative trait.

Key words: Recursive partitioning, random forests, logic regression, single nucleotide polymorphisms (SNPs), R tools.

1. Introduction

Genetic association studies typically involve collection of data on a large number of single nucleotide polymorphisms (SNPs) and a measure of disease progression or disease status. The goal of these investigations is to identify SNPs that, either singly or in combination with other SNPs and environmental or demographic factors, associate with the measured trait (*see* "Association mapping" in **Chapter 3**). The use of R tools for this data setting is increasingly popular and several introductory level reference texts are available that describe both key statistical principles and the application of associated software tools to this setting (1–3).

Specifically, these texts offer extensive coverage of the fundamental methods underlying R tools for (a) identification of genotyping errors, relatedness, and population substructure – including the cmdscale() and prcomp() functions in the R base installation; GenomicControl() and qqpval() in SNPassoc;

B. Yu, M. Hinchcliffe (eds.), *In Silico Tools for Gene Discovery*, Methods in Molecular Biology 760,
DOI 10.1007/978-1-61779-176-5_5, © Springer Science+Business Media, LLC 2011

ibs.stats() and qq.chisq() in snpMatrix; ibs() and estlambda() in GenABEL; and gcontrol() and gcontrol2() in the gap package; (b) estimation and testing for linkage disequilibrium and Hardy–Weinberg equilibrium – including the LD(), HWE.chisq(), and HWE.exact() functions in genetics; LD() and tableHWE() in SNPassoc; HWE.show() in GenABEL; ld.snp() and summary() in snpMatrix; and hwe(), hwe.cc(), hwe.hardy(), LD22(), and LDkl() in the gap package; (c) multiple testing adjustments – including p.adjust() in the R base installation; qvalue() in qvalue; qvaluebh95() in GenABEL; Bonferroni.sig() in SNPassoc; and mt.maxT() and mt.minP() in the multtest package; (d) analysis of unobservable haplotypic phase – including haplo.em() and haplo.glm() in haplo.stats; and htr() in gap; and (e) efficient design of experiments – including pbsize() and pbsize2() in the gap package.

In this chapter, we focus on the application of three exploratory, machine learning approaches – namely conditional inference trees (CITs), random forests (RFs), and logic regression (LR) – that are designed specifically for uncovering complex structures of association in high-dimensional data settings. Our investigations concentrate on quantitative traits, although discussion is provided on alternative outcomes in **Section 4**. Further, we assume the data under study arise from population-based investigations of unrelated individuals, so that observations are independent (*see* **Note 1**). Important considerations in population-based studies that are not addressed in this chapter include population substructure, missing data, and unobservable haplotypic phase (*see* **Notes 2** and **3**). We begin in **Section 2** by describing the genotype data and a range of underlying models of association that can be applied to derive the phenotype data used throughout this chapter. Both the simulated genotype and the phenotype data are publicly available at the URL noted below. In **Section 3** we demonstrate application of CITs, RFs, and LR to each of the simulated data sets using existing R packages and highlight the interpretation and relative advantages of each approach. Finally, in **Section 4**, we offer some additional notes on the application of these methods.

2. Materials

The data used throughout this chapter are publicly available at http://people.umass.edu/foulkes/asg/data.html and are generated based on data provided in the R snpMatrix package (4). All analyses presented are performed using R version 2.11.1 (2010-05-31). In order to install and upload the required R packages – party, randomForest, and LogicReg – for use in the programs described in this Chapter, the following commands can be typed at the R prompt:

```
> install.packages(c("party," "randomForest," "LogicReg"))
> library(party)
> library(randomForest)
> library(LogicReg)
```

Additional packages may be required for earlier versions of R. The genotype data are simulated according to data from the HapMap project as described in (5) and derived from data available through the snpMatrix package. Briefly, the data we consider are comprised of $n = 1000$ individuals and 449 SNPs across 12 genes on chromosome 10 that are potentially relevant to the study of cardiovascular disease. A sample of these data are provided in **Table 5.1**, where the rows represent the first 10 individuals and the columns correspond to 5 SNPs within the tumor necrosis factor receptor superfamily, member 6 (*FAS*) gene, and 2 SNPs within the nuclear factor-kappa-B2 (*NFKB2*) gene. All SNPs under study are bi-allelic, and thus genotypes are three-level factors for homozygous for the major (wild-type) allele, heterozygous, and homozygous for the minor (variant) allele.

To read the simulated genotype data into a current R session, the following commands can be typed directly at the R prompt:

```
> snpSIM <- read.table("http://people.umass.edu/foulkes/asg/data/
  snpSimCVDNum.txt")
```

Table 5.1
Sample simulated genotype data

	FAS					*NFKB2*	
ID	**rs1324551**	**rs6586164**	**rs7097467**	**rs9325603**	**rs6586165**	**rs7897947**	**rs11574851**
jpt.869	C/T	A/T	C/T	C/G	A/T	G/T	C/T
jpt.862	C/C	T/T	T/T	G/G	T/T	T/T	C/C
jpt.948	C/T	A/T	C/T	C/G	A/T	G/T	C/C
ceu.564	C/C	T/T	T/T	G/G	T/T	T/T	C/C
ceu.904	C/T		T/T	G/G	A/T	G/T	C/C
ceu.665	C/C	T/T	T/T	G/G	T/T	T/T	C/C
jpt.663	C/T	A/T	C/T	C/G	A/T	G/G	C/C
ceu.977	C/T	A/T	T/T	G/G	A/T	T/T	C/C
jpt.637	C/T	A/T	C/T	C/G	A/T	T/T	C/C
ceu.897	C/T	A/T	T/T	G/G	A/T	T/T	C/C

```
> snpSIMcvd <- read.table("http://people.umass.edu/foulkes/asg/
  data/snpSimCVD.txt")
```

The snpSIM data table contains a numeric representation of the data, in which 0, 1, and 2 represent the numbers of variant alleles at the corresponding SNP locus, while snpSIMcvd contains the genotypes in the form of nucleotides. In addition to the genotype data, multiple quantitative traits are generated according to a range of underlying models of association, labeled Models A–D and described below (*see* **Note 4**). These traits can be called into R using the following code or regenerated based on the details provided below. Note that in order for the examples used throughout this chapter to give the same results as presented, the original simulated data must be used.

```
> ySIM <- read.table("http://people.umass.edu/foulkes/asg/data/
  ySimCVD.txt")
> attach(ySIM)
```

We consider four scenarios (Models A–D below), and in each case we assume three genes – namely, nuclear factor-kappa-B2 (*NFKB2*), tumor necrosis factor receptor super family, member 6 (*FAS*), and conserved helix-loop-helix ubiquitous kinase (*CHUK*) – are relevant predictors of the variability in a quantitative trait (*see* **Note 5**). A complete list of the observed SNPs within each of these genes is given in **Table 5.2**. Models A and D are both additive models of association with dominant SNP effects; however, Model A assumes a single SNP within each gene as a significant predictor, while Model D assumes all of the observed SNPs in each gene are relevant. Model B assumes a multiplicative association while Model C involves both an additive and multiplicative relationship between the SNPs and the trait.

Table 5.2
SNP names (rs numbers) within each of three genes

Gene	SNPs
NFKB2	rs7897947 rs11574851
FAS	rs1324551 rs6586164 rs7097467 rs9325603 rs6586165 rs6586167 rs2147420 rs4406738 rs9658727 rs9658741 rs9658750 rs2031613 rs9658761 rs982764 rs2234978 rs9658767 rs1977389
CHUK	rs11597086 rs6584350 rs12764727 rs17729417 rs7923726 rs7909855 rs12269373 rs7922090 rs11591741 rs11190430 rs12247992

Simple Additive Model (Model A). The first model of association is an additive model with a single important SNP within each of the three genes. Each of these SNPs is assumed to have a dominant effect on the trait so that one or more variant alleles at the corresponding locus will induce an increase (or decrease) in the value of the trait. For simplicity, we let the first SNP within each gene be the relevant one (respectively given by rs7897947, rs1324551, and rs11597086) and apply the following code to create a binary indicator for the presence of at least one variant allele at this SNP locus. These new variables are labeled x*NFKB2*, x*FAS*, and x*CHUK* for the respective genes.

```
> xNFKB2 <- snpSIM[,is.element(colnames(snpSIM),rsNFKB2)]
  [,1]>0
> xFAS <- snpSIM[,is.element(colnames(snpSIM),rsFAS)][,1] >0
> xCHUK <- snpSIM[,is.element(colnames(snpSIM),rsCHUK)]
  [,1]>0
```

A normally distributed trait, yA, is then generated using the following code: Suppose for example that yA is triglyceride (TG) level, measured in mg/dL. This model implies that the mean TG level among individuals in our population who are homozygous for the major alleles at rs7897947, rs1324551, and rs11597086 is $\mu = 85$ mg/dL with a standard deviation of sd = 4. Further, the presence of at least one variant allele at the rs7897947 locus will lead to an average increase in TG level of 5 mg/dL. Similarly, at least one variant allele at either the rs1324551 or rs11597086 locus will increase the TG level an average of 5 mg/dL. Finally, these effects are assumed to be additive in nature as they will occur regardless of whether or not variant alleles are present at any other SNP loci.

```
> yA <- 85 + 5*xNFKB2 + 5*xFAS + 5*xCHUK+ rnorm
  (1000,0,4)
```

Multiplicative Model (Model B). The second model we consider is a multiplicative model of association in which polymorphisms across all three genes must be present in order to impact the trait. Again, each SNP is assumed to have a dominant genetic model. Specifically, we assume the mean value of the trait increases by 10 units if at least one variant allele is present at each of the three SNPs rs7897947, rs1324551, and rs11597086 in *NFKB2*, *FAS*, and *CHUK*, respectively. In this case, the trait is generated using the following code:

```
> yB <- 85 + 10*xNFKB2*xFAS*xCHUK + rnorm(1000,0,4)
```

Combined Additive and Multiplicative Model (Model C). The third model assumes a combination of additive and multiplicative associations and a dominant genetic model. Specifically, the presence of at least one variant allele at rs11597086 is assumed to increase the mean of the trait by 10 units and the presence of a variant allele at both rs7897947 and rs1324551 increases this mean an additional 4 units. The following code is used to simulate the trait under this model:

```
> yC <- 85 + 4*xNFKB2*xFAS + 10*xCHUK+ rnorm(1000,0,4)
```

Additive Model with Multiple Informative SNPs Within Each Gene (Model D). Finally, the fourth model we consider assumes an additive effect of the three genes; however, under this model the effect is present if at least half of the SNPs within the gene have one or more variant alleles. These data are simulated as follows, where again x*NFKB2*, x*FAS*, and x*CHUK* represent the newly created indicator variables:

```
> xNFKB2 <-
  apply(snpSIM[,is.element(colnames(snpSIM),rsNFKB2)]!=0,1,
  sum,na.rm=T)>=2/2
> xFAS <-
  apply(snpSIM[,is.element(colnames(snpSIM),rsFAS)]!=0,1,sum,
  na.rm=T)>=(17/2)
> xCHUK <-
  apply(snpSIM[,is.element(colnames(snpSIM),rsCHUK)]!=0,1,
  sum,na.rm=T)>=(11/2)
> yD <- 85 + 5*xNFKB2 + 5*xFAS + 5*xCHUK+ rnorm
  (1000,0,4)
```

3. Methods

3.1. Conditional Inference Trees (CIT)

Recursive partitioning (RP) is a well-described exploratory data analysis approach for uncovering complex underlying structure in high-dimensional data settings (2, 6, 7), with corresponding R tools within the rpart, tree, and party packages. A detailed description of the rpart package, including functions for growing and pruning classification and regression trees (CARTs), is provided in (2). Here we demonstrate application of an alternative approach involving generation of conditional inference trees (CITs) (8, 9), based on the ctree() function within the party package in R (*see* **Note 6**).

A CIT is generated through application of the following three-step procedure: (a) Test formally for a global association between the potential predictor variables and the outcome and, if statistically significant, identify and select the most important predictor variable; (b) Split data into groups based on the values of this selected variable; and (c) Recursively split according to steps (a) and (b) until a significant association is not detectable.

Importantly, implementation of a multiple comparison adjustment at each stage of the splitting algorithm obviates the need for subsequent pruning of the resultant tree to ensure reproducibility. We begin in the following example by fitting a CIT to the simulated outcome described by ModelA in **Section 2**.

Example 1: Fitting a CIT in R to Model A data. First we define the variable yA to be our trait and subset the data with complete information on this variable. Notably, the ctree() function requires no missing data on the outcome variable.

```
> trait <- yA
> snpSIM.c <- subset(snpSIM, !is.na(trait))
> trait.c <- subset(trait, !is.na(trait))
```

In order to avoid making an a priori assumption about the underlying genetic model (e.g., additive, dominant, or recessive), we define the SNPs as factor variables:

```
> snpSIMfact <- data.frame(apply(snpSIM.c,2,as.factor))
```

Finally, we generate a corresponding CIT and plot the results. Here we specify type ="simple" to return the means at each of the terminal nodes.

```
> ctreeSIM <- ctree(trait.c~.,data=snpSIMfact)
> plot(ctreeSIM,type="simple")
```

A visual representation of the resulting tree is given in **Fig. 5.1a**. To understand the output from this analysis, consider first the data arising from Model A and the corresponding CIT given in **Fig. 5.1a**. In this case, the first split is on the rs1324551 SNP within the *FAS* gene. Among individuals with 1 and 2 variant alleles at this SNP locus – left daughter node, indicated by the symbol [2] – and individuals with no variant alleles at this locus – right daughter node, indicated by the symbol [9] – the next best predictor variable is rs7897947 within *NFKB2*. Among all resulting groups – child nodes, represented by the symbols [3], [6], [10] and [13] – the best predictor is rs11597086 within the *CHUK* gene. As expected, the predicted mean response for individuals with no variant alleles at these three SNPs – node [15] – is approximately equal to 85. On the other hand, the means for those individuals with 1 or 2 variant alleles at exactly one of the three SNPS – nodes [8], [12] or [14] – are approximately 85+5=90. Individuals with variants at exactly two of these SNPs – nodes [5], [7] or [11] – have a mean response of approximately 85+2*5=95, and finally those individuals with variants at all three SNPs – node [4] – have a mean of approximately 85+3*5=100.

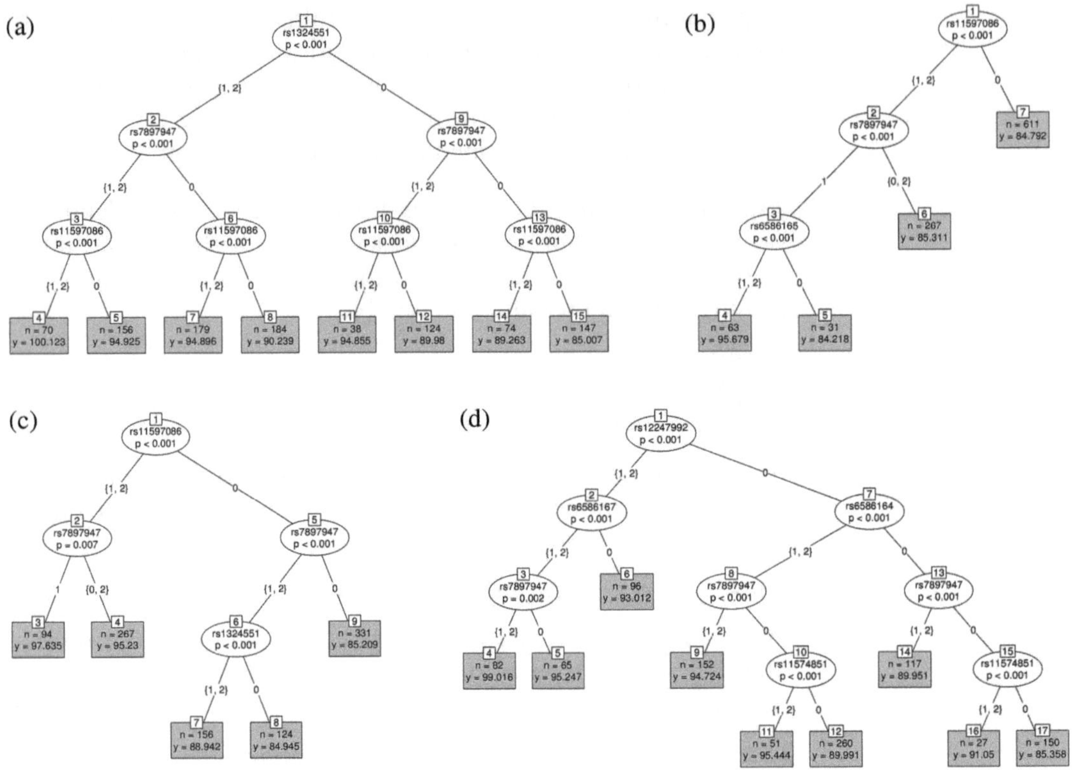

Fig. 5.1. Conditional inference tree with unspecified genetic model. (**a**) Model A: simple additive model with single informative SNP within each gene. (**b**) Model B: multiplicative model. (**c**) Model C: additive and multiplicative model. (**d**) Model D: additive model with multiple informative SNPs within each gene.

Example 2: Fitting a CIT in R to Model B data (assuming a dominant genetic model). A CIT from Model B data can be generated using the same code as in Example 1, with the trait defined as yB. The resulting tree is illustrated in **Fig. 5.1b** and similarly identifies all three important SNPs: rs11597086, rs7897947, and rs6586165. In this case, however, as expected, we see an asymmetrical tree. That is, the rs7897947 SNP is a significant predictor of the trait only among individuals with at least one variant allele at rs11597086 – node [2] – and is not a significant predictor among individuals who are homozygous wild type at this SNP locus – node [7]. Notably, the best split on the rs7897947 SNP differentiates between individuals with exactly one variant allele – node [3] – and those with either no variant alleles or two copies of the variant allele – node [6]. If we, alternatively, specify the genotype data as binary indicators for the presence of one or more variant alleles (i.e., a dominant genetic model), then the tree illustrated in **Fig. 5.2a** would result. The following code is used to generate this tree:

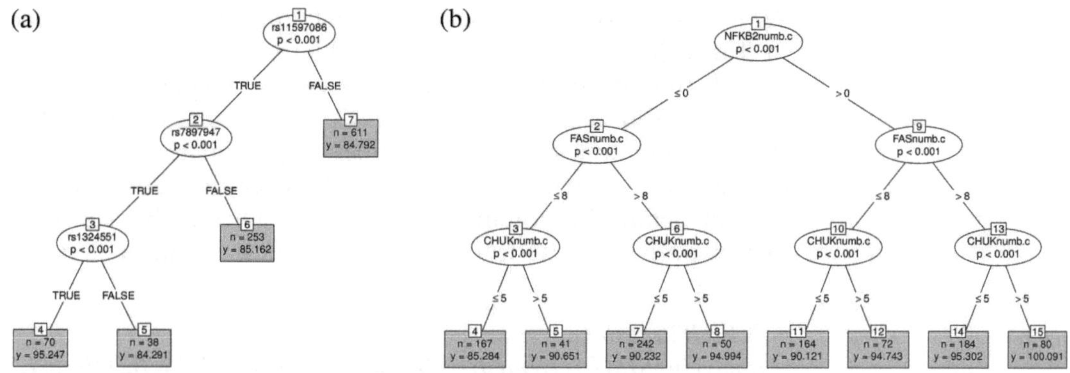

Fig. 5.2. Conditional inference trees with alternative genetic models. (**a**) Model B: dominant genetic model. (**b**) Model D: threshold genetic model.

```
> snpSIMfact <- data.frame(apply(snpSIM.c>=1,2, as.factor))
```

In this figure, "TRUE" corresponds to one or two variant alleles, given by {1,2} **Fig. 5.1b**, while "FALSE" corresponds to no variant alleles or {0}. In this example, the same result is obtained if genotypes are treated as numeric so that the only possible splits are {0} versus {1,2} and {0,1} versus {2}.

Example 3: Fitting a CIT in R to Model C data. Next we fit a CIT to data arising from Model C, illustrated in **Fig. 5.1c**, for the more general genetic model. Similar to the results we saw in **Fig. 5.1b**, this tree is generally consistent, with the exception of the split based on rs7897947 at node 2. Recall Model C includes a main effect of rs11597086, and as expected, in both cases the first split is on this variable such that individuals with at least one variant allele belong to node 2 while individuals who are homozygous wild type are in node 5. Additional splits reveal the existence of an interaction between rs7897947 and rs1324551, although the precise nature of the interactions is less clear than we saw for Model B. Specifically, the interaction between these two SNPs is discovered among individuals who are homozygous wild type at rs11597086 – node 5 – but not among those individuals with a variant allele at this SNP locus – node 2.

Example 4: Fitting a CIT in R to Model D data (assuming a threshold genetic effect). Finally, the CIT generated based on Model D, illustrated in **Fig. 5.1d**, suggests multiple SNPs within each gene are informative. Similar to **Fig. 5.1a**, the near symmetry in this tree suggests an underlying additive model of association, as expected. However, the selected SNPs – namely, rs12247992 in *CHUK*, rs6586167 in *FAS*, rs7897947 and rs11574851 in

NFKB2 – are only a subset of the truly informative SNPs listed in **Table 5.2**. Interestingly, if Model D is truly the underlying model, this approach to fitting the tree favors genes with fewer observed SNPs, in this case *NFKB2*. This results from the fact that splitting on a single SNP will best approximate the true predictor variable when there are fewer SNPs per gene. Alternatively, we can define the potential predictor variables to be the number of SNPs with at least one variant allele within a gene, as follows:

```
> NFKB2numb <-
  apply(snpSIM[,is.element(colnames(snpSIM),rsNFKB2)]!=0,1,
  sum,na.rm=T)
> NFKB2numb.c <- subset(NFKB2numb, !is.na(trait))

> FASnumb <- apply(snpSIM[,is.element(colnames(snpSIM),
  rsFAS)]!=0,1,sum,na.rm=T)
> FASnumb.c <- subset(FASnumb, !is.na(trait))

> CHUKnumb <-
  apply(snpSIM[,is.element(colnames(snpSIM),rsCHUK)]!=0,1,
  sum,na.rm=T)
> CHUKnumb.c <- subset(CHUKnumb, !is.na(trait))
```

The ctree() function is then applied as follows:

```
> ctreeSIM <- ctree(trait.c~NFKB2numb.c + FASnumb.c
  + CHUKnumb.c)
> plot(ctreeSIM,type="simple")
```

The corresponding tree that results in is given in **Fig. 5.2b**. Here we again see a symmetric tree, suggesting an additive model, and this approach is able to identify with reasonable precision, the true underlying thresholds defined in the Model D simulation.

3.2. Random Forests

Random forests (RFs) are comprised of an ensemble of classification or regression trees and result in a measure of variable importance for each potential predictor variable (2, 10–12). The RF algorithm proceeds as follows: after initializing $b = 1$: (a) Randomly sample with replacement n_1 (approximately equal to $2n/3$) individuals, and call this the learning sample (LS). Let the remaining $n_2 = n - n_1$ individuals represent the out-of-bag (OOB) data. (b) Using the LS data only, generate an unpruned tree by randomly sampling a subset of the p predictors (denoted $\mathbf{x}_1,\ldots, \mathbf{x}_p$) at each node to be considered as potential splitting variables. (c) Based on the OOB data only: (i) Record the overall tree impurity, and let this be denoted π_b; (ii) Permute $\mathbf{x}_j$, and record overall tree impurity using the permuted data for each $j = 1,\ldots, p$. Denote this π_{bj} and define the variable importance for the jth predictor as $\delta_{bj} = \pi_{bj} - \pi_b$. (d) Repeat steps (a)–(c) for $b = 2, \ldots,$

B to obtain $\delta_{1j}, \ldots, \delta_{Bj}$ for each j. (e) Record the overall variable importance score for $\mathbf{x}_1, \ldots, \mathbf{x}_p$, defined for the jth predictor as $\hat{\theta}_j = \frac{1}{B}\sum_{b=1}^{B}\delta_{bj}$. The mean decrease in accuracy (denoted %IncMSE in R) is given by $\hat{\theta}_j/SE(\hat{\theta}_j)$ and is typically reported as a standardized measure of variable importance for each j. In the following example we illustrate fitting a RF to each of the data sets derived from Models A–D.

Example 5: Fitting a RF in R to Model A–D data. Using the snpSIM.c and trait.c objects described in Example 1 of **Section 3.1**, we fit a RF using the randomForests() function in R as follows. We begin by replacing the missing data with "0," representing homozygous wild type, which constitutes a single imputation. The variable importance scores are returned by applying the importance() function to the resulting tree object and plotted using the generic dot chart() function:

```
> snpSIM.c[is.na(snpSIM.c)] <- 0
> snpSIMfact <- data.frame(apply(snpSIM.c,2,as.factor))
> forestSIM <- randomForest(snpSIMfact,trait.c, importance=
  TRUE)
> imp <- importance(forestSIM)
> ord <- order(imp[,1],decreasing=TRUE)[30:1]
> dotchart(imp[ord,1],label=row.names(imp)[ord], xlab="%Inc
  MSE," cex=0.8,xlim=c(0,60))
```

The resulting ordered variable importance scores and corresponding SNP names are illustrated in **Fig. 5.3a–d**. Consider first the additive model (Model A) depicted in **Fig. 5.3a**. As expected, the SNPs with the highest corresponding variable importance scores are rs7897947, rs1159086, and rs1324551. Interestingly, the first of these SNPs has a much greater %IncMSE than the remaining SNPs, despite having the same underlying effect size as rs1159086 and rs1324551. Also of note, several additional SNPs in the same genes – including rs11591741, rs12269373 in *CHUK* and rs6586164, rs6586165, and rs6586167 in *FAS* – have relatively high importance scores. This ability of RF to detect correlated SNPs is a natural consequence of step (b) in the RF algorithm that involves sampling a subset of the p predictors. In turn, the smaller number of SNPs under study in the *NFKB2* gene, and thus fewer variables that are highly correlated with rs7897947 (as compared with rs1159086 and rs1324551 for which there are several correlated potential predictor variables – *see* **Table 5.2**) may explain the relatively high importance score associated with rs7897947.

Similar to the additive model setting, the variable importance scores for Model B data illustrated in **Fig. 5.3b** implicate rs7897947 in *NFKB2* as the strongest predictor of the trait. Based

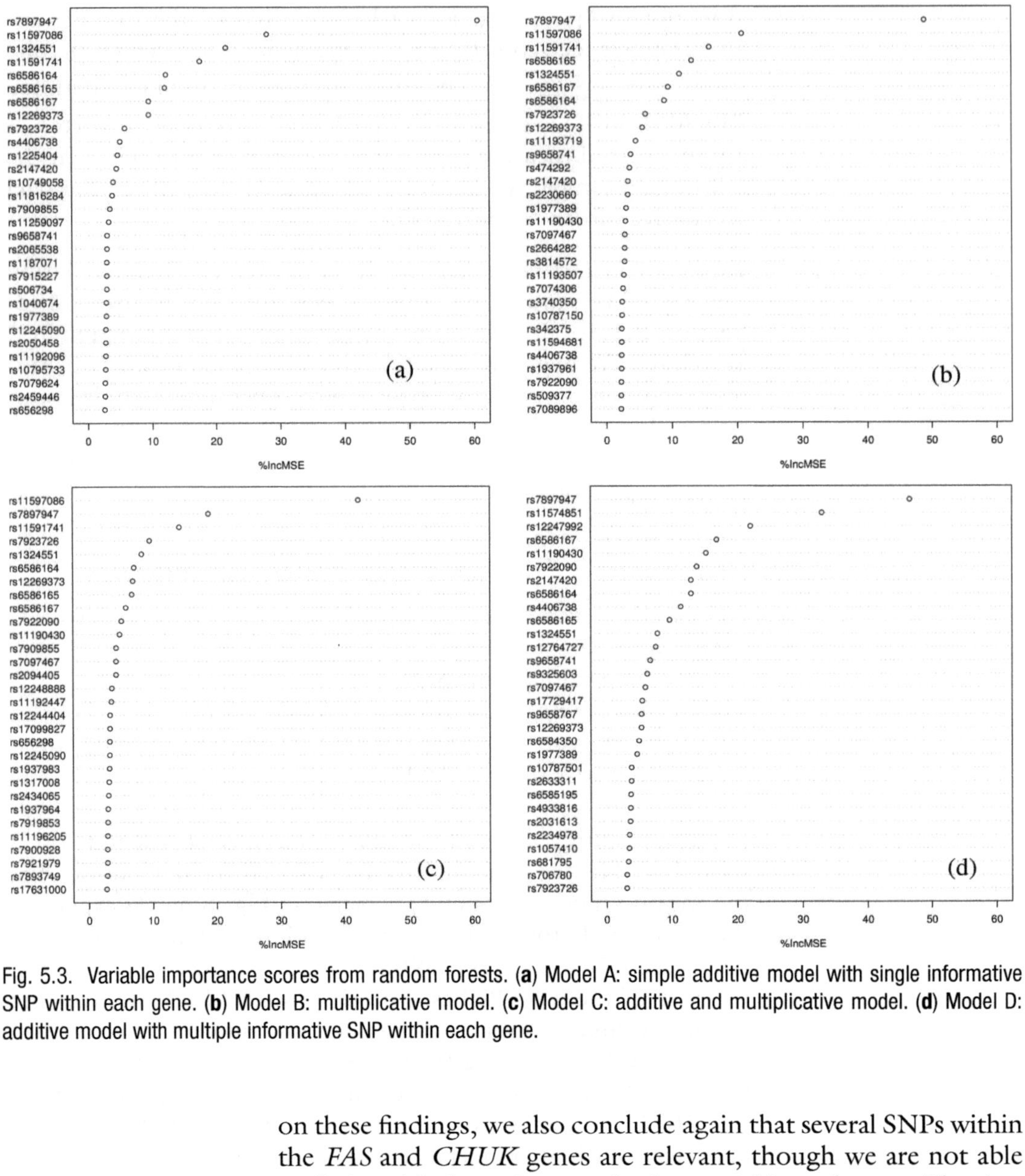

Fig. 5.3. Variable importance scores from random forests. (**a**) Model A: simple additive model with single informative SNP within each gene. (**b**) Model B: multiplicative model. (**c**) Model C: additive and multiplicative model. (**d**) Model D: additive model with multiple informative SNP within each gene.

on these findings, we also conclude again that several SNPs within the *FAS* and *CHUK* genes are relevant, though we are not able to distinguish the truly causative locus within each gene. The similarity in the results presented in **Fig. 5.3a, b** suggests that application of a RF yields important information about the relative importance of sets of SNPs but does not uncover the underlying model of association. That is, we cannot distinguish between the additive and the multiplicative model based on the resulting variable importance scores.

The results of fitting a RF to Model C data are given in **Fig. 5.3c**. In this case, as expected, the most important predictor is rs11597086 in the *CHUK* gene, which has the largest underlying effect size. The next highest importance score corresponds to rs7897947 in *NFKB2* which contributed to the trait through an interaction term with rs1324551 in *FAS*; however, rs1324551 is ranked with the fifth highest importance score and SNPs in *CHUK* (and thus correlated with rs11597086) surpass it in rank. Again, overall we identify all three genes as relevant, though the precise underlying model is indecipherable. Finally, fitting a RF to Model D data yields the results illustrated in **Fig. 5.3d**. In this case, almost all of the 30 SNPs listed belong to the three relevant genes. Comparing this figure to **Fig. 5.3a–c**, we see that the importance scores tend to be slightly larger, suggesting more of the SNPs within each gene are indeed impacting the trait (*see* **Notes 5, 6**).

3.3. Logic Regression

Logic regression is an alternative approach that searches for the best predictor variables in the form of a linear combination of Boolean expressions (13) and has been described for use with SNP data (2, 14–19). For example, suppose $\mathbf{x}_1$, $\mathbf{x}_2$, and $\mathbf{x}_3$ represent indicators for at least one variant allele at SNPs rs7897947, rs1159086, and rs1324551, respectively. A Boolean expression takes on the value 0 or 1 and is a logical function of these variables that involves "and," "or," and "complement" statements. For example, if $L_1 = \mathbf{x}_1 \wedge \mathbf{x}_2 \wedge \mathbf{x}_3$, read "$\mathbf{x}_1$ and $\mathbf{x}_2$ and $\mathbf{x}_3$," then L is a Boolean expression that equals 1 if there is at least one variant allele at all three SNPs, i.e., $\mathbf{x}_1 = \mathbf{x}_2 = \mathbf{x}_3 = 1$, and equals 0 otherwise. On the other hand $L_1 = \mathbf{x}_1 \vee \mathbf{x}_2 \vee \mathbf{x}_3$, read "$\mathbf{x}_1$ or $\mathbf{x}_2$ or $\mathbf{x}_3$," is an indicator for at least one variant allele at one or more of the three SNPs. A logic tree can be comprised of a single Boolean expression, such as $\beta_1 L_1$, or a combination of two or more Boolean expressions, such as $\beta_1 L_1 + \beta_2 L_2$.

The score of a logic tree is defined according to the type of outcome under study. In the case of a quantitative trait, the residual sum of squares is used as the measure of model fit while deviance is used for a binary outcome. To avoid over fitting, a tenfold cross-validation (CV) procedure is applied to arrive at the number of trees and leaves in the final model. Finally, a permutation test is applied to determine whether this model is statistically different than a null model of no association. This approach is illustrated in the following example.

Example 6: Logic regression applied to Model A–D data. We begin by specifying parameters for the simulated annealing algorithm using the logreg.anneal.control() function and then fit a logic tree using the logreg() function in R. Here, as our trait is quantitative, we specify type=2 to indicate that a regression model should be fitted. Further specifying select=2 results in fitting multiple models with the numbers of trees ranging, in this example, from 1 to 2 (as indicated by ntree) and the number of leaves ranging from 1 to 10 (as indicated by nleaves.) Notably, logic regression requires that the potential predictor variables are binary, and so we create the data matrix snpSIMbin, which contains binary indicators for the presence of at least one variant allele at the corresponding locus, consistent with a dominant genetic model.

```
> myanneal <- logreg.anneal.control(start = -1, end = -4,iter
  = 25000, update = 0)
> snpSIMbin <- data.frame(apply(snpSIM.c>=1,2, as.numeric))
> fitSIM1 <- logreg(resp = trait.c, bin=snpSIMbin, type = 2, +
  select = 2, ntrees = c(1,2), nleaves =c(1,10), anneal.control =
  myanneal)
```

Next we apply a CV procedure to determine the number of trees and leaves that result in the best cross-validated score. We do this by specifying select=3 in the logreg() function and plotting the resulting object. The resulting plots are illustrated in **Fig. 5.4a–d** for Models A–D, respectively.

```
> fitSIM2 <- logreg(select = 3, oldfit = fitSIM1)
> plot(fitSIM2)
```

We see, for example, in **Fig. 5.4a**, **c** for Model A and C data, the lowest cross-validated score is given by 2 trees and 3 leaves. For Model B data, illustrated in **Fig. 5.4b**, the cross-validated score for 2 trees decreases sharply as the model size increases from 1 to 5 nodes, and then begins to level with increasing model size. Thus, 2 trees with 5 leaves appears to be the optimal model. Finally, for Model D data, 3 trees with 8 leaves is optimal.

Once the number of trees and leaves is determined, we can fit the final model again using the logreg() function with select=2. Corresponding trees are illustrated in **Fig. 5.5a–d**. In these figures, unshaded boxes indicate "TRUE" (i.e., the presence of at least one variant allele at the corresponding site) while shaded boxes indicate "FALSE" or the complement (i.e., homozygous for the wild-type allele at the corresponding site). Consider, for example, the Model A data. Here an optimal model includes 2 trees and 3 leaves, and so we specify ntrees=2 and nleaves=3 as shown below.

```
> lrFinal <- logreg(resp=trait.c,bin=snpSIMbin,select=2,ntrees=2,
  nleaves=3)
> lrFinal
2 trees with 3 leaves: score is 4.395
+5.56 * (rs7897947 or rs11597086) + 5.26 * rs1324551
```

As expected, the final model, shown in the above output and **Fig. 5.5a**, includes indicators for the presence of a variant allele at each of the three SNPs rs7897947, rs11597086, and rs1324551. The "or" and "+" in this model suggest additive associations and the estimated coefficients 5.56 and 5.26 are close to the true value of 5.

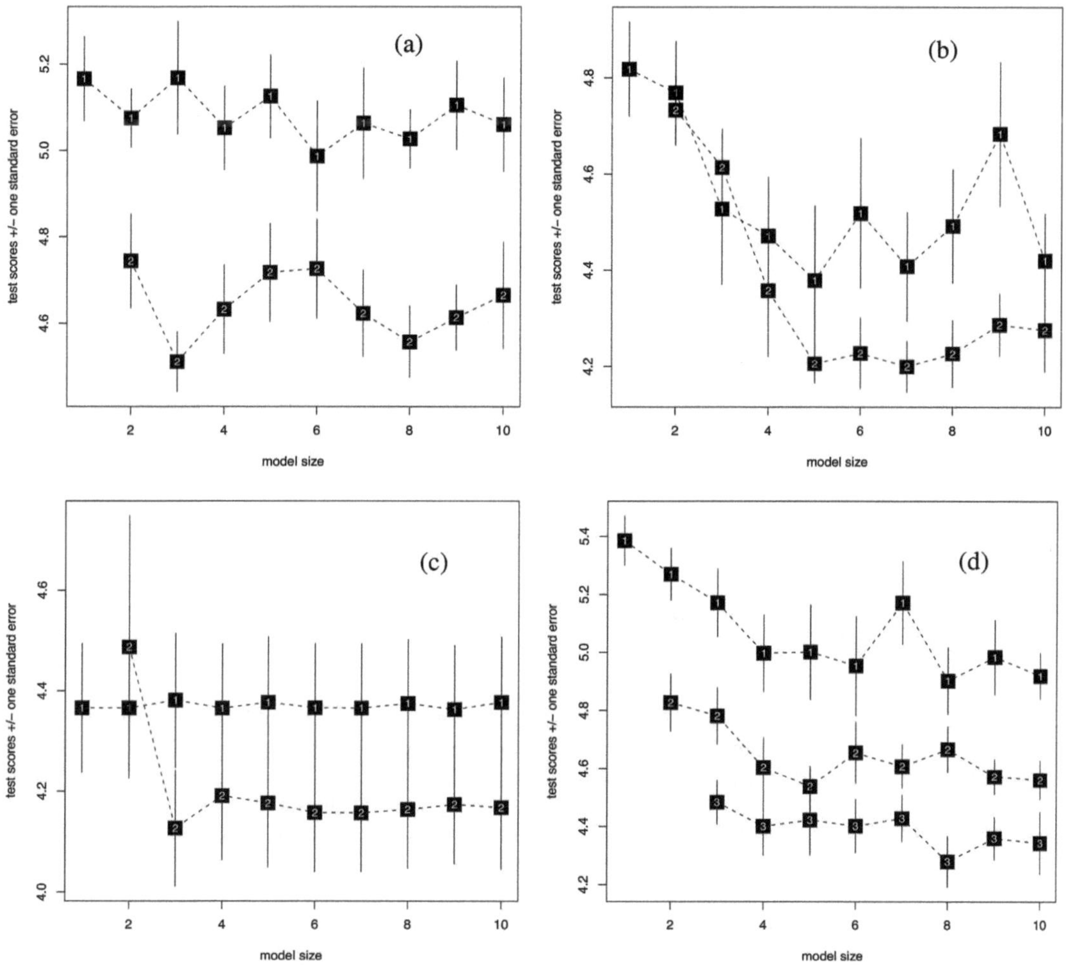

Fig. 5.4. Logic regression cross-validation results. (**a**) Model A: simple additive model with single informative SNP within each gene. (**b**) Model B: multiplicative model. (**c**) Model C: additive and multiplicative model. (**d**) Model D: additive model with multiple informative SNP within each gene.

Overall, the models corresponding to Models B–D data, illustrated in **Fig. 5.5b–d**, are reasonably consistent with the corresponding data generating model. The logic regression model with 2 trees and 5 nodes for Model B data is illustrated in **Fig. 5.5b**. Here the "and" in the first tree of this model and the corresponding coefficient estimate of 10.40 are both consistent with the underlying multiplicative effect used to generate the data. The second tree of this model, on the other hand, appears to over fit the data as the SNPs within this tree are unrelated to true causative loci.

The logic regression model for Model C data is illustrated in **Fig. 5.5c**. In the second tree of this model we see an additive effect of −10.0 for the presence of no variant alleles at rs11597086 in *CHUK* or equivalently an effect of 10.0 for at least one variant

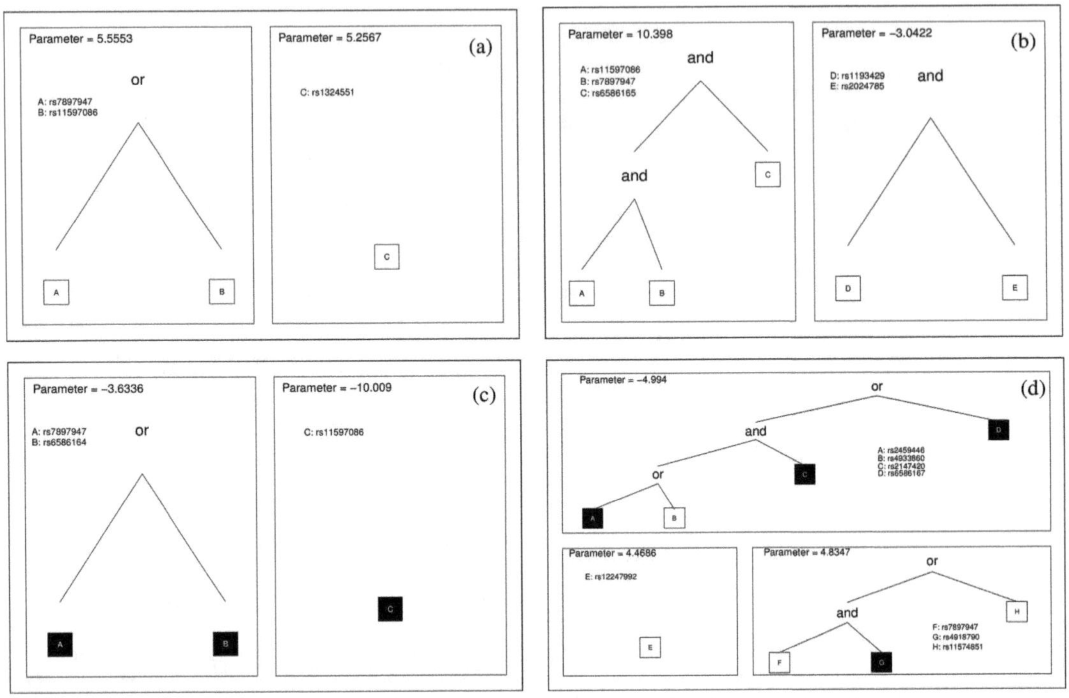

Fig. 5.5. Logic regression trees. (**a**) Model A data, 2 trees with 3 leaves: (score is 4.395) + 5.56 * (rs7897947 or rs11597086) + 5.26 * rs1324551. (**b**) Model B data, 2 trees with 5 leaves: (score is 4.045) + 10.4 * ((rs11597086 and rs7897947) and rs6586165) – 3.04 * (rs11193429 and rs2024785). (**c**) Model C data, 2 trees with 3 leaves: (score is 4.056) – 3.63 * ((not rs7897947) or (not rs6586164)) – 10 * (not rs11597086). (**d**) Model D data, 3 trees with 8 leaves: (score is 3.989) – 4.99 * ((((not rs2459446) or rs4933860) and (not rs2147420)) or (not rs6586167)) + 4.47 * rs12247992 + 4.83 * ((rs7897947 and (not rs4918790)) or rs11574851).

allele at this locus. Additionally, the first tree suggests the presence of an additional effect for being homozygous wild type at rs7897947 in *NFKB2* or rs6586164 (which is correlated with the true causative SNP rs1324551) in *FAS*, with a corresponding estimated coefficient of –3.63. Recall, in the true underlying model of association, the presence of variant alleles at both of these SNPs results in an increase in the trait by 4 units.

Finally, the model with 3 trees and 8 leaves fitted to Model D data is illustrated in **Fig. 5.5d**. Again the results are reasonably consistent with the true data generating distribution, in that multiple SNPs within the *NFKB2*, *FAS*, and *CHUK* genes are identified with corresponding estimated coefficients close to the true values of 5. Further, the relationship among the genes is additive in that each of the three trees contains SNPs from each of the three genes. Similar to the results for Models A–C, however, there appears to be some over fitting as some unrelated SNPs are also identified.

Example 7: Permutation testing. A permutation test can be applied to test formally whether the resulting logic regression model is statistically different than the null model of no association. This is performed in R again using the logreg() function and now specifying select=4, as shown below for the Model A data.

```
> fitPERM <- logreg(resp = trait.c, bin=snpSIMbin, type = 2, +
  select = 4, ntrees = 2, anneal.control = myanneal)
> fitPERM
```

```
Null Score 5.815 ; best score 4.363
Summary 25 Randomized scores
  Min. 1st Qu. Median Mean 3rd Qu. Max.
  5.506 5.559 5.572 5.583 5.600 5.780
0 randomized scores (0%) are better than the best score
```

In this example, 25 permutations of the trait are performed and the score from a corresponding logic regression model is recorded. The resulting output gives us information on the distribution of these 25 scores. In addition, we see that these permuted scores (reflecting the null distribution) are better than the best scoring model based on the observed data in 0/25=0% of the permutations. In conclusion for the Model A data, we would reject the null hypothesis of no association in favor of the logic regression model. A similar approach can be applied to the simulated data arising from each of the alternative data generating distributions (*see* **Note 5**).

4. Notes

1. For studies that involve paired and unevenly spaced longitudinal data, further extensions for correlated data settings are required.
2. Potential population substructure is an important consideration in population-based investigations of genetic association. The simplest approach to handling this issue is to perform stratified analysis, though some verification of self-declared race/ethnicity is needed and power may be adversely affected.
3. While some missing data approaches, including single and multiple imputations in the randomForest package, have been implemented, further methodological extensions are required to handle unobservable haplotypic phase.
4. Simulated effect sizes presented in this chapter are large and may not be seen in practice. In general, characterizing power for detecting higher order effects with machine learning methods requires additional research.
5. Methods for non-quantitative traits are also straightforward to implement with the R functions described. The ctree()

function is most flexible in that it can handle both quantitative and binary traits, as well as censored, ordered, and multivariate responses. Both the logreg() and randomForest() functions are also amenable to quantitative and binary traits while the logreg() function additionally handles censored outcomes.

6. The R functions with each of the three approaches considered in this chapter report predicted values for new observations. See for example the predict.logreg() function in the LogicReg library. The predict() function can also be applied to randomForest and ctree objects.

References

1. Broman, K. W., Sen, S (2009) *A Guide to QTL Mapping with R/qtl.* Springer, New York, NY.
2. Foulkes, A. S. (2009) *Applied Statistical Genetics with R: For Population-Based Association Studies.* Springer, New York, NY.
3. Ziegler, A., Koenig, I. R. (2007) *A Statistical Approach to Genetic Epidemiology.* Wiley-VCH, Weinheim.
4. Clayton, D., Leung, H. T. (2007) An R package for analysis of whole-genome association studies. Human Heredity, 64, 45–51.
5. Clayton, D., Wallace, C. (2008) snpMatrix vignette: Example of genome-wide association testing. http://bioconductor.org/packages/2.6/bioc/html/snpMatrix.html, pages 1–18
6. Breiman, L., Friedman, J. H., Olshen, R. A., Stone, C. J. (1993) *Classification and Regression Trees.* Chapman and Hall/CRC, Boca Raton, FL.
7. Zhang, H., Singer, B. (1999) *Recursive Partitioning in the Health Sciences.* Springer, New York, NY.
8. Hothorn, T., Hornik, K., Zeileis, A. (2006) Unbiased recursive partitioning: A conditional inference framework. Journal of Computational and Graphical Statistics, 15, 651–674.
9. Hothorn, T., Hornik, K., van de Wiel, M. A., Zeileis, A. (2006) A lego system for conditional inference. The American Statistician, 60, 257–263.
10. Breiman, L. (2001) Random forests. Machine Learning, 45, 5–32.
11. Breiman, L. (2003) Manual – Setting up, using and understanding random forests v4.0 http://oz.berkeley.edu/users/breiman/Using random forests v4.0.pdf.
12. Bureau, A., Dupuis, J., Falls, K., Lunetta, K. L., Hayward, B., Keith, T. P., Van Eerdewegh, P. (2005) Identifying SNPs predictive of phenotype using random forests. Genetic Epidemiology, 28, 171–182.
13. Ruczinski, I., Kooperberg, C., LeBlanc, M. (2003) Logic regression. Journal of Computational and Graphical Statistics, 12, 475–511.
14. Kooperberg, C., Ruczinski, I., LeBlanc, M., Hsu, L. (2001) Sequence analysis using logic regression. Genetic Epidemiology, 21, S626–S631.
15. Ruczinski, I., Kooperberg, C., LeBlanc, M. (2004) Exploring interactions in high dimensional genomic data: An overview of logic regression. Journal of Multivariate Analysis, 90, 178–195.
16. Kooperberg, C., Ruczinski, I. (2005) Identifying interacting SNPs using Monte Carlo logic regression. Genetic Epidemiology, 28, 157–170.
17. Schwender, H., Ickstadt, K. (2008) Identification of SNP interactions using logic regression. Biostatistics 9, 187–198.
18. Fritsch, A., Ickstadt, K. (2007) *Comparing Logic Regression Based Methods for Identifying SNP Interactions. Bioinformatics in Research and Development 2007,* LNBI 4414, Springer, Berlin, pp. 90–103.
19. Schwender, H., Ickstadt, K. (2008) Quantifying the importance of genotypes and sets of single nucleotide polymorphisms for prediction in association studies. Technical report, Dortmund University of Technology.

Chapter 6

In Silico PCR Analysis

Bing Yu and Changbin Zhang

Abstract

In silico PCR analysis is a useful and efficient complementary method to ensure primer specificity for an extensive range of PCR applications from gene discovery, molecular diagnosis, and pathogen detection to forensic DNA typing. In silico PCR, SNPCheck, and Primer-BLAST are commonly used web-based in silico PCR tools. Their applications are discussed here in stepwise detail along with several examples, which aim to make it easier for the intended users to apply the tools. This virtual PCR method can assist in the selection of newly designed primers, identify potential mismatches in the primer binding sites due to known SNPs, and avoid the amplification of unwanted amplicons so that potential problems can be prevented before any "wet bench" experiment.

Key words: Polymerase chain reaction, primer binding site, single nucleotide polymorphism (SNP), specific amplification.

1. Introduction

Polymerase chain reaction (PCR) is an in vitro method for the amplification of a target segment of DNA. This "molecular photocopying" technique, in theory, can produce a million copies from a single template through 20 cycles (i.e., 2^{20}) of template denaturing, primer annealing, and product extension. PCR was first described by Saiki et al. and perfected by Kary Mullis (1–3). The adoption of thermostable *Taq* polymerase in 1988 greatly simplified the process and enabled the automation of PCR (4). Since then, PCR has been extensively used in gene discovery, molecular diagnosis, pathogen detection, and forensic DNA typing. PCR sensitivity originates from its exponential amplification, while PCR specificity is determined by a pair of oligonucleotide

B. Yu, M. Hinchcliffe (eds.), *In Silico Tools for Gene Discovery*, Methods in Molecular Biology 760,
DOI 10.1007/978-1-61779-176-5_6, © Springer Science+Business Media, LLC 2011

sequences, known as primers (3). As calculated with four "building blocks" (dATP, dTTP, dCTP, and dGTP) for DNA synthesis, a primer of 16 nucleotides in length should be specific for one location in 3.2 billion (i.e., 4^{16}) base pairs (bp) of the human genome. PCR can be used to isolate a specific fragment of DNA from a complex genome. In practice, PCR primers are usually 18–30 nucleotides in length giving them high specificity. However, this theoretical prediction may not always be true in diverse and complicated biological genomes. Non-specific amplification with unexpected amplicons is not uncommon and the trial-and-error testing is laborious and time consuming. More seriously, PCR can be misleading in DNA diagnosis if there is an allele drop due to polymorphism-induced mismatches in primer binding sites. Publication errors in primer sequences can lead to amplification failure or even wrong amplification of an unwanted target.

In silico PCR refers to a virtual PCR executed by a computer program with an input of a pair or a batch of primers against an intended genome that is stored in a silicon media (e.g., a database server). In silico PCR aims to test PCR specificity including the target location and amplicon size in one or multiple target genome(s). It can identify the mismatches in primer binding sites due to known single nucleotide polymorphisms (SNPs) and/or unwanted amplicons from a homologous gene or a pseudogene (*see* **Note 1**). With the development of sequencing technology and rapid cost reduction, many genomes have been sequenced and annotated in databases. Such a wealth of genomic information makes in silico PCR possible. In silico PCR analysis can assist in the selection of newly designed primers and avoid potential problems before primer synthesis or a "wet bench" experiment. This analysis is also useful to validate the published primers before being blindly adopted. In this chapter, we introduce three publically available in silico tools for PCR analysis (*see* **Chapter 18** for additional in silico tools for quantitative PCR). These tools can be used individually or in combination for different purposes (*see* **Note 2**).

2. Materials

Personal computer and the Internet access are required for in silico PCR analysis. Three web-based in silico PCR tools that are discussed in this chapter include (i) "In silico PCR" from UCSC (University of California, Santa Cruz) Genome Browser (http://genome.cse.ucsc.edu/) (5); (ii) "SNPCheck" from the National Genetics Reference Laboratory (Manchester, http://ngrl.manchester.ac.uk/SNPCheckV2/); and (iii) primer-BLAST from the National Center for Biotechnology Information (NCBI, http://www.ncbi.nlm.nih.gov/tools/primer-blast/).

3. Methods

3.1. UCSC "In Silico PCR" Program

The performance of this program is fast since an indexing strategy is used in the program.

3.1.1. Program Application

The in silico PCR program can be initiated by clicking on either "PCR" in the top menu bar or "In silico PCR" in the left pane (*see* "Home Page" in **Fig. 6.1**). The required input items can be grouped into three parts.

1. *Primer sequences to be tested*: The "Forward Primer" and "Reverse Primer" can be typed in or pasted into two text boxes as indicated. If both primer sequences are originated from the same strand, the "Flip Reverse Primer" box should be ticked ☑ (*see* "Input Page" in **Fig. 6.1**). The program will automatically take the reverse and complement sequence before analysis. The default minimal length is 15 nucleotides for any input primers.

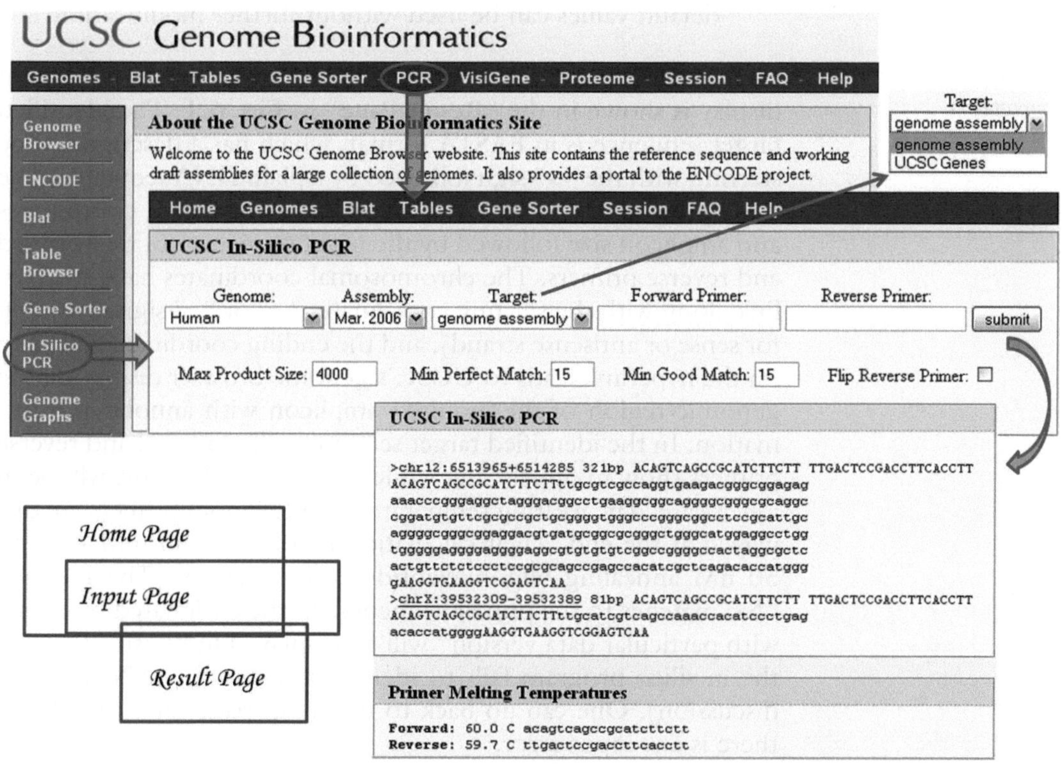

Fig. 6.1. Application of in silico PCR from UCSC Genome Browser. Access and input contents of the program are illustrated in the two different sections. The human genome is selected among other genomes from 47 organisms (*see* **Table 6.1**). The assembly is chosen from March 2006 and its target can be "genome assembly" or "UCSC Genes." The example results are shown in the analysis of a pair of *GAPDH* primers as a reference gene. This set of primers can result in two amplicons with 321 bp and 81 bp on chromosomes 12 and X, respectively.

2. *Selection of target genomes*: There are two dropdown menus of "Genome" and "Assembly." One can select a target genome from 47 organisms (**Table 6.1**) and a particular version of the genome assembly (6). Additional target options of "genome assembly" and "UCSC Genes" are available only for the human and mouse genomes. One can choose PCR template as either genomic DNAs or cDNAs (expressed transcripts) in these two species.
3. *PCR parameters*: The box of "Max Product Size" has the default value of 4000 bp allowing users to define the maximal size of the expected PCR product. Any amplicon larger than a defined value will be filtered out. Both "Min Perfect Match" and "Min Good Match" define the stringency of primers. The former refers to the minimal number of nucleotides ($\geq$15) on the 3′ ends of primers that must exactly match the template target. "Min Good Match" is only relevant to the nucleotides beyond the number defined by "Min Perfect Match," among which they should have two-thirds matching to the template target. Both "Min Perfect Match" and "Min Good Match" are not critical and the default values can be used without further modification.

3.1.2. Result Interpretation

Click on "summit" button after all inputs are completed. A typical display is shown in the "Result Page" in **Fig. 6.1**. The identified target sequence is in FASTA format, which has a description line starting with the ">" sign followed by a plain DNA sequence. The description line provides the target's chromosomal coordinates and amplicon size followed by the input sequences of the forward and reverse primers. The chromosomal coordinates have a hyperlink along with the starting coordinate, "+" or "–" sign (standing for sense or antisense strand), and the ending coordinate. Clicking on the hyperlink leads to UCSC's genome browser displaying the genomic region of the inquired amplicon with annotated information. In the identified target sequence, the forward and reverse primers show in upper case, while mismatch(es), if any, will be in lower case. The melting temperatures of the input primers are displayed at the end. Their calculation is based on 50 mM salt and 50 nM annealing oligonucleotide concentrations. The message "No matches to the primer sequences in the designated organism with particular data version" will be displayed in "Result Page" if the in silico program fails to identify any target (*see* **Note 3** for discussion). One can go back to the input page for correcting if there is any input error.

3.2. SNPCheck Tool

It is a web-based tool designed for checking if there are any SNPs in primer binding sites as well as total SNPs in a predicted amplicon. This program was launched by the National Genetics Reference Laboratory (Manchester) in 2005 and was updated to

Table 6.1
Available genomes in 47 organisms for in silico PCR analysis

Species	Release Date	Species	Release Date
VERTEBRATES			
Human[a]	Feb. 2009	Marmoset	Jun. 2007
	Mar. 2006	Medaka	Oct. 2005
	May 2004	Mouse[a]	Jul. 2007
	Jul. 2003		Feb. 2006
Cat	Mar. 2006		Aug. 2005
Chicken	May 2006	Opossum	Oct. 2006
	Feb. 2004		Jan. 2006
Chimp	Mar. 2006		Oct. 2004
	Nov. 2003	Orangutan	Jul. 2007
Cow	Oct. 2007	Platypus	Mar. 2007
	Aug. 2006	Rat	Nov. 2004
	Mar. 2005		Jun. 2003
Dog	May 2005	Rhesus	Jan. 2006
	Jul. 2004	Stickleback	Feb. 2006
Fugu	Oct. 2004	Tetraodon	Feb. 2004
	Aug. 2002	*X. tropicalis*	Aug. 2005
Guinea pig	Feb. 2008		Oct. 2004
Horse	Sep. 2007	Zebra finch	Jul. 2008
	Jan. 2007	Zebrafish	Jul. 2007
Lamprey	Mar. 2007		Mar. 2006
Lizard	Feb.2007		May 2005
DEUTEROSTOMES			
C. intestinalis	Mar. 2005	*S. purpuratus*	Sep. 2006
	Dec. 2002		Apr. 2005
Lancelet	Mar. 2006		
INSECTS			
A. mellifera	Jan. 2005	*D. mojavensis*	Aug. 2005
	Jul. 2004		Aug. 2004
A. gambiae	Feb. 2003	*D. persimilis*	Oct. 2005
D. ananassae	Aug. 2005	*D. pseudoobscura*	Nov. 2004
	Jul. 2004		Aug. 2003
D. erecta	Aug. 2005	*D. sechellia*	Oct. 2005
D. grimshawi	Aug. 2005	*D. simulans*	Apr. 2005
D. melanogaster	Apr. 2006	*D. virilis*	Aug. 2005
	Apr. 2004		Jul. 2004
	Jan. 2003		
NEMATODES			
C. brenneri	Feb.2008	*C. japonica*	Mar. 2008
	Jan. 2007	*C. remanei*	May 2007
C. briggsae	Jan. 2007		Mar. 2006
	Jul. 2002	*P. pacificus*	Feb. 2007
C. elegans	May 2008		
	Jan. 2007		
	Mar. 2004		
OTHER			
Yeast	Oct. 2003		
	Jun. 2008		

[a]Both genome assembly and USSC transcript databases are available

version 2 in August 2009. The database of SNPCheck is limited to the human genome from NCBI with weekly updates. This tool uses the BLAST function to identify the position in the sequence where the primers bind and allow multiple primer pairs (up to 1000 pairs) to be inputted and checked simultaneously.

3.2.1. Preparation of Primer Input for SNPcheck

The in silico tool SNPcheck can be freely accessed through the Internet. The large text box is for primer pair input (**Fig. 6.2**). A first-time user can click "Sample Input" to load a demonstration sample batch of primers and get oneself familiar with the valid input format. Each pair of primers occupies a single row with four fields of information including "name of primer pair," "sequence of primer 1," "sequence of primer 2," and "chromosome identifier." Each field is separated either by spaces or by tabs. In case of a batch input, many rows can stack together to

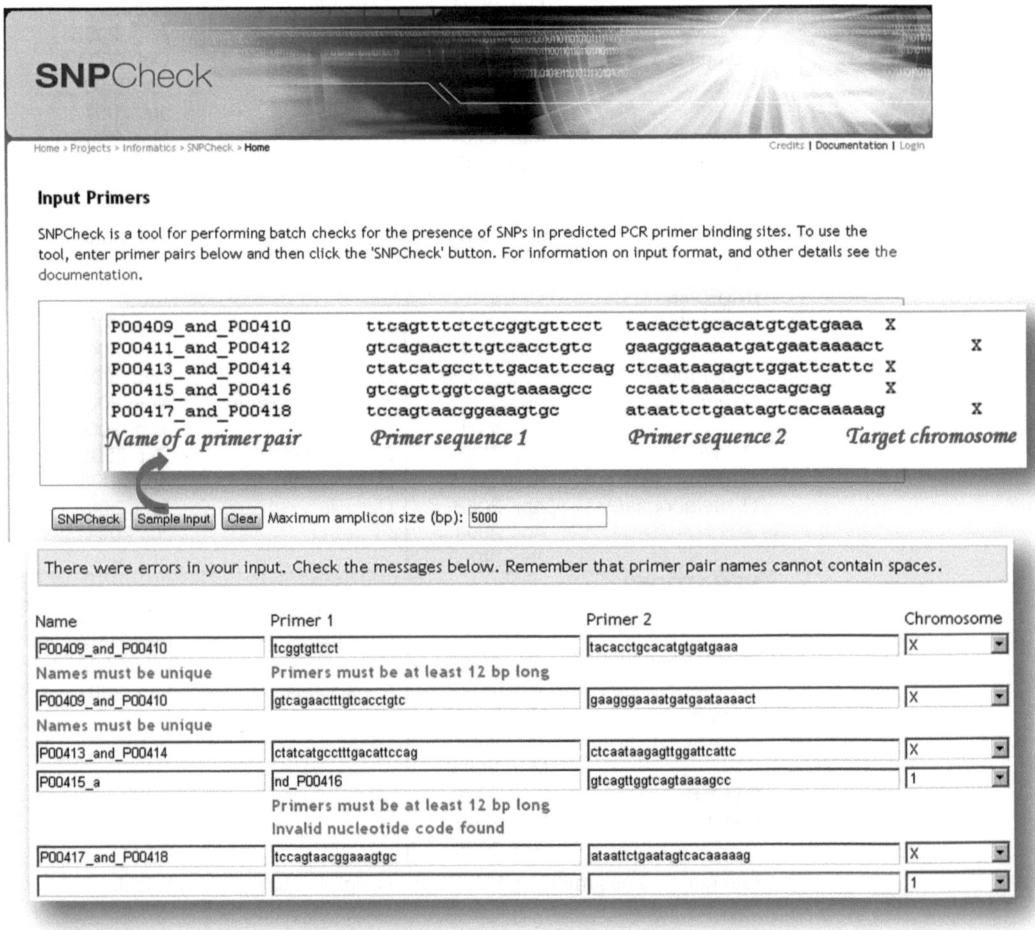

Fig. 6.2. SNPCheck input page and its input modification table. The primer input contains four parts including the name of a primer pair, primer sequence 1, primer sequence 2, and target chromosome. If any input error occurs, a modification table will appear with the explanation under the error field allowing the correction and/or adding of more data.

form a four-columned table, but these four parts are not necessarily well aligned (**Fig. 6.2**). All input data can be reset by clicking "Clear" button. Users can modify the default value of 5000 bp for "Maximum amplicon size" in order to filter out larger amplicons. The "SNPCheck" button is for data submitting and analysis. It is important to ensure the following requirements for a valid input.

1. Duplicated names of primer pairs in the same batch are not valid. No space is permitted in any name of a primer pair or sequence string. The program recognizes a field by a continuous string flanked by spaces/tabs. It only reads the first four fields from left most onward in a row and regards them as the requested information. Other parts will be ignored and hence, any unwanted space/tab within the input will cause an error in reading.
2. Only A, T, C, and G are valid codes for primer sequences. Degenerate bases are not accepted. The minimum primer length is 12 nucleotides written from 5′ to 3′ direction. Only 1–22, X, Y, and MT (for mitochondrial chromosome) are valid target chromosomal identifiers.
3. If any error is encountered after submission, a table will display as shown in the lower part of **Fig. 6.2**. Error descriptions are under fields where problems were found. One can correct the errors and provide additional new data into the last empty row of the table if necessary. The last empty row will be regenerated automatically after the data are entered. In addition to error correction and data entry, this table provides users with an overview of how the raw input has been allocated to the relevant fields. This table won't be seen if the input is correct. When correction and input are completed, click "SNPCheck" button again for resubmitting.

3.2.2. Result Layout

The results of SNPCheck are illustrated with an "Overview" part (**Fig. 6.3a**) and the detailed result sections (**Fig. 6.3b**). On the top right corner of the "Overview," there are three icons for bookmarking the results' web page, converting the results into a PDF file and printing the results in the computer default printer.

1. The "Overview" presents as a table with nine columns and each primer pair occupies a single row (**Fig. 6.3a**). Columns 1, 2, 4, and 6 are "Name," "Primer1," "Primer2," and "Chr," respectively, which are derived from the input. A dynamic rolling icon will initially show under the "Result" column indicating the running status. The results will replace the icon and fill with other fields once the analysis is completed. Each primer name acts as a hyperlink, which can lead to its own detailed result section under the "Overview" table. Sometimes the program recognizes that a particular pair of primers was checked previously and the

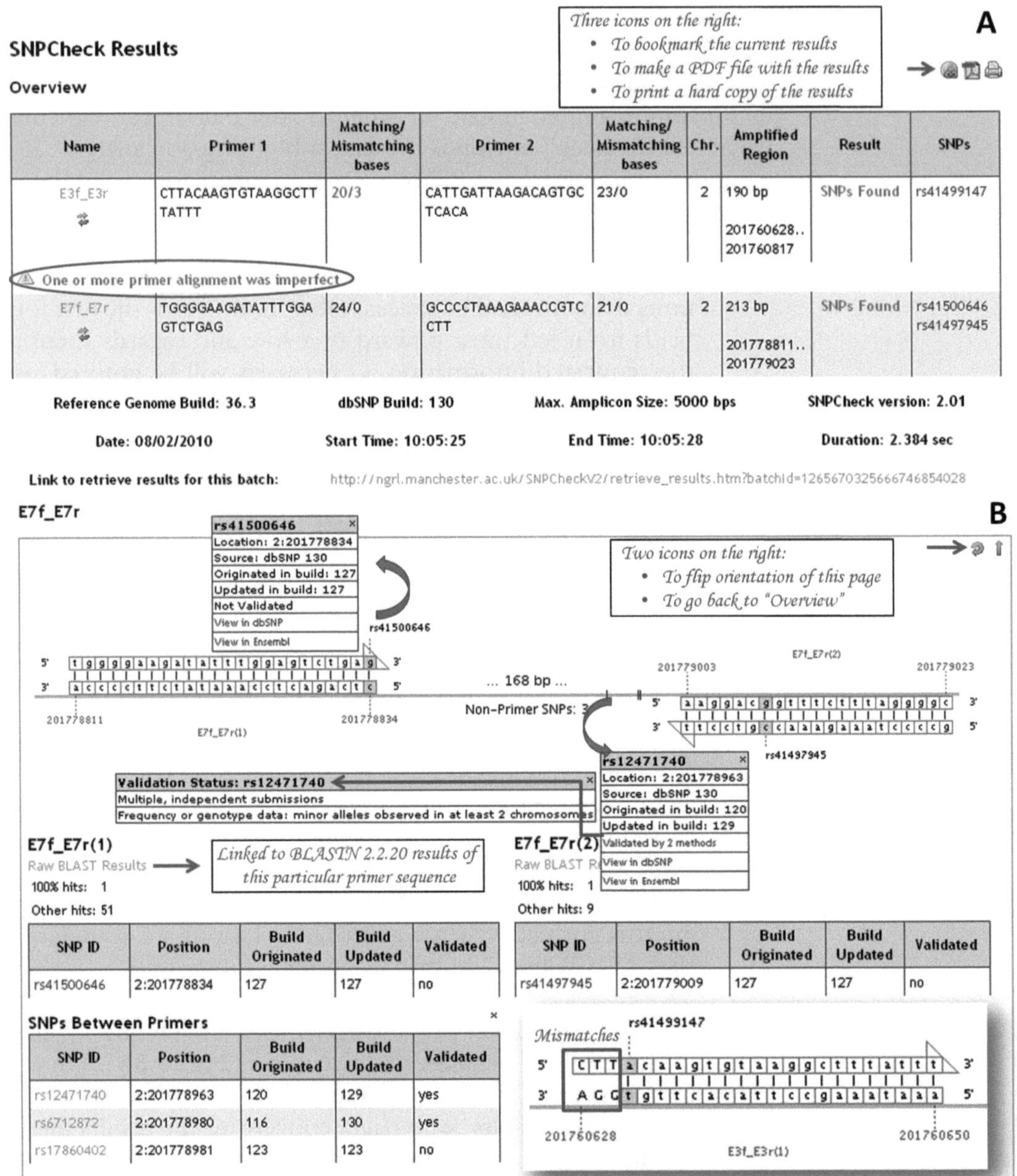

Fig. 6.3. SNPCheck results. Partial results of the "Overview" table are shown on the *top* (**a**). A refresh icon (*double arrows*) under the name of a primer pair can force the program to reanalyze the primer set or to consider the remaining matches if there are a large number of matches. This "Overview" table has nine columns including the primer pair "Name," "Primer" sequence, "Matching/Mismatching bases," "Chromosome" identifier, "Amplified Region," "Results," and "SNPs." An imperfect alignment warning can appear as circled. Detailed results of a primer pair are displayed within a framed section (**b**). A diagram of the primer-template binding is shown with the presence of SNPs highlighted and its accession number listed above with the hyperlink to its database. Clicking on the hyperlinks (*curved arrows*) will display the SNP details. The mismatches of the primer-template binding are demonstrated in the insert at the right lower corner. The amplicon size and non-primer SNPs with the hyperlinks are indicated on the diagram. There are two hyperlinks under the primers below the diagram. Three tables list the SNP details with the hyperlinks for the forward and reverse primer binding sites as well as between primers.

result is still available. In this case the results will be reloaded rather than perform a de novo analysis. In such a case, a refresh icon (double arrows) under the name of that particular primer pair appears. One can force the reanalysis process by clicking the refresh icon, which could be critical when a primer has many matches (*see* **Note 2**). The column next to primer sequence indicates "Matching/Mismatching bases," i.e., the numbers of perfect matches and mismatch(es) to their genomic targets, respectively. The amplicon size and its chromosomal coordinates of 5′ and 3′ ends are provided under the column "Amplified Region." The "Result" column shows whether any SNPs are found in the primer binding sites. The last column will display the NCBI SNP database rs number(s), if any, in the primer binding sites with the hyperlink(s) to the original database record(s). A warning message under a row of paired primers can appear if there is any problem during alignment such as an imperfect alignment (see the circle in **Fig. 6.3a**) or when both primers originated from the same strand. Under the "Overview" table, the target database, analysis parameters, analysis date, and time as well as the URL for the results retrieved will be listed. All these analysis results remain in the server for approximately 1 month.

2. Detailed results are displayed in a framed section with a primer pair name as the section heading (**Fig. 6.3b**). This part can be accessed by scrolling down in the web browser or by clicking the primer pair "Name" in the "Overview" table. The latter is particularly useful for a large batch analysis. Within each framed section, there are two green icons on the top right. A circular arrow can flip the diagram 180°. Most users are used to reading the sequence along the direction of the sense strand, but diagrams of detailed results show the direction according to that of the contigs assembled in the source database. Such horizontal flips will be possible by clicking on the circular arrow. An upward arrow can bring one back to the "Overview" part. It avoids an excessive amount of page scrolling in order to achieve a switch from "Overview" to the detailed result sections, particularly in a large batch analysis. The framed result section is arranged with one diagram, some hyperlinks and several tables.

In the diagram, elongation directions of the primers are indicated by a half-arrow on their 3′ ends (**Fig. 6.3b**). Nucleotides of primer binding sites on the genomic targets are boxed and linked by an alignment bar to their perfectly matched counterparts on the primer. If there are mismatches, the unmatched nucleotides on the genomic sequence are not boxed and do not have an alignment bar (see the insert on the right lower corner of

Fig. 6.3b). The chromosomal coordinates of the 5′ and 3′ ends of the primers and the amplicon size are displayed in the diagram. In addition, the total number of non-primer SNPs is indicated under the amplicon size, and these SNPs are marked by vertical lines with their relative locations between the two primers (**Fig. 6.3b**). Clicking on the rs number of an identified SNP in the primer binding site (e.g., rs41500646) or the tiny vertical line of non-primer SNP (e.g., first vertical line) can popup more SNP information as shown by the curved arrows in **Fig. 6.3b**. The popup information includes the validation status of the query SNP and further clicking on its hyperlink will lead to the validation details such as the validation methods applied to this particular SNP (e.g., Validation Status: rs12471740 in **Fig. 6.3b**). Any popup can be turned off by clicking the cross on its top right.

There are hyperlinks under the two primers below the diagram. Clicking on the hyperlink will lead to a raw BLAST result page for the chosen primer (7). If SNPs are found in both of the primer binding sites and of the non-primer binding sites, there will be three summary tables displayed as shown in **Fig. 6.3b**. Each SNP's rs number, genomic position, database build information, and validation status are listed in every table. It may be difficult to distinguish non-primer SNPs represented by tiny vertical lines in the diagram since they tend to be tightly packed together. One can select them from the table "SNPs Between Primers" in the left lower corner of **Fig. 6.3b**. These non-primer SNPs could indicate a potentially hemizygous status for an amplicon (*see* **Note 4**).

3.3. NCBI Primer-BLAST

This tool is publicly available. It includes the primer design and the primer specificity check. Only the latter part is discussed here. Primer-BLAST uses a heuristic approach to generate the alignment (8). Multiple organisms can be searched simultaneously.

3.3.1. Setup of Analysis Parameters

The relevant input interface of Primer-BLAST is shown in **Fig. 6.4**, which mainly includes three parts.

1. *Primer Parameters*: Primer sequences can either be typed in or pasted into the fields of "Use my own forward/reverse primer (5′->3′ on plus/minus strand)" (the top panel of **Fig. 6.4**). A valid input includes the A, T, C, G nucleotides, and N for any of the four, whereas other degenerate nucleotides are invalid. The built-in maximal number of nucleotides of a primer is 36, while no minimal number is imposed. Any input fields can be reset by clicking on the label of "Clear." The defaults for "Min" and "Max" amplicon size are 100 and 1000, respectively. These values can be redefined with the minimal size more than the length of two primers. Neither of these two values is indispensible for

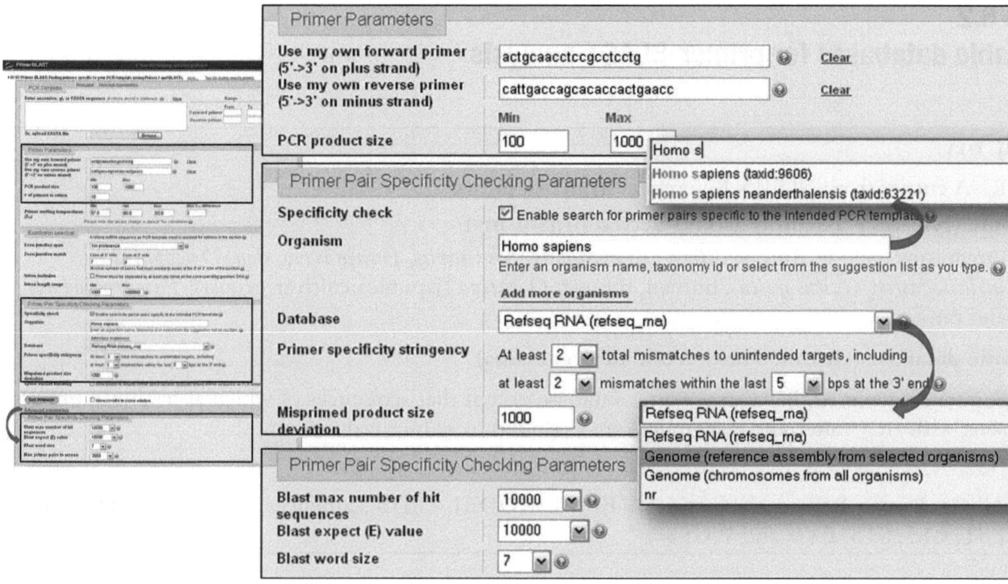

Fig. 6.4. Input of NCBI Primer-BLAST. The full input page is shown on the *left* with the three relevant sections enlarged on the *right*. Primer-BLAST allows testing multiple target genomes simultaneously. There are more options for the selected database including "Refseq RNA (refseq_rna)," "Genome (reference assembly from selected organisms)," "Genome (chromosomes from all organisms)," and "nr (all sequences available)." Clicking on the "Advance Parameters" as indicated by a *curved arrow* on the left lower corner can modify the maximal number of hit sequences, *E* value, and word size of BLAST analysis.

BLAST analysis, although the modification can help users to filter those amplicons that exceed chosen limits.

2. *Primer Pair Specificity Checking Parameters*: Genomic target organisms and the type of reference databases can be selected for a BLAST search. A suggestion list will display while typing, as indicated by the top curved arrow in the middle panel of **Fig. 6.4**. It is convenient to select from the list rather than to type in the full name or taxonomy identification. If necessary, one can add more organisms by clicking the hypertext "Add more organisms." Particular reference databases can be selected from the "Database" dropdown list, of which four options are available (**Table 6.2**). The assembled genome database contains minimal redundancy and will be the database of choice for specificity checking on a target genomic DNA due to the fast search speed.

   There are four primer stringency definitions. These parameters will assist the Primer-BLAST program to sort out possible amplicons. The first dropdown field defines total mismatches between primers and their potential templates. The second one defines how many mismatches can be tolerated within a defined segment of the 3′ ends of the primers. Only 1, 2, 3, or 4 can be chosen for these two fields. When querying one's own primer pair in Primer-BLAST, the larger

Table 6.2
Available databases for primer-BLAST analysis

refseq_rna	
	RNA entries from NCBI's Reference Sequence project
Genome (reference assembly from selected organisms)	
	Organisms include *Apis mellifera*, *Arabidopsis*, *Bos taurus*, *Danio rerio*, *dog*, *Drosophila melanogaster*, *Gallus gallus*, human, mouse, *O. sativa* (japonica cultivar-group), *Pan troglodytes*, and rat.
Genome database (chromosomes from all organisms)	
	Sequences from NCBI chromosome database except that sequences of which accession numbers start with AC_ (alternate assemblies) are excluded to reduce redundancy.
nr	
	All GenBank + RefSeq Nucleotides + EMBL + DDBJ + PDB sequences (excluding HTGS0,1,2, EST, GSS, STS, PAT, and WGS)

the value selected, the more possible hits/amplicons will be retrieved for visual analysis. The last dropdown defines the distance from the 3′ end of the primers in which the mismatches that are defined in the previous field are taken into account. This distance ranges from 1 to 20. The "Misprimed product size deviation" field specifies the size variation of the off-target PCR products relative to that of the intended PCR product.

3. *Advanced Parameters*: These parameters are intended to be modified by experienced users, and new users can leave these fields unchanged since the defaults work well in most situations. They can be accessed by clicking on "Advanced Parameters" (the left curved arrow in **Fig. 6.4**). Only the first three fields are relevant. The first field is "Blast max number of hit sequences" with the dropdown range from 10 to 100000. The second "BLAST expect (E) value" dropdown contains seven options ranging from 1 to 100000. The E value gives the expected number of chance matches in a random model. In principle, the higher the values chosen for these two fields, the more predicted amplicons will be given in the search results. The last dropdown "Blast word size" stands for the minimal number of contiguous matches of nucleotides between the query and the target sequences that are needed for BLAST to detect the targets. A lower value of "Blast word size" results in more hits, but consumes more time for the search.

The modified items can be identified by yellow highlight in Internet browser. If one wants to save all these settings as a whole for later use, he/she can just bookmark this page.

All the settings can be reset to their defaults by clicking the "Reset page" at the top of this page. The output results can be displayed in a new window if "Show results in a new window" is ticked on the right side of the "Get Primers" button. Once all inputs are completed, the analysis can be initiated by clicking on "Get Primers." The running time for a Primer-BLAST query can last up to several minutes depending on the parameter settings and local Internet speed. When the query has been successfully submitted, a status page will be displayed immediately. This page will automatically refresh at a regular interval until the results return. One can click "Cancel" to call off the query or click "Check" to force a page refresh during the BLAST analysis process.

3.3.2. Search for Useful Information from the Output

Figure 6.5 is an example page of BLAST results with a summary at the top followed by details. In the summary, "Input PCR template" would be "none" since there is no entry of any PCR

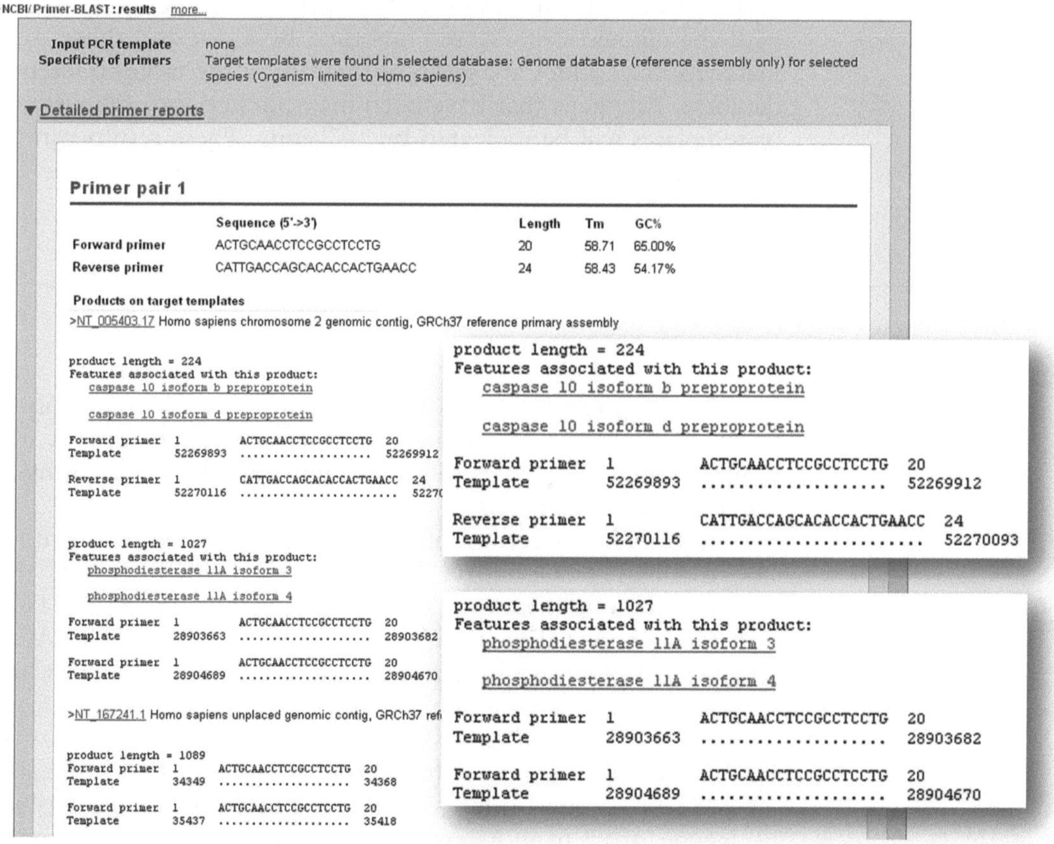
NCBI/Primer-BLAST : results
Input PCR template none
Specificity of primers Target templates were found in selected database: Genome database (reference assembly only) for selected species (Organism limited to Homo sapiens)
Detailed primer reports
Primer pair 1
Sequence (5'->3') Length Tm GC%
Forward primer ACTGCAACCTCCGCCTCCTG 20 58.71 65.00%
Reverse primer CATTGACCAGCACACCACTGAACC 24 58.43 54.17%
Products on target templates
>NT_005403.17 Homo sapiens chromosome 2 genomic contig, GRCh37 reference primary assembly
product length = 224
Features associated with this product:
caspase 10 isoform b preproprotein
caspase 10 isoform d preproprotein
Forward primer 1 ACTGCAACCTCCGCCTCCTG 20
Template 52269893 52269912
Reverse primer 1 CATTGACCAGCACACCACTGAACC 24
Template 52270116 52270093
product length = 1027
Features associated with this product:
phosphodiesterase 11A isoform 3
phosphodiesterase 11A isoform 4
Forward primer 1 ACTGCAACCTCCGCCTCCTG 20
Template 28903663 28903682
Forward primer 1 ACTGCAACCTCCGCCTCCTG 20
Template 28904689 28904670
>NT_167241.1 Homo sapiens unplaced genomic contig, GRCh37
product length = 1089
Forward primer 1 ACTGCAACCTCCGCCTCCTG 20
Template 34349 34368
Forward primer 1 ACTGCAACCTCCGCCTCCTG 20
Template 35437 35418

Fig. 6.5. An example of Primer-BLAST results. The input is an E5 primer pair for the amplification of exon 5 of *CASP10* gene (*see* **Table 6.3**). There are two perfect hits (see two blow-up inserts). The first hit with both forward and reverse primers is expected for the *CASP10* gene with a 224 bp amplicon, while a second hit with only the forward primer is unexpected to the phosphodiesterase 11A gene with a 1027 bp amplicon.

template. "Specificity of primers" summarizes whether any templates have been found from the designated target (organism and database). Detailed results are reported in an amplicon-oriented manner. First, features of the query primer pair including their sequences (5′> 3′), lengths, T_m (melting temperatures), and percentage contents of GC in primers are listed at the top. Then the identified products follow. The products are grouped by the target template they are found in. A description line of a template begins with a ">" sign followed by its unique identification. In a query using genomic DNA as a target, the chromosome number and version of the assembly are displayed after the GenBank accession number. There are some annotations of the template if the query target database is Refseq_RNA. The unique identifications of templates and the related features overlapping or flanking the products have the hyperlinks to the relevant target database in NCBI. One or multiple products can be found with the product size(s) under each description. Alignment of primers to their target template will be shown along with their starting and ending coordinates. Nucleotides on the template which perfectly match with the aligned primer are embodied by a dot and those mismatched nucleotides are given as they are in the target reference database. Any gaps that have been incorporated into the primers or templates will be indicated by "–" signs. These results can be saved using the "save as . . ." function in the browser.

4. Notes

In silico PCR can be useful and efficient in the identification of potential problems before any "wet bench" experiment. A few examples are discussed as follows to illustrate the applications of the in silico PCR analysis.

1. *GAPDH* is a commonly used reference gene in quantitative PCR (*see* **Chapter 18** for more on qPCR design) and can be amplified with the pair of primers (5′-ACAGTCA GCCGCATCTTCTT-3′, 5′-TTGACTCCGACCTTCACC TT-3′) (9). It is quite unexpected to see the two perfect hits using "genome assembly" instead of "UCSC genes" from the in silico PCR analysis (**Fig. 6.1**). This primer pair has an unexpected target on the chromosome X with a same size (81 bp) amplicon, as would be expected for its transcribed gene, apart from its expected genome target 321 bp amplicon on chromosome 12. Therefore, the contamination of genomic DNA in the preparation of total RNA for reverse transcription and quantitative PCR could influence this reference gene's level.

Table 6.3
Primers used for mutational analysis of *CASP10* gene[a]

Name	Sense primer sequence (5′-3′)[b]	Antisense primer sequence (5′-3′)	Amplicon size (bp)
E2A	gggccatatgtcctcactctc	AAACTTGAGGTTCTCCACATCTTG	184
E2B	CTTTCGTGAGAAGCTTCTGATTAT	TTCTGCCGTATGATATAGAGGAGT	210
E2C	TGCTGAGTGAGGAAGACCCTTTCT	ctccca tctccaccacagacc	169
E3	cttacaagtgtaaggctttattt	cattgattaagacagtgctcaca	191
E4	tgagtgga taa tcaa taggcaagt	ctccaagttagcaatcacaagc	217
E5	actgcaacctccgcctcctg	cattgaccagcacaccactgaacc	224
E6	gtccttccctgcatcaagtc	ccctaccataccga tctaagttgt	173
E7	tggggaaga ta tttggagtctgag	gcccctaaagaaaccgtcctt	213
E8	Aaggattcctactaagtggctcta	gcttttgataaactgttccaga	177
E9A	tgtgcccggccttgtttcag	GGGCTGGATTGCACTTCTGCTTCT	214
E9B	CGAAAGTGGAAATGGAGATGGT	CAGGCCTGGATGAAAAAGAGTTTA	220
E9C	GGGAGATCATGTCTCACTTCACA	CCACATGCCGAAAGGATACA	234
E9D	CTACTTGGTCTGGCCACTGT	taccaaaggtgttgaatgagagta	189
E10	aaattttgttttcttctttgttgc	caatgattcgtttgaggtctaag	222
E11	ttccccttttatttctctttgtgc	gtcaatctcaggcgatgtgg	237

[a]The primer sequences are obtained from Oh et al. (12)
[b]Upper case letters correspond to exons and lower case letters correspond to introns

2. We ran a random snapshot analysis of 15 published primer pairs (**Table 6.3**, (12)), of which Oh et al. used for the mutational analysis of *CASP10* gene in several cancers. Two minor errors and one issue of an unknown nature have been found using the UCSC in silico PCR program. The amplicon size for the E2C primer pair should be 191 bp instead of 190 bp, and there is a mismatch at the third base from the 5′ end of E8 reverse primer. Interestingly, the E5 primer pair does not have any match in the human genome. UCSC in silico PCR is quite good at verifying the target size and location, but it can only check one target genome at a time and can't look for all known DNA variants. SNPCheck has identified five mismatches in three primers (3/30, see an example of E3 forward primer in the insert of **Fig. 6.3b**) and three SNPs in total from the E3 and E7 pairs of primers (2/15, **Fig. 6.3a, b**). The identified SNP rs41500646 is located just at the 3′ end of E7 forward primer (**Fig. 6.3b**). SNPCheck also suggests that no PCR can be formed using the E5 primer pair. It is known that SNPCheck would only consider limited matches if a particular primer has too many hits. In such a case, it may initially miss the best pair. Therefore,

we clicked on the refresh icon and forced the program to consider the remaining matches. Then, the expected amplicon appears. It suggests that the E5 primers have a lot of matches and the expected target does not occur on the top of the list. This can explain the "no match" in both the UCSC in silico PCR and SNPCheck analyses and is further confirmed by NCBI Primer-BLAST analysis (**Fig. 6.5**). Primer-BLAST shows that the E5 primer pair can form a PCR with the expected size, but at the same time, the E5 forward primer itself can result in many unwanted amplicons (not shown in **Fig. 6.5**) including perfect matches of the phosphodiesterase 11A gene generating a 1027-bp amplicon. Primer-BLAST is useful for the explanation of one or multiple unwanted amplicon(s) besides the expected target. This combination of multiple in silico tools can complement one another to improve the detection sensitivity and explain some odd phenomena.

3. "No matches" can result from many underlying causes besides the wrong primer sequences. For example, an exon-over hanging primer won't find any target in a genome assembly database rather than in a gene transcript one. It is also possible that a primer has been designed on a polymorphic region that is absent from the database sequence. For example, the primer pairs (5′-TGGGATTACAGGCG TGATACAG-3′; 5′-ATTTCAGAGCTGGAATAAAATT-3′) are commonly used for the genotyping of a deletion/insertion polymorphism of the angiotensin-I converting enzyme (*ACE*) gene (10). However, the forward primer falls in the 287 bp Alu repeat sequence in intron 16 of the *ACE* gene and the genotype of the human genome in the UCSC Genome Browser is the homozygous absence of this Alu repeat. "No matches" would be the warrant result in the in silico PCR analysis, although this pair of the primers is widely applied in *ACE* genotyping.
4. Direct sequencing of PCR amplified coding regions has become more and more common for mutation screening in molecular diagnosis (11, 12). A well-known shortcoming of this method is that deletion fragments larger than the amplicon sizes can be ignored due to the diploid nature of the human genome. In this case only hemizygous PCR amplification of the undeleted fragment may occur. Therefore, it is quite useful to know how many SNPs are expected in an amplicon through an in silico analysis such as SNPCheck. Absence of heterozygotes in these expected common SNPs should ring a bell to look for a potential hemizygous status in the sample using other methods. More importantly, SNPCheck can exclude the potential miss-diagnosis due to the failed primer binding caused by known polymorphisms.

References

1. Mullis, K., Faloona, F., Scharf, S., et al. (1986) Specific enzymatic amplification of DNA in vitro: the polymerase chain reaction. *Cold Spring Harb Symp Quant Biol* 51 Pt 1, 263–273.
2. Saiki, R. K., Scharf, S., Faloona, F.,et al. (1985) Enzymatic amplification of beta-globin genomic sequences and restriction site analysis for diagnosis of sickle cell anemia. *Science* 230, 1350–1354.
3. Bartlett, J. M., and Stirling, D. (2003) A short history of the polymerase chain reaction. In Bartlett, J. M., and Stirling, D., (Eds.) *PCR protocols,* 2nd ed. In Methods in Molecular Biology, Vol. 226. Humana, Totowa, NJ.
4. Saiki, R. K., Gelfand, D. H., Stoffel, S., et al. (1988) Primer-directed enzymatic amplification of DNA with a thermostable DNA polymerase. *Science* 239, 487–491.
5. Kent, W. J., Sugnet, C. W., Furey, T. S., et al. (2002) The human genome browser at UCSC. *Genome Res* 12, 996–1006.
6. Rhead, B., Karolchik, D., Kuhn, R. M., et al. (2010) The UCSC Genome Browser database: update 2010. *Nucleic Acids Res* 38, D613–619.
7. Altschul, S. F., Madden, T. L., Schaffer, A. A., et al. (1997) Gapped BLAST and PSI-BLAST: a new generation of protein database search programs. *Nucleic Acids Res* 25, 3389–3402.
8. Sayers, E. W., Barrett, T., Benson, D. A., et al. (2010) Database resources of the National Center for Biotechnology Information. *Nucleic Acids Res* 38, D5–16.
9. Pinhu, L., Park, J. E., Yao, W., and Griffiths, M. J. (2008) Reference gene selection for real-time polymerase chain reaction in human lung cells subjected to cyclic mechanical strain. *Respirology* 13, 990–999.
10. Evans, A. E., Poirier, O., Kee, F., et al. (1994) Polymorphisms of the angiotensin-converting-enzyme gene in subjects who die from coronary heart disease. *Q J Med* 87, 211–214.
11. Fouchier, S. W., Kastelein, J. J., and Defesche, J. C. (2005) Update of the molecular basis of familial hypercholesterolemia in The Netherlands. *Hum Mutat* 26, 550–556.
12. Oh, J. E., Kim, M. S., Ahn, C. H.,et al. (2010) Mutational analysis of CASP10 gene in colon, breast, lung and hepatocellular carcinomas. *Pathology* 42, 73–76.

Chapter 7

In Silico Analysis of the Exome for Gene Discovery

Marcus Hinchcliffe and Paul Webster

Abstract

Here we describe a bioinformatic strategy for extracting and analyzing the list of variants revealed from an exome sequencing project to identify potential disease genes. This in silico method filters out the majority of common SNPs and extracts a list of potential candidate protein-coding and non-coding RNA (ncRNA) genes. The workflow employs Galaxy, a publically available Web-based software, to filter and sort sequence variants identified by capture-based target enrichment and sequencing from exomes including selected ncRNAs.

Key words: Exome capture, next generation DNA sequencing (NGS), single-nucleotide variant (SNV), single-nucleotide polymorphism (SNP), Galaxy, BED file.

1. Introduction

Exome capture followed by massively paralleled DNA sequencing and bioinformatic filtering of discovered variants is an effective new methodology for the detection of novel Mendelian genes. A significant number of Mendelian conditions, both rare and common, remain to have their molecular basis identified (1). The Online Mendelian Inheritance in Man (OMIM) Web site lists over 1,700 Mendelian conditions that have either a described phenotype or a chromosomal locus recognized but no molecular cause discovered (http://www.ncbi.nlm.nih.gov/Omim/mimstats.html).

Exome sequencing has significant advantages for the discovery of new disease genes including the following: (i) no prior knowledge of a candidate gene's function is necessary, (ii) only a small number of affected individuals are required (*see* **Table 7.1**), and (iii) common, rare, and family-specific, protein-coding

B. Yu, M. Hinchcliffe (eds.), *In Silico Tools for Gene Discovery*, Methods in Molecular Biology 760,
DOI 10.1007/978-1-61779-176-5_7, © Springer Science+Business Media, LLC 2011

Table 7.1
Examples of published exome or whole genome sequencing gene discovery cases

Disease	Mode of inheritance	No. of individuals sequenced (method)	Gene discovered	References
Freeman–Sheldon syndrome	AD	4 (Exome)	MYH3 (confirming earlier gene discovery)	(4)
Bartter syndrome	AR	1 (Exome)[a]	SLC26A3	(5)
Schinzel–Giedion syndrome	AD	4 (Exome)	SETBP1	(6)
Miller syndrome	AR	4 (Exome)	DHODH	(7)
Non-syndromic, X-linked intellectual disability (XLID)	XLR	4 (Exome of X chromosome)	IQSEC2	(8)
Charcot–Marie–Tooth disease	AR	1 (whole genome sequencing)[b]	SH3TC2	(9)
Fowler syndrome	AR	2 (Exome)	FLVCR2	(10)
Metachondromatosis	AD	1 (whole genome sequencing)[b]	PTPN11	(11)

AD, Autosomal dominant; AR, autosomal recessive; XLR, X-linked recessive
[a]Followed by targeted Sanger sequencing in other affected individuals
[b]Followed by segregation analysis

variants can be readily discovered, thereby allowing the examination of a large spectrum of allelic heterogeneity. Indeed, evidence from genome-wide association studies has indicated that a significant fraction of rare or family-specific variation may explain an important fraction of heritable risk for common diseases (2). Bioinformatic assessment of exomes and genomes is poised to play a significant role in disease gene discovery and also in the genetic clinic for establishing a genetic diagnosis (3).

Targeted exome hybridization and capture followed by next generation sequencing (NGS) makes the examination of individual exomes accessible (12). A few prior considerations need to be made before embarking (*see* **Section 3.1**). The great majority of Mendelian conditions to date have been linked to protein-coding genes (1). This is despite the fact that the Encode pilot project has demonstrated widespread transcription of the human genome beyond the fraction of protein-coding exons (13–14). However, as the list of identified functional non-coding RNAs (ncRNAs) grows, it will be necessary to include them in any disease gene discovery project (15). The exome therefore should be the initial location to investigate a Mendelian disease gene but using a capture-based system that includes known ncRNA sites should be considered in future. The 38 MB Agilent SureSelect Human All Exon Kit includes close to 1000 identified ncRNAs

(16). Analysis of these ncRNAs has been incorporated into the following Galaxy-based workflow.

Galaxy is a Web-based software portal (http://galaxy.psu.edu/) that provides a diverse toolkit of functions that can coordinate the manipulation and analysis of large volume genomic data sets typical of NGS projects (17–18). This software allows molecular geneticists without programming skills to perform genome-scale analysis by building stepwise workflows. Most of its tools include explanatory text and examples. There are also video tutorials which explain how to use the Web site. For example, click on the "Help" button on the top toolbar, select "video tutorials," and then "Generating a workflow from a history." A video tutorial is available that demonstrates how to save a workflow for use with another exome sequencing file. A written step-by-step tutorial can be accessed via the GMOD Web site (http://gmod.org/wiki/Galaxy_Tutorial).

This chapter does not cover measures of statistical significance such as Bonferroni corrections for multiple sampling of variants. Rather, the stepwise process whittles down the large number of variants by filtering them against the dbSNP database and eight previously sequenced HapMap individuals.

2. Materials

1. An exome file in gff3 format of variants output by the Applied Biosystems Bioscope SNP finder program.
2. A personal computer connected to the Internet to access the Galaxy Web site (http://galaxy.psu.edu/). Register or login (http://main.g2.bx.psu.edu/) to the site on the top toolbar so that the workflow history can be automatically saved as it is created.
3. It is also possible to download the Galaxy software to be run on a local server. This may be useful for performance or data security considerations but it is not a requirement.

3. Methods

3.1. Project Design and Planning

Factors to consider when designing a gene discovery project using exome sequencing include the following:

1. *Mode of inheritance*: Given that costs and bench time for exome capture and sequencing are reasonably substantial,

genetic conditions with a clear Mendelian mode of inheritance will be more likely to uncover a disease gene. Complex and polygenic diseases may be tackled in the future when routine genome sequencing becomes feasible.

2. *Number of subjects* to process is dependent on the mode of inheritance and availability of subjects for segregation analysis. Previous studies indicate that you can expect to find 300–600 *novel* nonsynonymous and splice site variants per individual (*see* **Table 7.1**). Recessive conditions (autosomal or X-linked) have been identified using two to four individuals. One individual may be all that is required if subsequent segregation analysis is available for confirmation of identified double heterozygote or homozygote variants in all affected family members. Dominant conditions will usually require more subjects as only a single mutation will usually be present in the affected gene unlike recessive conditions where there will be two mutations per subject and hence will be easier to spot against the large number of novel nonsynonymous variants.
3. *Clear phenotypes*: It is critical to have a well-defined phenotype that can be objectively measured to avoid potential phenocopies.

3.2. Sample Preparation

3.2.1. DNA Preparation

High-quality genomic DNA from either blood or tissue is preferred (specifically, a non-degraded and high *A*260/*A*280 ratio (1.8–2.0) sample). Relatively high concentration is required to ensure 3 μg of DNA in 120 μL of 10 mM Tris, 1 mM EDTA buffer (16).

3.2.2. Exome Capture and DNA Sequencing

Exome capture using the SureSelect system targets 38 MB of the genome. Refer to the protocol manual for details (16). Greater sequencing coverage will result in less false-positive and false-negative variant calls. Successful studies to date have typically used approximately 50× coverage of mappable reads (4–5).

3.3. NGS Data Analysis

3.3.1. Base Calling, Sequence Alignments, and Identification of Subject Variants

Primary and secondary bioinformatic analysis of NGS fragment sequence data is done with software appropriate to the sequencing platform. For example, color space reads from a SOLiD sequencer are typically analyzed with the Bioscope software package (19). Bioscope includes "SNP finder" and "Find Indels" tools for identifying variants (**Fig. 7.1**). The output of these programs is in gff3 format (discussed in **Section 3.4**, Step 7).

3.3.2. Annotation

Annotation involves comparing the SNVs identified in the exomes of studied subjects to identify the characteristics of each SNV. This data will form the basis for decisions on which SNVs should be prioritized for investigation. Key features include the following:

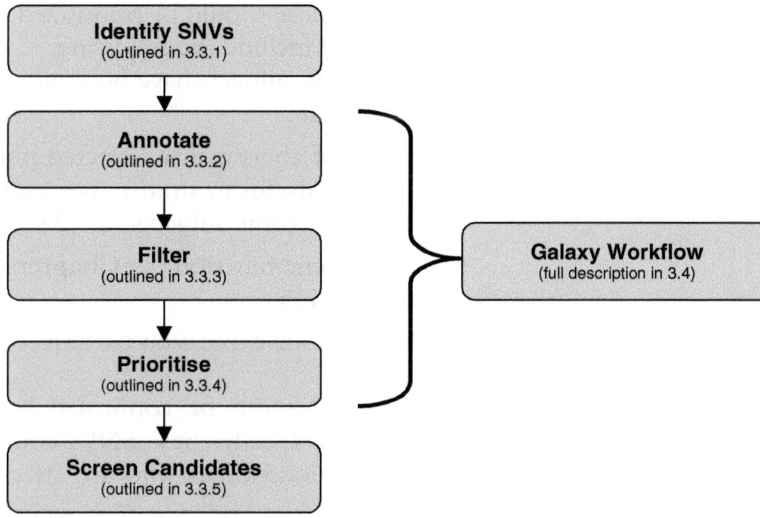

Fig. 7.1. Flowchart of the downstream filtering and prioritizing of discovered SNPs using Galaxy as a third-party tool.

- Variant frequency (rare/novel?).
- Type of DNA site – coding/intronic/splice site/regulatory/miRNA.
- Effect of variant – synonymous/nonsynonymous.
- Name/function of gene associated with this SNV.

3.3.3. Filtering

Sequencing an exome will identify ~20,000 SNVs compared with the human reference genome, and a full genome sequence would identify ~3,500,000 SNVs (4–6, 20). Most of these SNVs have a low probability of causing disease and are of low priority. For a rare disease, this would include many non-coding SNVs, SNPs in dbSNP, and SNPs in published genomes.

At least 90% of all SNVs found in an individual are likely to be previously documented (4–7, 20). For rare disorders, it will be appropriate to initially consider only novel SNVs, but it should be remembered that published databases are not without error. Mitchell et al. (21) estimated that dbSNP has a false-positive rate of 15–17% due to genotyping errors inherent in balancing false-positive and false-negative rates for heterozygous loci. Musumeci et al. (22) found that up to 8% of SNPs reported in dbSNP may be due to misaligned paralogous sequences. Of the 24 million SNPs recorded in dbSNP131, only 15 million have been verified in population studies (23).

3.3.4. Prioritizing

Previous studies indicate that a small number of genes, probably less than 50, will share nonsynonymous SNVs across the subjects in the study (depending on the number of individuals sequenced)

(4, 20, 24). These should be prioritized for investigation. Criteria to apply could include the following:

- How many subjects have nonsynonymous SNVs in each particular gene.
- Degree of abnormality/affected phenotype in subjects (i.e., it may be useful to stratify the quality of phenotypes seen in the list of exome subjects, *see* (24)).
- Known gene function (*see* **Chapters 11** and **12** for candidate prioritization).
- Known tissue expression patterns of the gene product.

3.3.5. Screening Candidate Genes

Candidate SNVs can be confirmed by Sanger sequencing the study subjects. Ideally these SNVs could be confirmed in additional related individuals who are affected (*see* Step 35 below).

3.4. Galaxy Workflow

Galaxy's main page is divided into three sections: tools (left side), analysis window (middle) where data files can be perused, and the workflow history page on the right side (**Fig. 7.2**). Each of the 35 workflow steps for exome SNP filtering and sorting is numbered and italicized. The following method runs through the creation of a workflow so that the reader can understand and therefore potentially modify some of the filtering stringencies

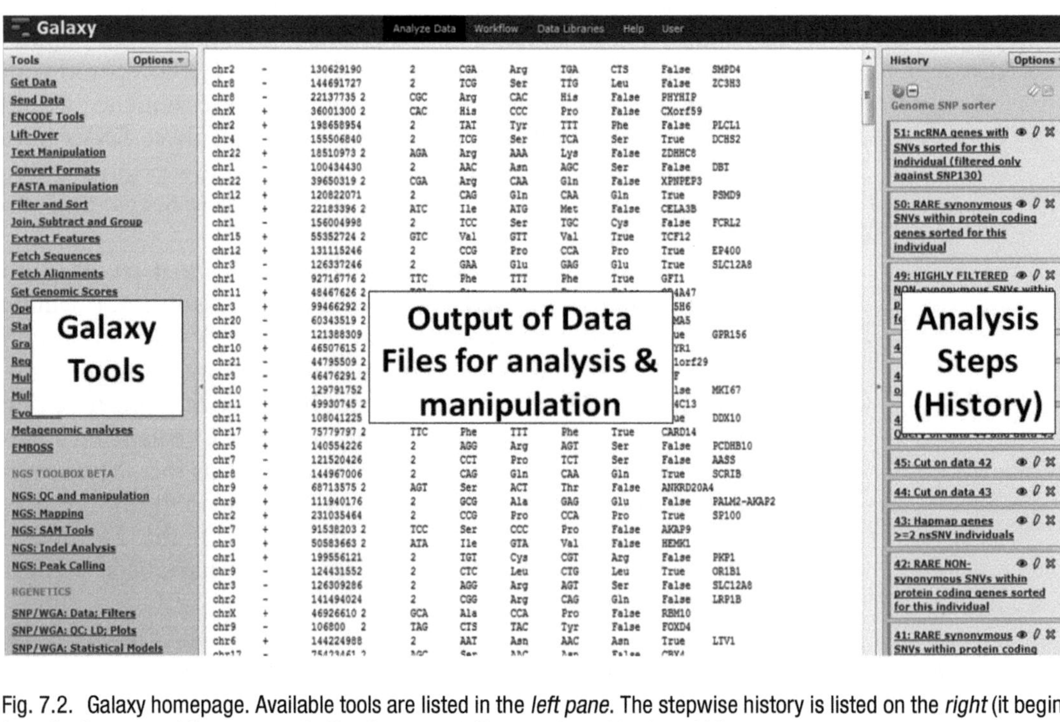

Fig. 7.2. Galaxy homepage. Available tools are listed in the *left pane*. The stepwise history is listed on the *right* (it begins from the bottom and flows upward). The data output files are viewed in the middle.

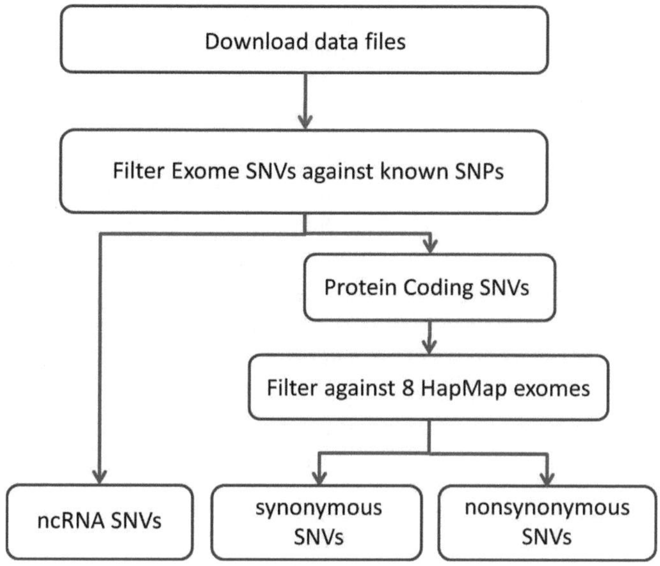

Fig. 7.3. Galaxy workflow for filtering and sorting exome SNVs.

and initial input files to suit the particular question being asked (**Fig. 7.3**).

1. *Download BED file of known genes into Galaxy*

   Select "Get Data" link on the left toolbar panel on the main page. Click on "Bx main browser" and choose the following parameters (**Fig. 7.4**):

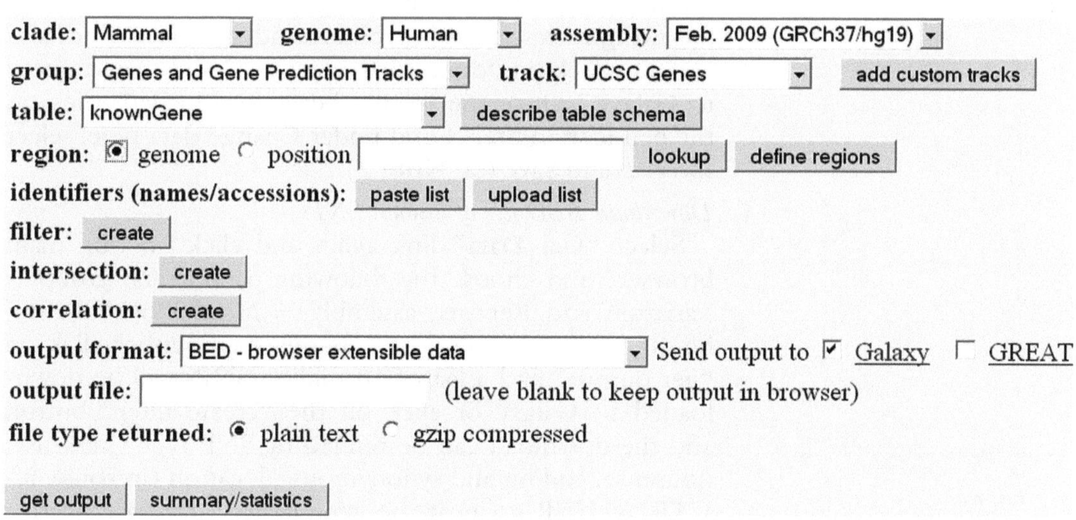

Fig. 7.4. UCSC Gene track download page options.

Clicking the "get output" button sends you to the "Output knownGene as BED" page. Click on "Send query to Galaxy" button. This runs a query against the UCSC database and returns a file which appears in your Galaxy history panel on the right side of the screen. This will send chromosomal locations and unique identifiers for the entire complement of known protein-coding isoforms (about 78,000 in Feb.2009(GRCh37/hg19)) to Galaxy (*see* **Notes 1, 2**, and **3**).

2. *Download BED file of known miRNAs and snoRNAs*

   Select "Get Data" link on the left toolbar panel on the main page. Click on "UCSC Main table browser" and choose the following parameters: group = Genes and Gene Prediction Tracks, assembly = Mar.2006(NCBI36/hg18), track = sno/miRNA. Click "get output," then click "Send query to Galaxy."

3. *Download BED file of known RNA genes*

   This is another ncRNA file list which will be concatenated with the miRNA and snoRNA data file in Step 9 below. Go through the same steps as in Step 2 but substitute track = RNA genes.

4. *Download tabular file of RefSeq gene names and convert to an interval file*

   Select "Get Data" link again and select "UCSC Main table browser." Choose the following parameters: group = Genes and Gene Prediction Tracks, assembly = Mar.2006(NCBI36/hg18), track = RefSeq Genes, and in the "output format," field pick "selected fields from primary and related tables." Click on "get output" and in the table "Select Fields from hg18.knownGene," tick the following boxes: name, chrom, strand, txStart, txEnd, and name2. Click on "done with selections" and "Send query to Galaxy." Once the file has been downloaded, click on the pen icon in Step 4 and under Change data type, select *interval* and Save (*see* **Note 2**).

5. *Download BED file of known SNPs*

   Select "Get Data" link again and click on "Bx main browser" and choose the following parameters: group = Variation and Repeats, assembly = Mar.2006(NCBI36/hg18), track = SNPs(130). At this stage, either click on "get output" and a list of 18 million SNPs will be downloaded to Galaxy or click on the "create filter" button and the download can be refined by SNP type (missense, nonsense, coding and synonymous), location (intronic, 5′-UTR, 3′-UTR, or near the gene limits), database overlap (HapMap, 1000 genomes), and average heterozygosity of the minor allele (*see* **Note 4**).

6. *Create and upload a tabular genetic code file*

   In a text document, create a tabulated file of codons and their 64 respective amino acid translations. This will be used in a later step to distinguish between synonymous and nonsynonymous coding SNVs:

```
TTT    Phe
TTC    Phe
TTA    Leu
TTG    Leu
CTT    Leu     etc. for 64 codons.
```

Upload this file to Galaxy by clicking "Get Data" and "Upload file."

7. *Convert and upload the Exome Sequencing file*

The SOLiD NGS output file from the Bioscope "SNP finder" software program will be in gff3 format (*see* **Note 5**). This is a tabulated file with nine columns. Each line gives the details for one SNV and the following *bolded* columns and attributes can be extracted using the PERL script below: (1) **Chromosome**, (2) Source (SOLiD_diBayes), (3) Type (SNP), (4) **Start position** (numbering corresponds to Mar.2006(NCBI36/hg18)), (5) **End position**, (6) Score, (7) **Strand** ("." only from SNP finder), (8) Phase. Column 9 contains multiple attributes of the SNV separated by semicolons including the following: **genotype** (IUPAC code), **reference base** (IUPAC code), coverage, refAlleleCounts, refAlleleStarts, refAlleleMeanQV, novelAlleleCounts, novelAlleleStarts, novelAlleleMeanQV, and whether the SNV is calculated (by coverage and counts) to be **heterozygous** (het=1) or **homozygous** (het=0).

Use the following PERL script to convert the gff3 SNP finder output file to a tabulated file suitable for use in Galaxy:

PERL Script

```
# parsegff.pl
# Reads GFF3 file from ABI Bioscope SNP finder
  tool
# Extracts SNV genotype and reference allele
  from attributes field
# outputs columnar format file suitable for
  processing in galaxy
# example usage:
# perl parsegff3.pl infile.gff outfile.txt
$tab="\t";
$eol="\n";
$infile = $ARGV[0];
$outfile = $ARGV[1];
#hash table for translating heterozygous
```

```
 genotypes to bases
$code{"R"} = {"G", "A", "A", "G"};
$code{"Y"} = {"C", "T", "T", "C"};
$code{"S"} = {"G", "C", "C", "G"};
$code{"W"} = {"A", "T", "T", "A"};
$code{"K"} = {"G", "T", "T", "G"};
$code{"M"} = {"A", "C", "C", "A"};

open(INFILE, $infile);
open(OUTFILE, ">$outfile");
print OUTFILE "chr\tstart\tend\tstrand\tSNP\thet
  \tvar\tref\n";
while (<INFILE>) {
  chomp;
  @columns = split("\t");
  $columns[3]-=1;
  $columns[8] =~/type=(\w);reference=(\w).+het=
   (.)/;
  $genotype=$1;
  $reftype=$2;
  if($genotype ne "N"){
    if (index("RYSWKM",$genotype)>=0) {$genotype
     =$code{$genotype}{$reftype}};
    print OUTFILE $columns[0],$tab,$columns[3],
     $tab,$columns[4],$tab,$columns[6],$tab;
    print OUTFILE $var,"/",$reftype,$tab,$3,$tab,
     $genotype,$tab,$reftype,$eol;
  }
}
close INFILE;
close OUTFILE;
exit;
```

Three SNVs in tabulated format from a HapMap individual are shown here:

chr	start	end	strand	SNP	het	var	ref
chr1	871489	871490	.	A/G	0	A	G
chr1	873761	873762	.	T/T	0	T	T
chr1	877663	877664	.	G/A	0	G	A

This file can be uploaded to Galaxy by clicking "Get Data" and "Upload file." In the "File Format" box, select *interval* and in the Genome box, select "Human Mar. 2006 (NCBI36/hg18) (hg18)" and click "execute."

8. *Convert coordinates of BED file of known genes to Mar.2006 (NCBI36/hg18)*

   Click on "Lift-Over" in Galaxy tools and select "Convert genome coordinates." Choose file from Step 1, click on Hg18, and accept the default 0.95 as the minimum ratio of bases that must remap (*see* **Notes 3** and **6**).

9. *Combine both ncRNA files*

   Click "Operate on Genomic Intervals" in Galaxy tools and select "*Concatenate* two queries into on query." Select data files from Steps 2 and 3 for the first and second query and press "execute." This will combine both ncRNA data files into a single file for later use.

10. *Subtract database SNPs from exome sequencing SNV file*

    This step will remove all SNVs from the uploaded Exome SNV file (Step 7) that appear in the SNP data file uploaded in Step 5. Click "Operate on Genomic Intervals" in Galaxy tools and select "*Subtract* the intervals of two queries." Under "Subtract," select Step 5 and under "from" select Step 7. Select "Intervals with no overlap" in the "Return" box and keep the default setting of 1 bp for the minimal overlap. Press "Execute."

11. *Define heterozygosity and homozygosity columns*

    The "SNP finder" Bioscope program calculates the heterozygosity/homozygosity status of each SNV by counting the number of novel base reads against the reference base reads located at each base of the NCBI36/hg18 reference genome. It returns het=0 for a homozygous SNV and het=1 for a heterozygous SNV. This step simply creates a new data column (column 9) and converts the values to het=1 (heterozygous) and het=2 (homozygous). This is a practical counting method that can be usefully employed for recessive genetic conditions to quickly establish if an exome is either homozygous for a SNV or double heterozygous for two different SNVs in any particular gene. Click on "Text Manipulation" and then "Compute" in Galaxy tools. Type "2-c6" in the "Add expression" box, select the data file from Step 10 in the "as a new column to" box and select "YES" for rounding the result. Select "Execute." Column 6 is denoted as "c6" in the above expression. It is the original heterozygosity/homozygosity column.

12. *Identify SNVs that are located in ncRNAs*

    Click on "Operate on Genomic Intervals" in Galaxy tools and select "*Intersect* the intervals of two queries." Select "Overlapping Intervals" in the "Return" box, then choose the ncRNA data file (Step 9) in the "of" box and the filtered SNV data file (Step 11) in the "that intersect" box. Select 1 bp in the "for at least" box and press "Execute."

13. *Join SNV attributes to the ncRNA intersection*

    Step 12 just returns the locus and name of ncRNAs that intersect with the exome SNV data. This step re-joins each SNV's attributes to the file. Click on "Operate on Genomic Intervals" in Galaxy tools and select "*Join* the intervals of two queries side-by-side." Select Step 11 in the "Join" box and Step 12 in the "with" box, and keep the default 1 bp minimum overlap. Nominate to return "only the records that are joined (INNER JOIN)." Press "Execute."

14. *Identify all protein-coding genes that overlap with exome SNVs*

    Click on "Operate on Genomic Intervals" in Galaxy tools and select "*Intersect* the intervals of two queries." Select "Overlapping Intervals" in the "Return" box, then choose the "Known Gene Locations" data file (Step 8) in the "of" box and the filtered SNV data file (Step 11) in the "that intersect" box. Select 1 bp in the "for at least" box and press "Execute."

15. *Create a complete list of codons existing in genes with filtered SNVs*

    Click on "Extract Feature" in Galaxy tools and select "Gene BED To Exon/Intron/Codon BED expander." In the "Extract" box, select "Codons," in the "from" box, select Step 14 data file, and press "Execute." This will deliver a BED file including chromosome numbers and the start and end locations for each codon in the genome in genes with filtered SNVs.

16. *Narrow the codon list to those containing filtered SNVs*

    Click on "Operate on Genomic Intervals" in Galaxy tools and select "*Intersect* the intervals of two queries." Select "Overlapping Intervals" in the "Return" box, then choose the codon data file (Step 15) in the "of" box and the filtered SNV data file (Step 11) in the "that intersect" box. Select 1 bp in the "for at least" box and press "Execute."

17. *Extract the genomic DNA base sequences for the intersecting codons*

    Click on "Fetch Sequences" in Galaxy tools and select "*Extract* Genomic DNA." In the popup menu for "Fetch sequences corresponding to Query," select the data file output from Step 16 and select "Interval" format for the output data type. Press "Execute."

18. *Join SNV attributes to the intersecting codon list*

    Click on "Operate on Genomic Intervals" in Galaxy tools and select "*Join* the intervals of two queries side-by-side." Select Step 17 in the "Join" box, Step 11 in the "with" box, and keep the default 1 bp minimum overlap. Nominate to return "only the records that are joined (INNER JOIN)." Press "Execute."

19. *Add mutated codon DNA sequence column*

    Galaxy can return a single base codon change column with the DNA sequence for every codon with a SNV. Click on the "Evolution" tool, then "Mutate Codons" and in the "Interval file with joined SNPs" box, select the data file from Step 18. The following column selections should be made: Codon Sequence column = c7, SNP chromosome column = c8, SNP start column = c9, SNP end column = c10, SNP strand column = c11 (*see* **Note 7**), and SNP observed column = c12 (*see* **Note 8**).

20. *Add a reference amino acid column*
    Click on "Join, Subtract and Group" in galaxy tools and select "*Join two Queries* side by side on a specified field." Choose the data file from Step 19 for the "Join" box using column 7 (reference codon sequence) and the uploaded codon table file from Step 6 for the "with" box using column 1. Choose "Yes" for including all the lines from the first input that do not join with the second input as well as lines that are incomplete. Choose "No" to "fill empty columns." Press "Execute."

21. *Add a mutated amino acid column*
    Click on "Join, Subtract and Group" in galaxy tools and select "*Join two Queries* side by side on a specified field." Choose the data file from Step 20 for the "Join" box using column 17 (mutated codon sequence) and the uploaded codon table file from Step 6 for the "with" box using column 1. Choose "Yes" for including all the lines from the first input that do not join with the second input as well as lines that are incomplete. Choose "No" to "fill empty columns." Press "Execute."

22. *Determine whether base changes are synonymous or nonsynonymous*
    Click on "Text Manipulation" and then "*Compute*" in Galaxy tools. Type "c19 = = c21" in the "Add expression" box, select the data file from Step 21 in the "as a new column to" box and select "YES" for rounding the result. Select "Execute." Columns 19 and 21 should contain the three letter amino acid codes (or stop codon) determined in Steps 20 and 21 (column 19 = reference amino acid and column 21 = substituted amino acid (or nonsense mutation)). This step will output a new column with either "True" (which indicates a synonymous SNV (sSNV)) or "False" (which indicates a nonsynonymous SNV (nsSNV) or nonsense mutation) for each nucleotide change.

23. *Join reference gene names to data file*
    Click on "Operate on Genomic Intervals" in Galaxy tools and select "*Join* the intervals of two queries side-by-side." Select Step 22 data file in the "Join" box and Step 4 (RefSeq gene names linked to genomic loci data

file in interval format) in the "with" box and keep the default 1 bp minimum overlap. Nominate to return "only the records that are joined (INNER JOIN)." Press "Execute."

24. *Obtaining and uploading HapMap nsSNV data for further filtering*

At this stage, all the information from one individual's exome list of nsSNVs, sSNVs, and ncRNA SNVs filtered against the SNP database has been collated. The remaining steps in this workflow further filter this data file against eight HapMap individuals to remove commonly found SNVs (that are not listed in dbSNP) and then sort the final list into categories.

An excel file of nonsynonymous coding SNVs identified by sequencing eight HapMap individuals (7) was obtained from this Web site: http://krishna.gs.washington.edu/12_exomes/. There are a number of genes contained within these HapMap individuals that commonly contain nsSNVs (*see* **Table 7.2**), i.e., these genes have a high rate of containing nsSNVs (with significant allelic heterogeneity) between the eight individuals. Also, there is known to be a subset of genes that commonly contain nonsense mutations (20).

Filtering the SNV and linked gene data file (Step 23) against these confounding HapMap genes and SNVs will significantly reduce the false-positive rate of identification of potential disease gene SNV associations (7).

Table 7.2
Genes containing novel nsSNVs in multiple HapMap individuals

No. of HapMap individual exomes	No. of genes containing ≥ 1 nsSNV (not listed in public SNP databases)
8 out of 8	10[a]
7 out of 8	20
6 out of 8	31
5 out of 8	45
4 out of 8	75
3 out of 8	205
2 out of 8	638
1 out of 8	2928

[a]There are 10 genes shared by 8 HapMap individuals that contain at least 1 nsSNV (in *each* HapMap individual) not listed in dbSNP

From the excel file, a list of shared SNVs was extracted and formatted into interval file format suitable for use in Galaxy. This file can be accessed using the following link: http://main.g2.bx.psu.edu/u/mhin/h/hapmap-genome-filtering-input-files.

25. *Organize columns from protein-coding dataset*
    Click on "Text Manipulation" Galaxy tool and select "*Cut* columns from a table." Use the column numbering described in the last paragraph of Step 24. This should mean the order of columns to type into the "Cut columns" box is c1,c6,c10,c16,c18,c19,c20,c21,c22,c28. Nominate a "Tab delimited" output using the data file from Step 23.

26. *Subtract common HapMap SNVs from protein-coding SNV dataset*
    Click on "Join, Subtract and Group" Galaxy tool and select "*Subtract* Whole Query from another query." Select the Step 24 data file upload for the "Subtract" box and select the Step 25 data file for the "from" box. Restrict the subtraction to between (and including) c1 and c10. Press "Execute."

27. *Create data file with only nonsynonymous SNVs*
    Click on "Filter and Sort" Galaxy tool and select "*Filter* data on any column using simple expressions." Choose to filter Step 26 data file with the following condition: "c9 = = 'False'."

28. *Create data file with only synonymous SNVs*
    Click on "Filter and Sort" Galaxy tool and select "*Filter* data on any column using simple expressions." Choose to filter Step 26 data file with the following condition: "c9 = = 'True'."

29. *Count the filtered ncRNA SNVs*
    Click on "Statistics" Galaxy tool and select "*Count* occurrences of each record." Choose the ncRNA data file from Step 13 and count occurrences of values from the following columns:
    c1 (chromosome), c9 (het/homozygosity score), and c13 (gene name).

30. *Count the filtered protein-coding synonymous SNVs*
    Click on "Statistics" Galaxy tool and select "*Count* occurrences of each record." Choose the synonymous SNV data file from Step 28 and count occurrences of values from the following columns:
    c1 (chromosome), c4 (het/homozygosity score), c9 ("True"/ "False"), and c10 (gene name).

31. *Count the filtered protein-coding nonsynonymous SNVs*
 Click on "Statistics" Galaxy tool and select "*Count* occurrences of each record." Choose the nonsynonymous SNV data file from Step 27 and count occurrences of values from the following columns:
 c1 (chromosome), c4 (het/homozygosity score), c9 ("True"/"False"), and c10 (gene name).
32. *Create a sorted list of ncRNA genes containing filtered SNVs*
 Click on "Filter and Sort" Galaxy tool and select "*Sort* data in ascending or descending order." Sort the query from Step 29 on column 1 (counting column) using a numerical sort in descending order.
33. *Create a sorted list of ncRNA genes containing filtered synonymous SNVs*
 Click on "Filter and Sort" Galaxy tool and select "*Sort* data in ascending or descending order." Sort the query from Step 30 on column 1 (counting column) using a numerical sort in descending order.
34. *Create a sorted list of protein-coding genes containing filtered nonsynonymous SNVs*
 Click on "Filter and Sort" Galaxy tool and select "*Sort* data in ascending or descending order." Sort the query from Step 31 on column 1 (counting column) using a numerical sort in descending order.
 At this stage, there will be three separate sorted data files for perusal. Non-coding RNA gene and protein-coding gene sSNV and nsSNV chromosomal locations can be viewed in data files from Steps 13, 28, and 27 respectively.
35. *Further filtering of datasets to narrow down the contributing gene/s*
 If there remains a large number of candidate genes for the genetic condition being investigated, further filters excluding genes that commonly have nsSNVs should be done (*see* **Table 7.2** and Step 24). Upload sequential HapMap sorted files from Step 24 that contain 8, 7, 6, 5, 4, 3, and 2 genes that have nsSNVs until the list of possible disease candidate genes appears to be limited enough to further investigate. There is going to be a trade-off using these filters between the sensitivity and precision of determining which genes to pursue.
 Intronic SNVs can be analyzed by subtracting the SNVs in the data file from Step 18 from those in Step 11. Protein-coding indels can be sorted using the Small Indel Finder Bioscope program and then without filtering the gene names can be included in the list of possible pathogenic mutations. Most coding indels can be considered to have a high probability of altering protein function

and the number discovered for any single individual will be modest in size.

3.5. Other Annotation and Filtering Tools

The Galaxy workflow above is designed for experimentalists to understand how exome sequencing-discovered variants can be systematically filtered and sorted. The data bases for filtering can be varied (e.g., SNP minor allele frequency can be altered in Step 5, the filtering gene data base/s can specifically be chosen in Steps 1–3, heterozygosity and the HapMap data filtering stringency can be imported from Step 24) . There are also a range of other tools which can be used to analyze SNVs. These could be employed in tandem with the above Galaxy workflow.

`Sequence Variant Analyzer (SVA) (http://people.genome.duke.edu/~dg48/sva/index.php)`

It is a software program for analyzing genomic variants which can be downloaded and run on a Linux computer. SVA uses data from a range of sources to automate annotation, filtering, and prioritizing variants. SVA presents information in a variety of tabular and graphical formats.

`SeqAnt sequence annotator (http://seqant.genetics.emory.edu/)`

It is an open source software package for annotating variations. It is available for download and can also be run by uploading a list of variants to the SeqAnt Web site.

`SeattleSeq (http://gvs.gs.washington.edu/SeattleSeqAnnotation/)`

This program allows exome sequencing files to be uploaded in Maq, gff, CASAVA, VCF, and custom format. It returns an annotated file categorizing each SNV into a dbSNP rs number, gene name and accession number, function (e.g., missense), HapMap frequency, and Polyphen prediction. Caution should be used in the bioinformatic interpretation by Polyphen. We recommend using this Web site to compare results found using the Galaxy workflow above.

`Annovar (http://www.openbioinformatics.org/annovar/)`

It is a freely available Web-based tool for variant filtering and annotation of SNVs and indels. Gff3 files generated from SOLiD sequencing data are compatible. Annovar was successfully employed to discover a gene associated with Miller syndrome (25).

`Taverna Workbench (http://www.taverna.org.uk/)`

Taverna is another workflow tool. It is a Java application which is installed and run on the user's workstation. Taverna can access data from many online data services which offer a SOAP interface. Currently, Biocatalogue.org lists over 1600 services. It is highly extensible with support for BeanShell scripting and execution of R scripts. It can also run services on computational grids.

3.6. Characterize Candidate Genes

See **Chapters 13**, **14**, **15**, **16**, **17**, **18**, **19**, **20**, and **21** for characterization of candidate genes. Some preliminary characterization of candidate genes may be appropriate before embarking on confirmatory segregation analysis.

3.7. Segregation Analysis and Sequence Unrelated Subjects

Subsequent targeted resequencing of related subjects that are also affected by the genetic condition being investigated can quickly exclude a number of candidate genes. Only the genomic sequence/s with the identified SNV/s needs to be amplified and analyzed by Sanger sequencing.

4. Notes

1. The Galaxy Web site can occasionally be slow, depending on the workload it is receiving. It is possible to run a local Galaxy server by downloading the software from the Galaxy Web site. On the main page (http://galaxy.psu.edu/), click on the download link. Installation is available for UNIX/Linux and Mac OS X. Alternatively, there are a few mirror Web sites that can be found using Google.
2. All pending and completed jobs are displayed under "History" on the right-hand side (*see* **Fig. 7.2**). Clicking on the pen icon for each step allows you to change file attributes including the name of the file, assignment of column data, and importantly the file format (interval, tabular, or BED). Clicking on the file name gives you details of the file including assignment of data columns.
3. It is important to be consistent in Galaxy manipulations with genome reference numbers. All downloaded files in this workflow are from Mar.2006(NCBI36/hg18) except in Step 1 for the up-to-date list of currently known gene locations which has numbering from Feb.2009(GRCh37/hg19) and is converted to Mar.2006(NCBI36/hg18) in Step 8.
4. This last refinement may be important if the Mendelian condition being investigated is relatively common (e.g., >2% in population) and may be due to an SNV already in the SNP database.
5. In this description, Step 7 is the only step that is specific for the SOLiD system. The downstream bioinformatic

steps (Steps 8 to 35) can use sequencing data (FASTA format) from either a SOLiD or an Illumina system and can be completed on a personal computer with an Internet connection.

6. The "Convert genome coordinates" tool might run twice. If it does, delete the extra output from the history on the right-hand side of the Galaxy main page.
7. Galaxy is capable of interpreting which strand the SNV is located on relative to the codon sequence. Hence, although Bioscope SNP finder does not return a strand (+ or −), this does not matter. In Step 19, nominate column 11 for the strand despite it being empty.
8. The Galaxy nomenclature for each SNV is *variation/reference*. For example, A/G would mean the reference allele is G and the mutated allele is A.

References

1. McKusick, V. A. (2007) Mendelian inheritance in man and its online version, OMIM. *Am J Hum Genet* ***80***, 588–604.
2. Manolio, T. A., and Collins, F. S. (2009) The HapMap and genome-wide association studies in diagnosis and therapy. *Annu Rev Med* ***60***, 443–456.
3. Ashley, E. A., Butte, A. J., Wheeler, M. T., et al. (2010) Clinical assessment incorporating a personal genome. *Lancet* ***375***, 1525–1535.
4. Ng, S. B., Turner, E. H., Robertson, P. D., et al. (2009) Targeted capture and massively parallel sequencing of 12 human exomes. *Nature* ***461***, 272–276.
5. Choi, M., Scholl, U. I., Ji, W., et al. (2009) Genetic diagnosis by whole exome capture and massively parallel DNA sequencing. *Proc Natl Acad Sci USA* ***106***, 19096–19101.
6. Hoischen, A., van Bon, B. W., Gilissen, C., et al. (2010) De novo mutations of SETBP1 cause Schinzel–Giedion syndrome. *Nat Genet* ***42***, 483–485.
7. Ng, S. B., Buckingham, K. J., Lee, C., et al. (2010) Exome sequencing identifies the cause of a Mendelian disorder. *Nat Genet* ***42***, 30–35.
8. Shoubridge, C., Tarpey, P. S., Abidi, F., et al. (2010) Mutations in the guanine nucleotide exchange factor gene IQSEC2 cause nonsyndromic intellectual disability. *Nat Genet* ***42***, 486–488.
9. Lupski, J. R., Reid, J. G., Gonzaga-Jauregui, C., et al. (2010) Whole-genome sequencing in a patient with Charcot-Marie-Tooth neuropathy. *N Engl J Med* ***362***, 1181–1191.
10. Lalonde, E., Albrecht, S., Ha, K. C., et al. (2010) Unexpected allelic heterogeneity and spectrum of mutations in Fowler syndrome revealed by next generation exome sequencing. *Hum Mutat* ***31***, 918–923.
11. Sobreira, N. L. M. (2010) Whole-genome sequencing of a single proband together with linkage analysis identifies a Mendelian disease gene. *PLOS Genetics* ***6***, e1000991.
12. Herman, D. S., Hovingh, G. K., Iartchouk, O., et al. (2009) Filter-based hybridization capture of subgenomes enables resequencing and copy-number detection. *Nat Methods* ***6***, 507–510.
13. Birney, E., Stamatoyannopoulos, J. A., Dutta, A., Guigo, R., Gingeras, T. R., et al. (2007) Identification and analysis of functional elements in 1% of the human genome by the ENCODE pilot project. *Nature* ***447***, 799–816.
14. Henikoff, S. (2007) ENCODE and our very busy genome. *Nat Genet* ***39***, 817–818.
15. Taft, R. J., Pang, K. C., Mercer, T. R., et al. (2010) Non-coding RNAs: regulators of disease. *J Pathol* ***220***, 126–139.
16. Agilent (2010) *SureSelect Target Enrichment System Protocol.* Agilent Technologies, Santa Clara, CA, USA.
17. Blankenberg, D., Von Kuster, G., Coraor, N., et al. (2010) Galaxy: a web-based genome analysis tool for experimentalists. *Curr Protoc Mol Biol Chapter* ***19***, Unit 19 10 11–21.
18. Giardine, B., Riemer, C., Hardison, R. C., et al. (2005) Galaxy: a platform for interactive large-scale genome analysis. *Genome Res* ***15***, 1451–1455.

19. AppliedBiosystems (2010) *Bioscope Software for Scientists Guide*. Applied Biosystems, Foster City, CA, USA.
20. Pelak, K., Shianna, K. V., Ge, D., Maia, J. M., et al. (2010) The characterization of twenty sequenced human genomes. *PLoS Genet* ***6***, e1001111.
21. Mitchell, A. A., Zwick, M. E., Chakravarti, A., and Cutler, D. J. (2004) Discrepancies in dbSNP confirmation rates and allele frequency distributions from varying genotyping error rates and patterns. *Bioinformatics* ***20***, 1022–1032.
22. Musumeci, L., Arthur, J. W., Cheung, F. S., et al. (2010) Single nucleotide differences (SNDs) in the dbSNP database may lead to errors in genotyping and haplotyping studies. *Hum Mutat* ***31***, 67–73.
23. NCBI. (2010) dbSNP summary for build 131 http://www.ncbi.nlm.nih.gov/projects/SNP/snp_summary.cgi.
24. Ng, S. B., Bigham, A. W., Buckingham, K. J., et al. (2010) Exome sequencing identifies MLL2 mutations as a cause of Kabuki syndrome. *Nat Genet* ***42***, 790–793.
25. Wang, K., Li, M., and Hakonarson, H. (2010) ANNOVAR: functional annotation of genetic variants from high-throughput sequencing data. *Nucleic Acids Res* ***38***, e164.

Chapter 8

In Silico Knowledge and Content Tracking

Herman van Haagen and Barend Mons

Abstract

This chapter gives a brief overview of text-mining techniques to extract knowledge from large text collections. It describes the basis pipeline of how to come from text to relationships between biological concepts and the problems that are encountered at each step in the pipeline. We first explain how words in text are recognized as concepts. Second, concepts are associated with each other using 2×2 contingency tables and test statistics. Third, we explain that it is possible to extract indirect links between concepts using the direct links taken from 2×2 table analyses. This we call implicit information extraction. Fourth, the validation techniques to evaluate a text-mining system such as ROC curves and retrospective studies are discussed. We conclude by examining how text information can be combined with other non-textual data sources such as microarray expression data and what the future directions are for text-mining within the Internet.

Key words: Text-mining, data mining, information retrieval, disambiguation, retrospective analysis, ROC curve, prioritizer, ontology, semantic web.

1. Introduction

The amount of biomedical literature is growing tremendously. It has become impossible for researchers to read all publications in their moving field of interest, which forces them to make a stringent selection of relevant articles to read. For the actual knowledge discovery process, which is in essence a systematic association process over an expanding number of interrelated concepts, life scientists increasingly rely on the computer. This stringent reduction of the percentage of relevant articles that can actually be "read" has the disadvantage that relevant information from non-selected articles can be missed. The largest database of recorded biomedical literature is PubMed, which contains over 14 million articles published in the last 30 years (from 1980

B. Yu, M. Hinchcliffe (eds.), *In Silico Tools for Gene Discovery*, Methods in Molecular Biology 760,
DOI 10.1007/978-1-61779-176-5_8, © Springer Science+Business Media, LLC 2011

till 2010). Besides the literature, there are many other resources ranging from curated databases to online blogs, digital books recorded in libraries, and any text information that can be found via a search engine like Google.

The field that deals with automated information extraction from text is called text-mining. Text-mining on its own is a challenging field of research that intensively has been further developed over the last years. Computer systems have been developed based on natural language processing, a method of processing any sentence into its building blocks such as the subject, verbs, and nouns. Other methods are based on word tagging. PubMed, for instance, uses the words in a search query and matches it with words found in abstracts with no additional information on how the words are related with other words in text. In this chapter, we describe the concept-based method for automated information extraction from text.

2. Materials

When dealing with text data, the analysis is normally done in two stages. The first stage is the hard-core data processing of raw text data. The text data are downloaded from Medline and its capacity can be as big as 50 GB of hard disk space. The processing is done using a programming language such as Java or Perl (object oriented preferred). Any programming language that has a flexible syntax and is fast in executing scripts will do. The tagging of words and storage of the processed documents is done on a server with high computational power. The result of the first stage is processed text data in any suitable format (e.g., concept profiles or HashMaps) designed for further analysis. This is stored offline on a hard disk. This offline data can then be used for calculating scores or generating a network of concepts. This normally results in a tab-delimited text file. In the file, the columns are usually features and the rows are the samples (PPIs of random protein pairs) or the text file is a matrix describing the connectivity of a network and the weights of edges and nodes.

The second stage is to do a statistical analysis on the processed text file. For the analysis, a statistics package is needed such as R (http://www.r-project.org/) or Matlab.

3. Methods

3.1. Concept-Based Text-Mining

For concept-based text-mining, three "ingredients" are needed: (1) text data, (2) a word tagger, and (3) a terminology system, mostly controlled vocabulary or ontologies.

For biomedical text data, normally the abstracts recorded in PubMed are chosen. Reasons for this are that this is the greatest source of recorded literature, the abstracts are publically available and free to download, and the information density of abstracts is higher than that of full-text documents (1).

Words in text are recognized by a so-called word tagger and mapped to a concept identifier (2). In order to do so, we first need to understand what a concept is. A concept is a unit of thought, meaning that people agree that they share information about one and the same thing. A concept has terms and other "tokens" that "refer" to it. It can have synonyms, abbreviations, but also, for instance, uniform resource identifiers (URIs) or accession numbers.

For instance, there exists a protein called dystrophin. When the gene encoding this protein is mutated, it can cause diseases such as Duchenne muscular dystrophy or Becker muscular dystrophy. Dystrophin normally is abbreviated to DMD. DMD (either in italic) also refers to the gene or the disease. Dystrophin is stored in databases like Entrez Gene (http://www.ncbi.nlm.nih.gov/gene) with the accession number 1756 and UniProt Knowledge Database (http://www.uniprot.org/) with accession number P11532. The words dystrophin, DMD, 1756, and P11532 all refer to one and the same concept (we treat a gene and a protein as the same concept). The tagger maps the words to the concept identifier for dystrophin.

Lastly, the synonyms, abbreviations, accession numbers, and concept identifiers are stored in an ontology (*see* **Note 1**). The most common vocabulary for the biomedical field is the unified medical language system (UMLS) (3). An ontology may be field specific. If only drug information from text needs to be extracted, a drug vocabulary is used instead of the whole vocabulary with all medical concepts.

3.2. Classical Direct Relationship Detection

Once a text-mining system has been developed and concepts in text are recognized and stored in a database, the question becomes: What to do with this tagged text data? The main question is: Which are the two concepts significantly related? The relationship between two concepts can be of any kind. In biology, these are the most common ones we chose as examples: (1) two proteins that have a molecular interaction, (2) a mutated gene that causes a disease, (3) a protein that has a particular function, and (4) a drug that treats a disease or has a (adverse) side effect. Any relationship between two concepts can be seen as a triplet with a subject, predicate, and object. An example of a triplet is as follows: protein dystrophin (subject) interacts with (predicate) protein ankyrin 2 (object).

The statistical way to define the strength of relationship between two concepts is by making a 2×2 contingency table (or frequency table). The table below gives an example for concepts X and Y.

	X	**Not X**
Y	*A*	*B*
Not Y	*C*	*D*

A is the number of documents where both concepts X and Y are co-mentioned (*see* **Note 2**). *B* is the number of documents where concept Y occurs but not concept X. *C* is the reverse version of *B* and *D* is the number of documents where X and Y are not mentioned. Any statistical test can be applied to this table such as the likelihood ratio test, chi-squared test, or the uncertainty coefficient (*see* **Note 3**). If X and Y are frequently co-mentioned together (e.g., *A* is a relatively large number) and the concepts are not exceptionally generic so that they occur frequently in text (e.g., *B* and *C* are small), then the two concepts may be significantly related (*see* **Note 4**). There are many text-mining systems available based on direct relationship detection such as IHOP (4), PubGene (5), and systems where text-mining is an integral part such as STRING (6), FunCoup (7), and Endeavour (8).

3.3. Implicit Information Extraction via Concept Profiling

The classical direct relationship detection method has the disadvantage that concepts that are not co-mentioned together are missed, while they still might be related to each other. This could be due to the reason that related concepts are stored in full text (frequently not freely available for mining) and not in the abstract or that concepts are related but no one made the link yet. Via indirect links between terms in text, terms can still be related to each other even when they have never been co-mentioned (9). This we call implicit information extraction. Swanson (10) was the first to demonstrate that this approach works by linking the treatment of Raynaud's disease with fish oil. van Haagen et al. (11) demonstrated this idea further by predicting protein–protein interactions. They predicted the physical interaction between calpain 3, which causes a form of muscular dystrophy, and parvalbumin B, which is found mainly in skeletal muscle. Those two proteins were strongly linked via the intermediate concept dysferlin, which is a protein.

Concept profiling contains the following steps (*see* **Fig. 8.1**). First, for a concept X (e.g., a gene, a chemical, or drug), the documents are selected wherein X appears. Next all other concepts that are co-mentioned with X are processed using the direct relationship detection method described previously (**Fig. 8.1b**). The 2×2 table information for each concept pair is stored in a profile. This concept profile for X is basically a vector of *N* dimensions.

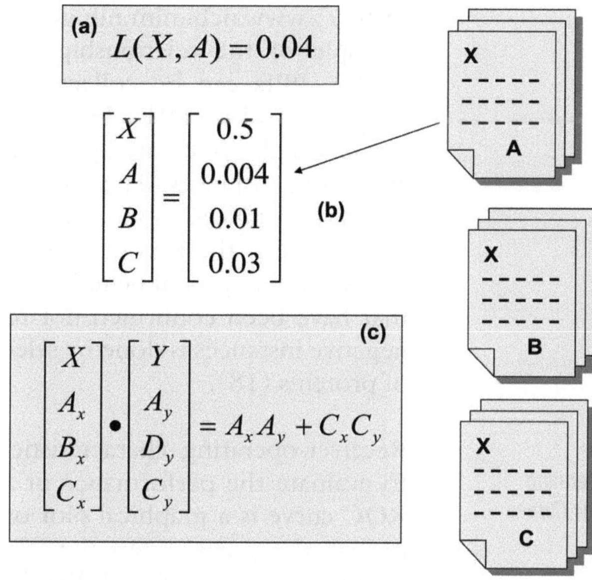

Fig. 8.1. Basic scheme for concept-based profiling. (**a**) Example of a likelihood function calculated between concept X and *A*. Information is taken from a 2×2 contingency table. The score reflects the strength of association between X and *A*. (**b**) Documents selected where concept X appears and is co-mentioned with other concepts. For a concept the documents are selected and transformed into a test statistic using a 2×2 contingency table. (**c**) The inner product score between two concept profiles. The score is only calculated over the concepts the two profiles have in common.

N is the number of concepts that are co-mentioned with X. Each entry in the vector is a number associating concept X with another concept (taken from a 2×2 table, **Fig. 8.1a**). Computation of the "conceptual association" between two concepts can now be performed by matching their respective concept profiles by vector matching (**Fig. 8.1c**). Any distance measure can be used for this matching (9) such as the inner product, cosine, angle, Euclidean distance, or Pearson's correlation. If two concept profiles have many concepts in their individual concept profiles in common, e.g., many implicit links, then the two concepts may be related to each other. A web tool is available, dubbed "Anni," for implicit information extraction by concept profiling (12). In the next section, we will describe how to validate text-mining approaches and the amount of relatedness.

3.4. Cross-validation Within Text-Mining and Other Performance Measures

3.4.1. Defining a Positive and a Negative Set

In the previous sections, we described how to extract relationships (content) between concepts from text with either direct relationship detection or concept profiling. Once a system is designed, it needs to be tested to evaluate its performance in extracting or predicting relationships. To enable this step, we need data to train the system and after training, testing it. For instance, data on protein function can be collected from the Gene Ontology (13) and data on gene–disease relationships from OMIM (http://www.ncbi.nlm.nih.gov/omim). Here we describe an example of the relationship type protein–protein interactions (PPIs). PPIs can be collected from electronic databases such as UniProt (14), DIP (15), BioGrid (16), and Reactome (17). These samples of curated protein–protein interactions are labeled as positive instances. These positive instances are compared with negative instances to see if the text-mining system can discriminate between the two groups. In biology research, no database that stores samples of negatives instances exists, e.g., two proteins that have been confirmed not to interact. Normally, generating negative instances is done by selecting random pairs from a group of proteins (18).

3.4.2. Receiver-Operating Characteristic Curves

Receiver-operating characteristic (ROC) curves are often used to evaluate the performance of a prediction algorithm (19). An ROC curve is a graphical plot of the true positive rate (sensitivity) on the *y*-axis versus the false-positive rate (1 − specificity) on the *x*-axis (*see* **Fig. 8.2b**). The ROC curve is defined for a binary classifier system (the positive and negative sets described in **Section 3.4.1**) as its discrimination threshold is varied. This measure is often used in information retrieval and it can be explained as a system design that collects as much information as possible (in terms of true positives) while at the same time reducing the noise (the false positives). An ROC curve is constructed as follows: in **Fig. 8.2a** the distributions of positive and negative instances are given and in **Fig. 8.2b** its corresponding ROC curve is given. The threshold that discriminates

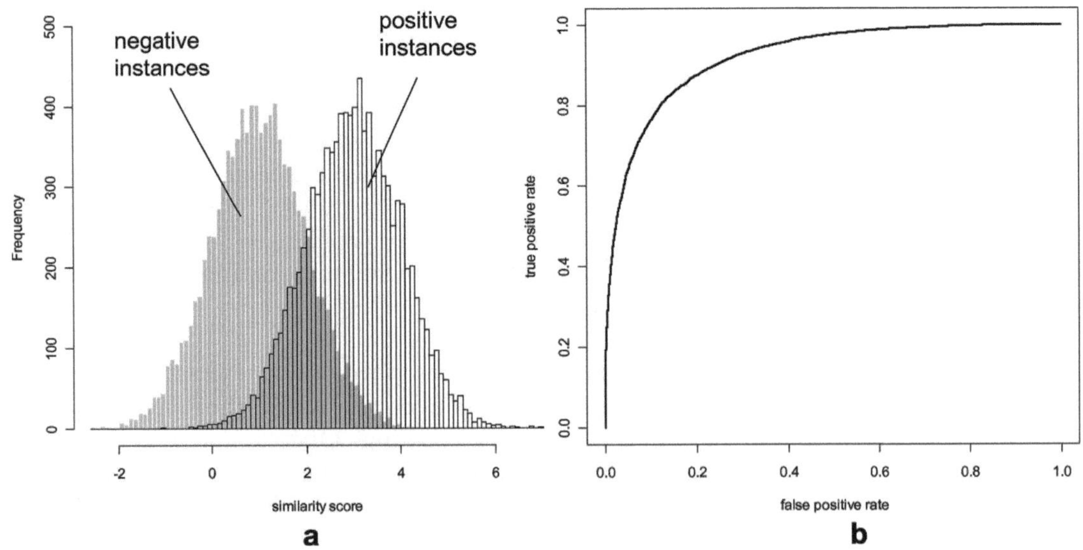

Fig. 8.2. Histogram and its corresponding ROC plot. (**a**) The distribution of the positive and negative sets. (**b**) An ROC curve with an AuC of 0.92.

between the two groups is varied from the highest match score (**Fig. 8.2a**, *x*-axis) value to the lowest. Each threshold corresponds to a true-positive and a false-positive rate in ROC space. In **Fig. 8.2a** all the way up to the right on the *x*-axis is the threshold (around 7) where no true or negative instances pass this threshold. Therefore, both the true-positive and false-positive rates are zero, resulting in the point (0,0) in ROC space (**Fig. 8.2b**, bottom left corner). Then the threshold as a slider is moved to the right. At each point, a number of positive and negative instances will pass the threshold, resulting in a point in ROC space anywhere between 0 and 1 on both axes. Finally, the threshold reaches the extreme left point on the *x*-axis (around –2, **Fig. 8.2a**). Here all positive and negative instances pass this threshold. This corresponds with the point (1,1) in ROC space (**Fig. 8.2b**, top right corner).

To translate the ROC space to a single measurement for performance, we calculate the area under the ROC curve (AuC). The AuC value normally varies between 0.5 and 1.

If a system shows a random behavior (e.g., two completely overlapping distributions, no discrimination between positive and negative sets), the ROC space results in a straight line from the point (0,0) to (1,1). This corresponds with an AuC of 0.5. If a system behaves like a perfect classifier, the ROC curve starts at point (0,0) and moves up to point (0,1) (e.g., first, all positive instances are predicted), then it moves from point (0,1) to point (1,1) (e.g., all negative instances are predicted). This corresponds with an AuC of 1. The AuC for the example in **Fig. 8.2** is 0.92.

3.4.3. Cross-validation and Bias

The performance of an associative in silico discovery system is tested using cross-validation (20). A system is first trained using training data. Then it is tested using test data. There is no explicit data for testing only, nor is their data used only for training. There is just data. Therefore, a part of the data is selected for training and the remaining part for testing. The way to select the training and test data is arbitrary. Here we describe the most common approach of cross-validation of the 10-fold CV. The first step (1) is to randomly shuffle the samples in your dataset (both positive and negative instances). (2) Then the dataset is divided into 10 equally sized subsets. Each piece contains samples of the positive and negative sets. (3) In one iteration, 9 of the 10 subsets are used for training and the remaining subset is used for testing. (4) Step three is repeated until each subset is used once for testing.

An extremely important step during cross-validation is to make sure that none of the test data is used during training. Else this would introduce a bias and gives an overestimation of the true performance. Within the field of text-mining and biology, this seems virtually impossible. Most of the data stored in curated databases, such as protein–protein interactions or gene–disease relationships recorded in OMIM, are based on published articles. This means that positive instances in the test set are based on articles that are also used to train a text-mining system. Other data sources also have this problem. For instance, the Gene Ontology contains functional descriptions for a protein that are normally also based on literature evidence. In order to evaluate prediction performance, it is therefore more appropriate to make use of a retrospective analysis.

3.4.4. Retrospective Validation

Before we explain the basics of retrospective validation, we need to distinguish between two types of prediction. The first one is prediction of current knowledge stored in databases. This knowledge is already known and the system recovers what is stored in these databases. For this, the cross-validation approach described above is useful.

The second one is the prediction of new and as yet unforeseen knowledge. This means "implicit" knowledge that is not recorded in any database cannot be explicitly found in text. To simulate the prediction of these "hidden associations," a retrospective validation is done. First, a time interval is defined when data are stored in a database. For PubMed, this could, for instance, be all the abstracts of articles published between 1980 and January 2010. The second step would be to select test data published after a certain date, for instance, all protein–protein interactions recorded in databases from January 2007 until January 2010. The third step is to train the text-mining system before that date using all data before January 2007. The last step is to evaluate what test samples were predicted before January 2007 that became only explicit (also in the literature) knowledge after January 2007. In other words, protein–protein interactions that could be found by simple co-occurrence before the "closure date", but were not added to the databases yet, should not be counted as true predictions. In this evaluation, there is no procedure to repeat these steps multiple times as with cross-validation. This means that no standard error on the performance can be calculated.

3.4.5. Prioritizers

Another way to view an ROC curve is as a prioritized list. The ROC curve is constructed by varying the threshold. The samples (e.g., protein pairs, either a PPI or random) are ranked from the highest match score to the lowest. Going down in this ranked list from the top prediction to the lowest is done by walking over the ROC curve from point (0,0) to point (1,1). Experimental biologists are mainly interested in what is predicted in the top, e.g., the most likely predictions. Prioritizers are useful to evaluate where your test samples rank in the top. An ROC curve can also be plotted on the absolute scales of true positives and false positives by translating a prioritized list in a graphical way. **Figure 8.3** shows an example of 20 ranked samples and its

sample	match score	label
s1	4.960111897	0
s2	4.662243252	0
s3	4.661449007	1
s4	4.589346313	0
s5	4.581602664	0
s6	4.438759168	0
s7	4.379399852	0
s8	4.377182023	0
s9	4.320084484	1
s10	4.303145807	0
s11	4.299505092	1
s12	4.259483679	0
s13	4.249962717	1
s14	4.230262428	1
s15	4.188873972	1
s16	4.179967181	1
s17	4.177931731	1
s18	4.176843766	0
s19	4.163993686	1
s20	4.118021526	1

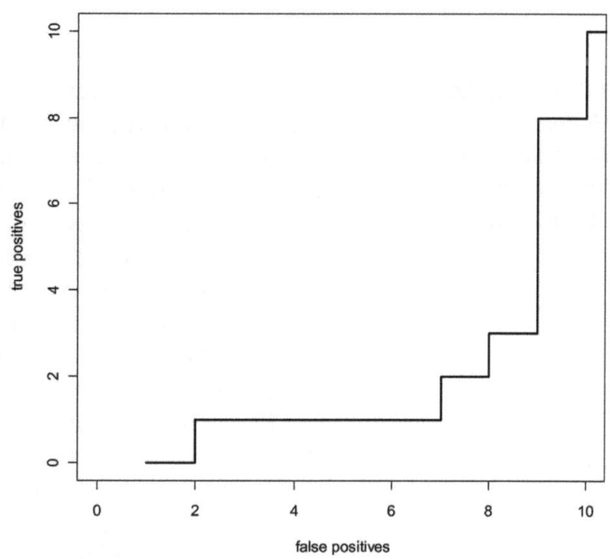

Fig. 8.3. Prioritized list of 20 samples and its corresponding ROC10 curve.

corresponding ROC curve. This curve is also called an ROC10 curve. It reflects the amount of true positive predictions (baits) at a fixed number of false positives (the costs), in this case 10. You can vary this threshold and define, for instance, an ROC50 or an ROC100 curve.

3.5. Extending Text-Mining Systems with Other Databases: Data Mining

Text-mining actually is a subdivision of the broader field of data mining. Data mining is the field of research to extract any kind of information from a variety of resources. For instance, there are many data sources available for proteins. Besides the literature, there exists information in curated databases, microarray expression data (21, 22), domain interaction databases (23), functional annotations from the Gene Ontology (*see* **Chapter 9**), phylogenetic trees, and sequence data. There are many tools and techniques available for data mining on databases but they all share a common idea. Combining all information from several distinct data sources into one should reveal more information than can be recovered by the mining of each data source alone (*see* **Note 5**). Data mining basically is a two-step approach. The first step is to define a match or an evidence score for every data source that is included in the system. For instance, a microarray dataset may be transformed into a data matrix by calculating Pearson's correlations between any two expression profiles for proteins or genes. The second step is to combine each evidence score for a data source into a single score. This can be done, for instance, using a Bayesian classifier. For protein–protein interactions, there are several resources available based on data-mining techniques such as STRING (6), FunCoup (7), IntNetDB (24), and Prioritizer (25).

3.6. Beyond Data Mining and Scalable Technology for the Internet: The Semantic Web

Data mining and text-mining are fields of technology that are used for the future web 3.0 technology: the semantic web (SW). The first trend in web technology (or web 1.0) included the static webpages that made the first version of the Internet. No information exchange was possible, just readable plain text pages. The second trend (web 2.0) made it possible for users to interact with the Internet. Think of uploading movies to YouTube, or writing your blog online and online shopping with a credit card. Web 2.0 is really the most unstructured and scattered form of information. Therefore, the new trend became web 3.0. It will structure the Internet into a network of concepts and relationships between these concepts. Other terms for web 3.0 are the concept web or the semantic web. One of the goals of the web is to present information in a computer-readable compact format instead of the current webpages that are retrieved after a search query. The predictions that are made using concept profiles or other technologies will be part of this SW.

The best known data model for the SW is RDF (resource description framework). RDF is used to translate any kind of date into a triple format. The ontologies used in web technology are mainly built using OWL (Web Ontology Language). The semantic web project is extremely large and it is very difficult to keep it scalable. There is now an ongoing project called the Large Knowledge Collider (LarKC). It builds the semantic web with all the current state-of-the-art technology that is out there (machine learning, information theory, pattern recognition, and first-order logic). All information on LarKC can be found on http://www.larkc.eu.

4. Notes

1. UMLS is poorly enriched with proteins. Therefore, we added protein information from other data sources to UMLS. Protein information such as accession numbers and synonyms can be found in Entrez Gene, OMIM, UniProt, and Hugo.
2. Co-occurrences between two concepts can be at the sentence level, abstract level, or full-document level. Some researchers have investigated what is the best option to use (26). Normally this is tagging at the sentence level. Two concepts appearing in the same sentence are more associated than when they appear in the same document in separate

paragraphs. We did an analysis (11) to investigate if there is a difference between sentence and abstract levels if only abstract information is used (no full-text information). In this case, the difference is negligible.

3. The type of test used in general is not very important. Match scores between profiles, classifiers (e.g., nearest mean or SVM), and 2×2 table tests more or less give the same results. The power of text-mining mostly lies within the correct tagging of words in text (recognition and disambiguation). Text-mining does not suffer from the curse of dimensionality where there are always more features to evaluate than samples (e.g., like in a microarray experiment). The large amount of text data gives stable statistical results.
4. Negations in text can influence the analysis of relationship detection. For example, a sentence could look like this: "Protein A does Not interact with Protein B." Using statistics only, the co-occurrence of A and B is counted without taking into account the negation. However, due to the large amount of text data, the negation effects are normally negligible. Furthermore, almost all published articles are on positive results. Published negative results are rare.
5. Adding other data sources besides text-mining not only has the advantage of more information but also can solve problems that are encountered in text-mining. Disambiguation is the biggest hurdle in text-mining that can be solved using other databases. For instance, when a protein pair is predicted as being interacting, this could be a false positive when one of the proteins suffers from a homonym problem (maybe the protein was mistakenly mapped to a disease concept). If a microarray experiment for this protein pair shows no correlation, the system could decide that this is a false positive.

References

1. Schuemie, M. J., Weeber, M., Schijvenaars, B. J., et al. (2004) Distribution of information in biomedical abstracts and full-text publications, *Bioinformatics* ***20***, 2597–2604.
2. Schuemie, M. J., Jelier, R., and Kors, J. A. (2007) Peregrine: lightweight gene name normalization by dictionary lookup, in *Biocreative 2 workshop*, pp. 131–140, Madrid.
3. Bodenreider, O. (2004) The Unified Medical Language System (UMLS): integrating biomedical terminology. *Nucleic Acids Res* ***32***, D267–270.
4. Hoffmann, R., and Valencia, A. (2004) A gene network for navigating the literature. *Nat Genet* ***36***, 664.
5. Jenssen, T. K., Laegreid, A., Komorowski, J., and Hovig, E. (2001) A literature network of human genes for high-throughput analysis of gene expression. *Nat Genet* ***28***, 21–28.
6. Jensen, L. J., Kuhn, M., Stark, M., et al. (2009) STRING 8 – a global view on proteins and their functional interactions in 630 organisms. *Nucleic Acids Res* ***37***, D412–416.
7. Alexeyenko, A., and Sonnhammer, E. L. (2009) Global networks of functional coupling in eukaryotes from comprehensive data integration. *Genome Res* ***19***, 1107–1116.

8. Aerts, S., Lambrechts, D., Maity, S., et al. (2006) Gene prioritization through genomic data fusion. *Nat Biotechnol 24*, 537–544.
9. Jelier, R., Schuemie, M. J., Roes, P. J., van Mulligen, E. M., and Kors, J. A. (2008) Literature-based concept profiles for gene annotation: the issue of weighting. *Int J Med Inform 77*, 354–362.
10. Swanson, D. R. (1986) Fish oil, Raynaud's syndrome, and undiscovered public knowledge. *Perspect Biol Med 30*, 7–18.
11. van Haagen, H. H. H. B. M., t Hoen, P. A. C., Botelho Bovo, A., et al. (2009) Novel Protein–Protein Interactions Inferred from Literature Context. *PLoS ONE 4*, e7894.
12. Jelier, R., Schuemie, M. J., Veldhoven, A., et al. (2008) Anni 2.0: a multipurpose text-mining tool for the life sciences. *Genome Biol 9*, R96.
13. Gene Ontology, C. (2000) *Gene Ontology: Tool for the Unification of Biology*, pp. 25–29.
14. UniProt (2009) The Universal Protein Resource (UniProt) 2009. *Nucleic Acids Res 37*, D169–174.
15. Salwinski, L., Miller, C. S., Smith, A. J., et al. (2004) The database of interacting proteins: 2004 update. *Nucleic Acids Res 32*, D449–451.
16. Stark, C., Breitkreutz, B. J., Reguly, T., et al. (2006) BioGRID: a general repository for interaction datasets. *Nucleic Acids Res 34*, D535–539.
17. Matthews, L., Gopinath, G., Gillespie, M., et al. (2009) Reactome knowledgebase of human biological pathways and processes. *Nucleic Acids Res 37*, D619–622.
18. Ben-Hur, A., and Noble, W. (2006) Choosing negative examples for the prediction of protein-protein interactions., p S2. *BMC Bioinformatics*.
19. Fawcett, T. (2003) *ROC Graphs: Notes and Practical Considerations for Data Mining Researchers.* Hewlett-Packard Company.
20. Wessels, L. F., Reinders, M. J., Hart, A. A., et al. (2005) A protocol for building and evaluating predictors of disease state based on microarray data. *Bioinformatics 21*, 3755–3762.
21. Obayashi, T., Hayashi, S., Shibaoka, M., et al. (2008) COXPRESdb: a database of coexpressed gene networks in mammals. *Nucleic Acids Res 36*, D77–82.
22. Su, A. I., Wiltshire, T., Batalov, S., et al. (2004) A gene atlas of the mouse and human protein-encoding transcriptomes. *Proc Natl Acad Sci USA 101*, 6062–6067.
23. Mulder, N. J., Apweiler, R., Attwood, T. K., et al. (2002) InterPro: an integrated documentation resource for protein families, domains and functional sites. *Brief Bioinform 3*, 225–235.
24. Xia, K., Dong, D., and Han, J. D. (2006) IntNetDB v1.0: an integrated protein–protein interaction network database generated by a probabilistic model. *BMC Bioinformatics 7*, 508.
25. Lage, K., Karlberg, E. O., Storling, Z. M., et al. (2007) A human phenome–interactome network of protein complexes implicated in genetic disorders. *Nat Biotechnol 25*, 309–316.
26. Ding, J., Berleant, D., Nettleton, D., Wurtele E. (2002) Mining medline: abstracts, sentences, or phrases, pp. 326–337, Pacific Symposium on Biocomputing.

Chapter 9

Application of Gene Ontology to Gene Identification

Hugo P. Bastos, Bruno Tavares, Catia Pesquita, Daniel Faria, and Francisco M. Couto

Abstract

Candidate gene identification deals with associating genes to underlying biological phenomena, such as diseases and specific disorders. It has been shown that classes of diseases with similar phenotypes are caused by functionally related genes. Currently, a fair amount of knowledge about the functional characterization can be found across several public databases; however, functional descriptors can be ambiguous, domain specific, and context dependent. In order to cope with these issues, the Gene Ontology (GO) project developed a bio-ontology of broad scope and wide applicability. Thus, the structured and controlled vocabulary of terms provided by the GO project describing the biological roles of gene products can be very helpful in candidate gene identification approaches. The method presented here uses GO annotation data in order to identify the most meaningful functional aspects occurring in a given set of related gene products. The method measures this meaningfulness by calculating an e-value based on the frequency of annotation of each GO term in the set of gene products versus the total frequency of annotation. Then after selecting a GO term related to the underlying biological phenomena being studied, the method uses semantic similarity to rank the given gene products that are annotated to the term. This enables the user to further narrow down the list of gene products and identify those that are more likely of interest.

Key words: Gene identification, gene ontology, protein functional annotation, semantic similarity, information content.

1. Introduction

Candidate gene identification is an active research topic that aims at associating genes to underlying biological phenomena, such as diseases and specific disorders. Many approaches have demonstrated their success in this topic but there are also many challenges to address (1). To address these challenges various computational methods have been proposed, which can be grouped

B. Yu, M. Hinchcliffe (eds.), *In Silico Tools for Gene Discovery*, Methods in Molecular Biology 760,
DOI 10.1007/978-1-61779-176-5_9,

into two approaches: genome-wide scanning and candidate gene approaches (2). The genome-wide scanning approach is normally based on expensive and resource intensive strategies. In contrast, the candidate gene approach is based on the knowledge about the functional characterization of the genes and therefore has been proven to be more effective when analyzing complex biological phenomena. For example, recent studies have shown that many classes of diseases with similar phenotypes are caused by functionally related genes (3).

Nowadays, a significant amount of knowledge about the functional characterization of the genes is already available in public databases. However, some of this knowledge is described through free-text statements that are normally ambiguous, domain specific, and context dependent. To cope with this, the research community is developing and using bio-ontologies for the functional annotation of genes (4). The GO project (5) is currently the major effort in this area, having developed a bio-ontology of broad scope and wide applicability that addresses the need for consistent descriptions of gene products in different databases (6).

GO provides a structured controlled vocabulary composed of terms that describe gene and protein biological roles, which can be applied to different species (5). Since the activity or function of a protein can be defined at different levels, GO has three different aspects: molecular function, biological process, and cellular component. This three-way partition is based on the following notions: each protein has elementary molecular functions that normally are independent of the environment, such as catalytic or binding activities; sets of proteins interact and are involved in cellular processes, such as metabolism, signal transduction, or RNA processing; and proteins can act in different cellular localizations, such as the nucleus or membrane.

Candidate gene approaches were quick to identify the potential of using GO annotations for the functional characterization of each candidate gene. Onto-Express was one of the first tools to use GO for creating functional profiles that improved the gene expression analysis (7). In 2005, at least 13 other tools have been proposed based on the same ontological approach, demonstrating the importance of this topic (8). These ontological approaches apply a large number of different statistical tests to identify whether a set of candidate genes represent an enrichment or depletion of a GO category of interest (9). Recently, semantic similarity has been proposed to cluster GO terms in order to identify relevant differentially expressed gene sets (10).

The method presented in this chapter uses GO annotation data to identify the most meaningful functional aspects in a set of related gene products, for example, identified from a gene expression experiment. It is based on the occurrence of each GO term in that set of gene products and on the global frequency of annotation of that GO term, which are used to calculate an e-value that measures the meaningfulness of that occurrence. The occurring GO terms are then ranked by e-value, and the user can select the term(s) found to be more relevant for the study being conducted by the user. Semantic similarity is then used to rank the proteins in the set that are annotated to the term(s) selected, to further narrow down the list of proteins and help the user identify those that are more likely of interest. This method is available through the web tool ProteInOn (http://xldb.di.fc.ul.pt/biotools/proteinon/).

The remainder of this chapter is organized as follows: **Section 2** provides a general theoretical background, **Section 3** describes the method, and **Section 4** presents useful notes on performing the method and interpreting the results obtained during its execution. The examples (*see* **Note 1**) presented along the chapter are derived from a proteomics analysis of cystic fibrosis that was performed using the proposed method (11).

2. Theoretical Background

2.1. Gene Ontology

The method here described will perform a functional analysis of gene products based on their GO annotations. The GO project aims at providing a controlled vocabulary for the description of molecular phenomena in which the gene products are involved. In order to achieve that it provides three orthogonal ontologies that describe genes and gene products in terms of their associated biological processes, cellular components, and molecular functions (5). Each ontology organizes the terms in a Directed Acyclic Graph (DAG), where each node represents a term and the edges represent a relationship between those terms. Each term is identified by an alphanumeric code (e.g., GO:0008150) and its textual descriptors, including its name, definition, and synonyms if they exist. Currently, the relationships between the terms can be of three main types: *is_a*, *part_of*, and *regulates.* Due to its broad scope and wide applicability, GO is currently the most popular ontology for describing gene and protein biological roles. Each of GO's ontologies describes the biological phenomena associated to gene products at different levels. Catalytic or binding activities are independent of the surrounding environment, and these are the kind of elementary molecular activities that are described by the *molecular function* ontology. On the other hand, activities of sets of proteins interacting and involved in cellular processes, such as metabolism or signal transduction, are described by the *biological process* ontology. Proteins can perform their functions in

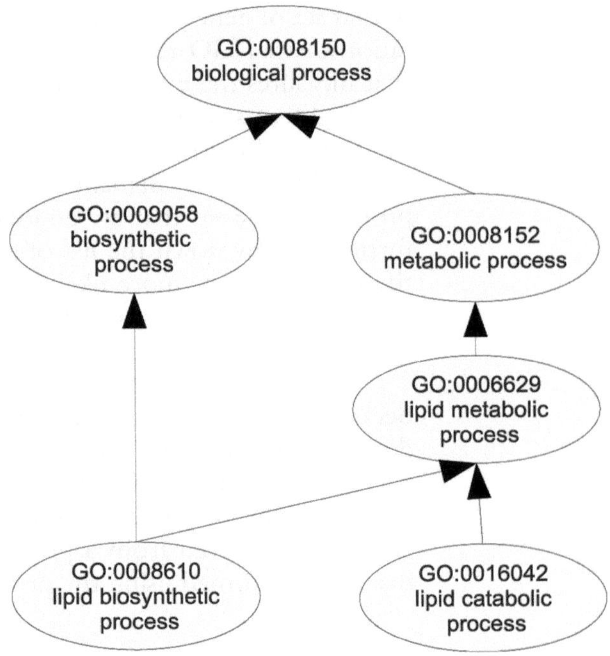

Fig. 9.1. Subgraph of GO's biological process ontology.

several cellular localizations, such as the Golgi complex or the ribosome, this aspect being then described by the *cellular component* ontology. All three biological aspects: biological process, molecular function, and cellular component, are each represented by an individual DAG. While *is_a* and *part_of* relations are only established within each hierarchy, *regulates* relations can occur across ontologies. **Figure 9.1** shows a subgraph of the GO ontology, where only *is_a* relationships are depicted.

Gene products are not actually incorporated into the Gene Ontology. The latter includes only terms that describe those gene products. However, the GO Consortium, through the Gene Ontology Annotation (GOA) project (12), does provide annotations, which are associations between gene products and the GO terms that describe them. A gene product can be annotated with as many GO terms as necessary to fully describe its function. Furthermore, because of GO's true path rule which states that "the pathway from a child term all the way up to its top-level parent(s) must always be true," a gene product which is annotated to a term such as *lipid catabolic process* is also automatically annotated to its parent term *metabolic process*.

Each annotation linking a GO term to a gene product is given an evidence code, which is an acronym that identifies the type of evidence that supports the annotation, i.e., the *IDA* code, which means *Inferred by Direct Assay* is assigned to annotations that are supported by that type of experiment. Two main types of annotations based on their evidence codes are usually considered: manual annotations and electronic annotations. Manual annotations correspond to annotations made through manual curation, whereas electronic annotations are made through automatic means. Although electronic annotations constitute over 97% of all annotations, many studies choose to disregard them due to a common notion that they are of low quality. However, their use greatly increases GO's coverage and some studies advocate their application (13).

2.2. GO-Based Gene Product Set Characterization

Using the GOA database (12), we can obtain the list of GO terms annotated to each gene product in a given set and therefore the global list of GO terms that characterizes that set. However, because GO is organized hierarchically, the number of occurrences of a given GO term in a set of gene products does not accurately reflect its relevance in that set. For instance, all annotated gene products are expected to be annotated (directly or by inheritance) to the root term *biological process*, and therefore the number of occurrences is not a synonym of relevance. Thus, in order to identify the GO terms that are relevant for the characterization of a set of gene products, we need not only the frequency of occurrence of the terms in that set but also a measure of how meaningful it is to observe such a frequency. One such measure is the probability of observing a frequency equal to or greater than the observed frequency in a random set of gene products of the same size as the set of interest, which results in an e-value of the observed frequency.

This e-value can be calculated using the global frequency of annotation of each GO term in the GOA dataset as an estimator of its probability of occurrence, $P(t)$. For each GO term t, a protein taken at random from the dataset can be considered a random event with two outcomes: success, if it is annotated to t, and failure otherwise. As such, the probability of observing at least k successes in a random set of n gene products is given by a cumulative binomial distribution with probability of success $P(t)$:

$$P(x_t \geq k) = \sum_{i=k}^{n} \left(i^n\right) P(t)^i \left(1 - p(t)\right)^{n-i}$$

The lower the e-value, the less likely it is that the observed frequency of the term is due to chance, and thus the more meaningful is the term in the set of gene products.

In addition to filtering GO terms by e-value, it is also necessary to exclude terms that are redundant. In this context, a GO term is considered redundant if one of its descendants annotates the exact same gene products in the set. While filtering by e-value naturally excludes many of these cases, there are cases where the ancestor and descendant terms are similar in specificity and thus have similar e-values. Despite being significant according to the e-value, the ancestor term is excluded because it is redundant since its annotations are already implied by the annotations of its descendant and thus does not contribute to the characterization of the set of gene products.

For instance, if the term *actin binding* occurs in 25% of the gene products in a given set, its parent term *cytoskeletal protein binding* will necessarily occur in the same gene products by inheritance and may or may not occur in additional gene products. If it does not, it is considered redundant and is excluded.

2.3. Semantic Similarity

Semantic similarity in the context of ontologies can be defined as a numerical value that reflects the closeness in meaning between two ontology terms or two sets of terms annotating two entities. Commonly, the semantic similarity between two gene products annotated with GO terms is called "functional similarity," since it gives a measure of how similar the gene products functions are.

The following sections focus first on semantic similarity applied to GO terms and then on semantic similarity for gene products annotated with GO terms.

2.3.1. Semantic Similarity for GO Terms

There are two main approaches for GO term semantic similarity measures: edge-based and node-based. Edge-based approaches use edges and their properties as data sources. Commonly, they rely on counting the number of edges between two terms on the ontology graph, which conveys a distance measure that can easily be converted to a similarity measure (14). The shorter the distance between two terms, the more similar they are. Taking the terms in **Fig. 9.1**, the distance between *lipid biosynthetic process* and *lipid catabolic process* is 2.

Alternatively to such distance metrics, the common path technique can be employed, which is given by the distance between the root node and the lowest common ancestor (LCA) the two terms share (15). In this case, the longer the distance between the root and the common ancestor, the more similar are the terms. Taking again **Fig. 9.1** to illustrate this technique, *lipid biosynthetic process* and *lipid catabolic process* are more similar than *biosynthetic process* and *metabolic process* since the former have *lipid metabolic process* as a LCA, which is at a distance of 2 from the root, whereas the latter have *biological process* as LCA, which is at a distance of 0 since it is the root. To increase the expressiveness of these measures, several properties of edges such as their type (i.e. *is_a*, *part_of*) and their depth can be used.

Node-based measures use nodes and their properties as data sources. These measures are better suited for ontologies, such as bio-ontologies, where nodes and edges are not uniformly distributed and where different edges convey different semantic distances. A commonly used node property is the information content (IC), which gives a measure of how specific a term is within a given corpus (16). The Gene Ontology is particularly well suited to this, since GO annotations can be used as a corpus. The IC of a term t can then be given by:

$$IC(t) = -\log_2 f(t)$$

where $f(t)$ is the frequency of annotation of term t. Consequently, terms that annotate many gene products have a low IC, while terms that are very specific and thus only annotate few gene products have a high IC. Additionally, the IC can be normalized so that it returns more intuitive values.

Semantic similarity measures can use the IC by applying it to the common ancestors that two terms have, under the rationale that two terms are as similar as the information they share. The two most general approaches to achieve this are the most informative common ancestor (MICA), which considers only the common ancestor with the highest IC (16), and the disjoint common ancestor (DCA) technique, which considers all common ancestors that do not incorporate any other ancestor (17). Popular node-based measures include Resnik's, which only considers the IC of the ancestor (16), and Lin and Jiang, and Conrath's, which consider the IC of both the ancestor and the terms themselves (19, 20). Consider the subgraph of GO given in **Fig. 9.2**. Using this subgraph, the Resnik similarity between *transcription factor activity* and *transcription co-factor activity* corresponds to the IC of their MICA, *transcription regulation activity*, which is 0.23.

2.3.2. Semantic Similarity for Gene Products

Semantic similarity for gene products is given by the comparison of the sets of GO terms that annotate each gene product within each GO ontology. There are two main approaches that can be used for this pairwise and groupwise (20).

Pairwise approaches are based on combining the semantic similarities between the terms that annotate each gene product. These approaches use only direct annotations and apply term semantic similarity measures to all possible pairs made between each set of terms. Variations within this type of approach include considering every pairwise combination (*all pairs* technique) or only the best-matching pair for each term (*best pairs* technique). Commonly, the pairwise similarity scores are combined by average, sum, or selecting the maximum to obtain a global functional similarity score between gene products. Consider the example in **Fig. 9.2** where two hypothetical proteins, A and B, and their annotations (direct and inherited) are shown. In this example, the *all pairs* technique would calculate the similarity for all four pairs of directly annotated terms, whereas the best pairs technique would only consider the pairs *transcription factor activity – transcription co-factor activity* and *transcription factor binding – DNA*

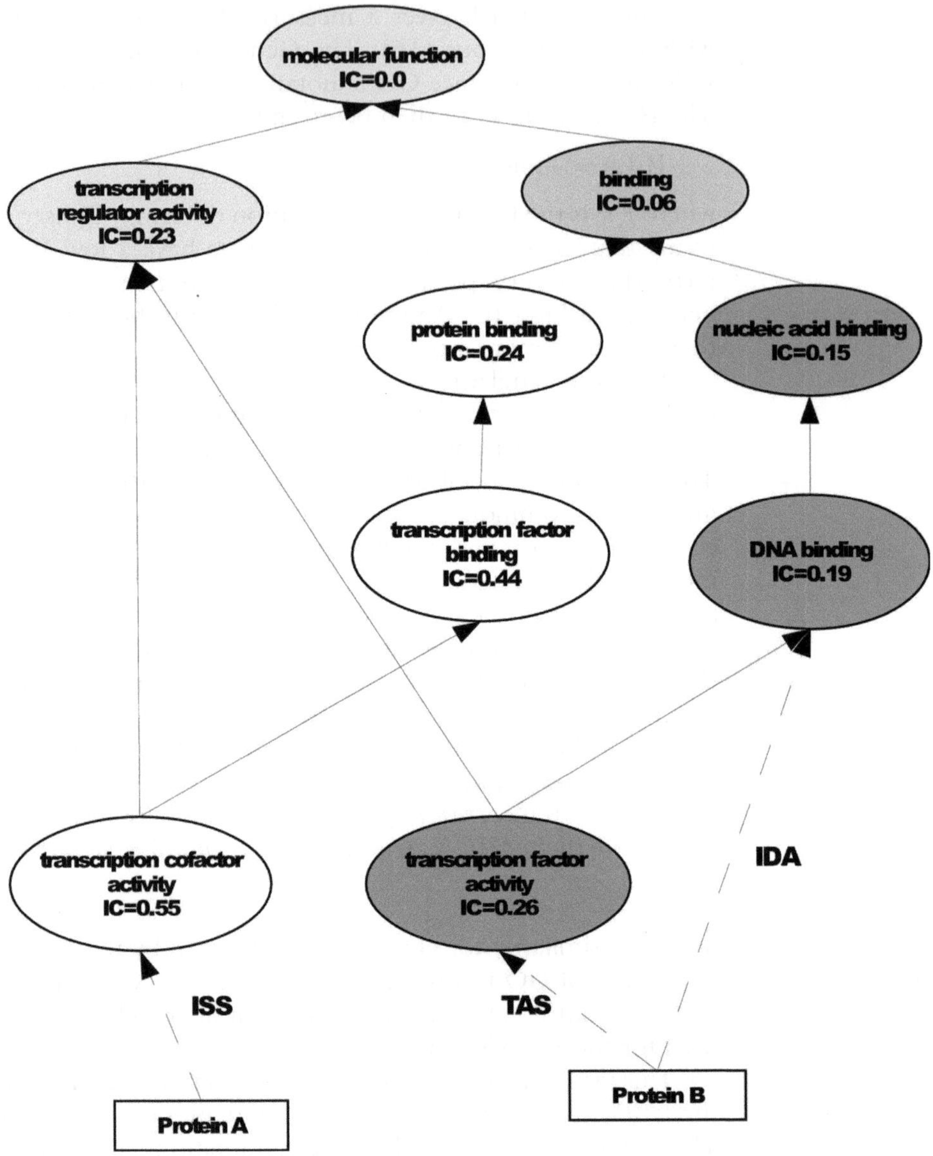

Fig. 9.2. Illustration of graph-based semantic similarity. *Full lines* are GO edges and *dashed lines* represent annotation identified with their evidence codes.

binding. The final value would then be given by the maximum, average, or sum of these similarities.

Groupwise approaches calculate similarity directly, without applying term similarity metrics. They fall into one of the three categories: set, vector, or graph. Set-based measures consider only direct annotations and use set similarity metrics, such as simple overlap. Vector-based measures consider all annotations and represent gene products as vectors of GO terms and apply vector similarity measures, such as cosine vector similarity. Graph-based measures represent gene products as the subgraphs of GO corresponding to all their annotations (direct and inherited). In this case, functional similarity can be calculated either by using graph matching techniques or, because these are computationally intensive, by considering the subgraphs as sets of terms and applying set similarity techniques. A popular set similarity technique used for this is the Jaccard similarity, whereby the similarity between two sets is given by the number of elements they share divided by the number of elements they have in total. The Jaccard similarity can be applied directly to the number of terms (simUI) (21) or be weighted by the IC of the terms (simGIC) (13) to give more preponderance to more specific terms. **Figure 9.2** illustrates this type of measure, since each node color identifies it as a term that strictly belongs to a single protein's annotations (white or dark gray) or to both (light gray). Using simUI, the similarity between the proteins would be 0.33, whereas using simGIC it would be 0.14.

The semantic similarity measures for GO terms have been developed and employed on various assessment studies. There is not one clear best measure for comparing terms or gene products. While a given measure can be suitable for one task it can perform poorly on another. Lord et al. (22) were among the first to assess the performance of different semantic similarity measures. In that assessment Resnik's, Lin's, and Jiang and Conrath's measures were tested against sequence similarity using the average combination approach. Pesquita et al. (13) also tested several measures against sequence similarity and found simGIC to provide overall better results. However, as stated before some measures perform better in some situations than in others. As an example, simUI was found by Guo et al. (23) to be the weakest measure when evaluated for its ability to characterize human regulatory pathways, while Pesquita et al. (13) found it to be fairly good when evaluated against sequence similarity.

3. Methods

3.1. The ProteInOn Web Tool

ProteInOn is a web tool that integrates GO-based semantic similarity, retrieval of interacting proteins, and characterization of gene product sets with meaningful GO terms. It uses GO, GOA, IntAct (24), and UniProt (25) as data sources.

ProteInOn implements several term and gene product semantic similarities:

- Resnik's measure calculates the similarity between two terms based strictly on the IC of their MICA (16).
- Lin's measure reflects how close the terms are to their MICA rather than just how specific that ancestor is (18).

- Jiang and Conrath's measure is based on a hybrid approach derived from edge-based notions with IC as a decision factor (19).
- SimUI defines semantic similarity as the fraction between the number of GO terms in the intersection of those graphs and the number of GO terms in their union. This measure accounts for both similar and dissimilar terms in a simpler way than finding matching term pairs (21).
- SimGIC also uses the fraction between the number of GO terms in the intersection of those graphs and the number of GO terms in their union, but weights each term by its IC, thus giving more relevance to more specific terms (22).

Every semantic similarity measure can be calculated using either the MICA or the DCA approach (26). They are also used to calculate gene product similarities using the best pairs technique and the average combination approach.

ProteInOn normalizes the IC to values between 0 and 1 so that all measures also return values between 0 and 1, which can be directly transformed to a percentage of similarity.

ProteInOn is also able to characterize a set of gene products with the top 100 most representative GO terms, by returning a list of the GO terms that annotate the set of gene products ordered by their e-value as discussed previously on **Section 2.2**.

3.2. Gene Finding Approach

This section describes how to use ProteInOn (**Fig. 9.3**) for gene finding, by combining several ProteInOn features.

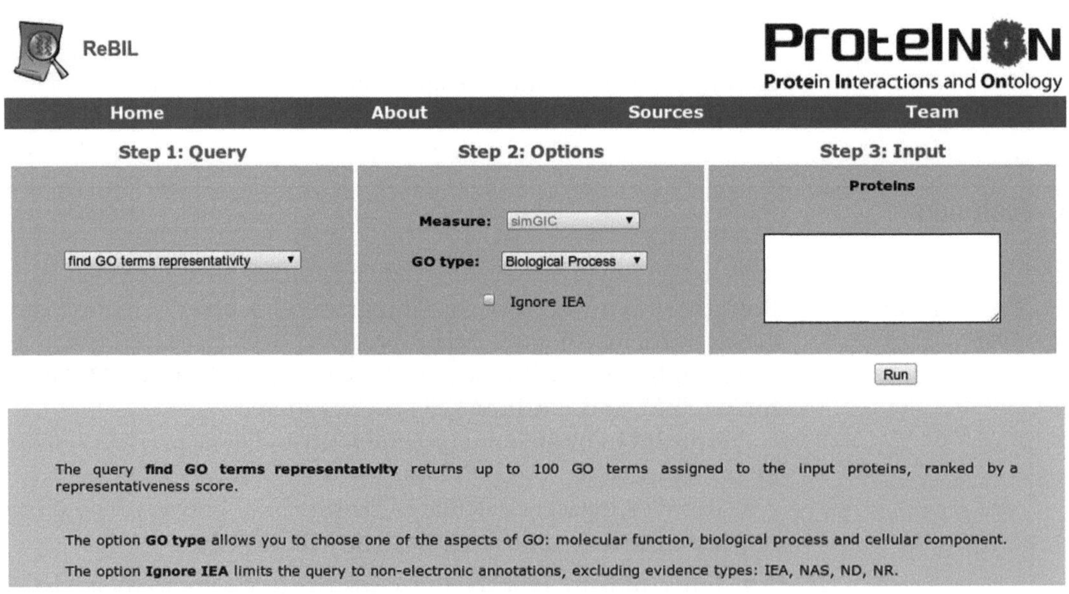

Fig. 9.3. ProteInOn web tool's homepage.

The input for this task is a set of gene products, which is used to generate a list of all GO terms annotated to the given gene products. The tool will calculate the e-value for each of these GO terms and display the sorted list to the user, who may then select the GO terms better related to the biomedical problem being studied. The selected GO terms are then used to select only the gene products from the input set that are annotated with them and the remaining can thus be disregarded. Finally, the semantic similarity between all remaining gene products is calculated to further support the identification of relevant gene products.

3.3. How to Use ProteInOn for Gene Finding

3.3.1. Input Preparation

Candidate gene approaches are normally based on a list of differentially expressed genes. Our method, however, only requires a set of gene products, regardless of their expression values, thus any mechanism able to produce a list of gene products is suitable to generate the input set.

The input set consists of a list of UniProtKB accession numbers for the gene products to be analyzed, which consist of six alphanumeric characters, for example: P23508, O00559, Q4ZG55. However, if your gene products are not identified by UniProtKB accession numbers, you can use UniProtKB mapping service (http://www.uniprot.org/mapping/) to convert common gene IDs and protein IDs to UniProtKB accession numbers and vice versa (**Fig. 9.4**).

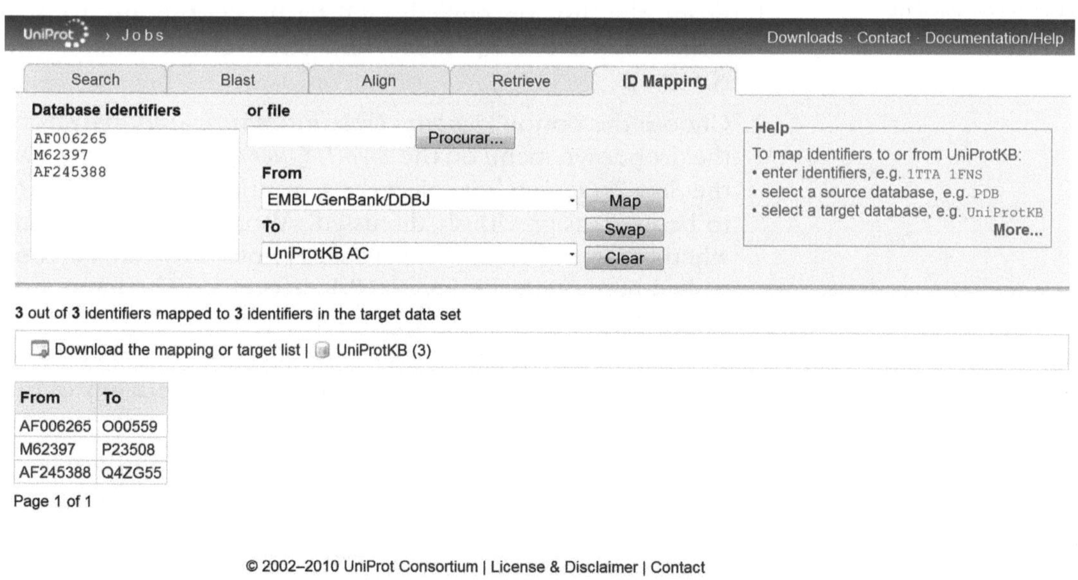

Fig. 9.4. Web tool for mapping external database identifiers into UniProt identifiers. Source: http://www.uniprot.org.

3.3.2. Finding Relevant Gene Ontology Terms

After preparing your input set, you can start using the ProteInOn tool.

1. Go to http://xldb.fc.ul.pt/biotools/proteinon/ and choose *find GO term representativity* from the dropdown menu on *Step 1: Query* (**Fig. 9.3**).
2. On *Step 2: Options*, you will be presented with another dropdown menu where you are able to choose the GO type (*see* **Note 2**) on which you want to focus your analysis: *molecular function*, *biological process*, or *cellular component*.
3. In *Step 2: Options* you can also choose to ignore electronic annotations by checking the *ignore IEA* box.
4. On *Step 3: Input* insert the protein list on the input box, taking notice it shouldn't be more than 1000 proteins long and press *Run*.
5. A list of the GO terms (*see* **Note 3**) annotated to the input set of gene products is displayed, with the GO terms ordered by e-value (**Fig. 9.5**).
6. This resulting list can be saved in either XML or TSV (under the *Step 3: Input box*) enabling posterior analysis on ProteInOn or other software.
7. You can also save a bar chart that shows the occurrence of the top 10 most representative GO terms (**Fig. 9.6**).

3.3.3. Gene Product Semantic Similarity Based on Selected GO Terms

You can continue your analysis by calculating the semantic similarity between the most relevant gene products:

1. From the list of ranked GO terms choose up to ten terms by checking their respective check boxes (*see* **Note 4**).
2. Choose the option *compute protein semantic similarity* from the dropdown menu on the *Step 1: Query* box (**Fig. 9.5**). On the *Step 2: Options* box select the semantic similarity measure to be used, as previously discussed. Also, the decision about whether or not to use electronic annotations can be controlled here (with the *ignore IEA* checkbox). The input area on the *Step 3: Input* box will be locked, since the gene products that will be used in the current query, correspond to the subset of the original query that is annotated with any of the previously selected GO terms.
3. After clicking the *Run* button, a list of gene product pairs (*see* **Note 5**) with their respective functional similarity scores is displayed (**Fig. 9.7**). As before, this list can also be saved either in XML or in TSV format for posterior or external use.

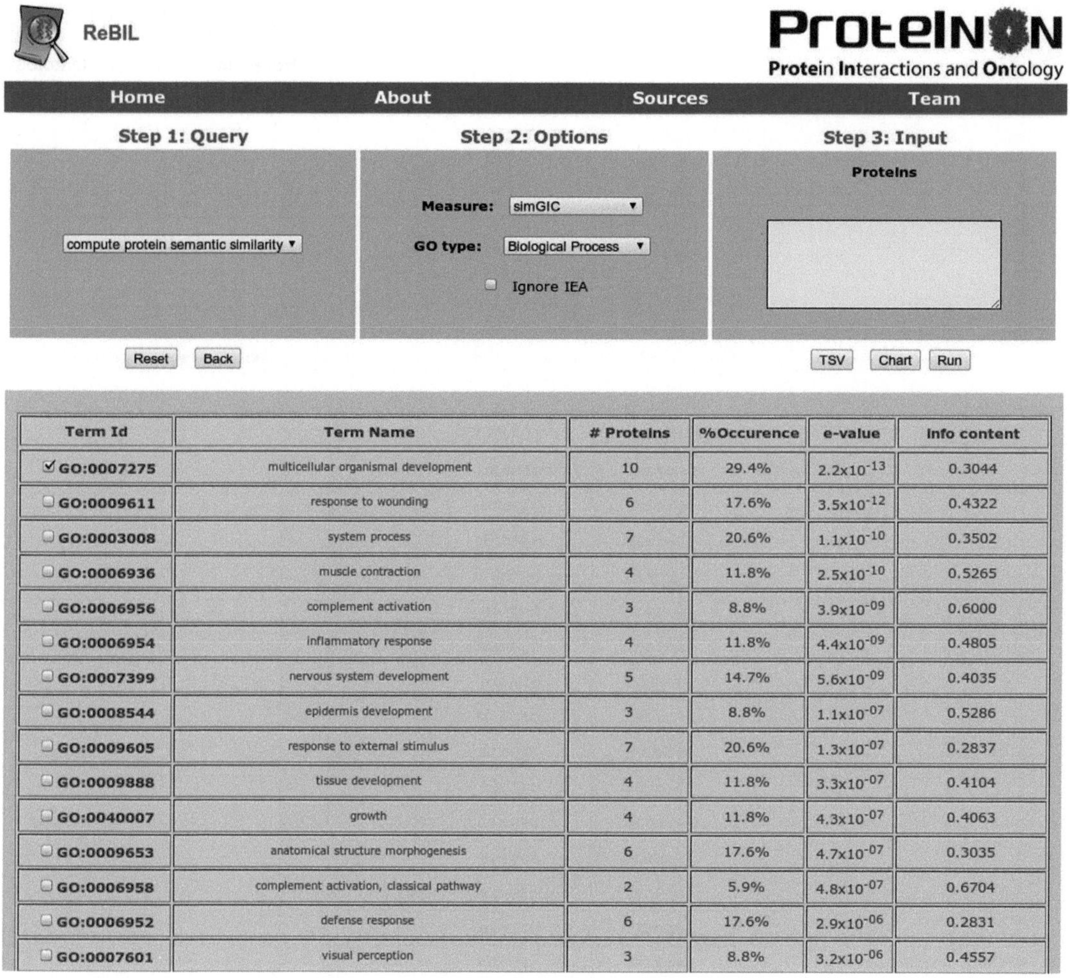

Term Id	Term Name	# Proteins	%Occurence	e-value	Info content
GO:0007275	multicellular organismal development	10	29.4%	$2.2x10^{-13}$	0.3044
GO:0009611	response to wounding	6	17.6%	$3.5x10^{-12}$	0.4322
GO:0003008	system process	7	20.6%	$1.1x10^{-10}$	0.3502
GO:0006936	muscle contraction	4	11.8%	$2.5x10^{-10}$	0.5265
GO:0006956	complement activation	3	8.8%	$3.9x10^{-09}$	0.6000
GO:0006954	inflammatory response	4	11.8%	$4.4x10^{-09}$	0.4805
GO:0007399	nervous system development	5	14.7%	$5.6x10^{-09}$	0.4035
GO:0008544	epidermis development	3	8.8%	$1.1x10^{-07}$	0.5286
GO:0009605	response to external stimulus	7	20.6%	$1.3x10^{-07}$	0.2837
GO:0009888	tissue development	4	11.8%	$3.3x10^{-07}$	0.4104
GO:0040007	growth	4	11.8%	$4.3x10^{-07}$	0.4063
GO:0009653	anatomical structure morphogenesis	6	17.6%	$4.7x10^{-07}$	0.3035
GO:0006958	complement activation, classical pathway	2	5.9%	$4.8x10^{-07}$	0.6704
GO:0006952	defense response	6	17.6%	$2.9x10^{-06}$	0.2831
GO:0007601	visual perception	3	8.8%	$3.2x10^{-06}$	0.4557

Fig. 9.5. GO terms annotated to the list of proteins used in the proteomics analysis of cystic fibrosis. The terms are ordered by relevance as determined by their e-value. Additionally, the occurrence (absolute and percentage) and the information content of each term are presented.

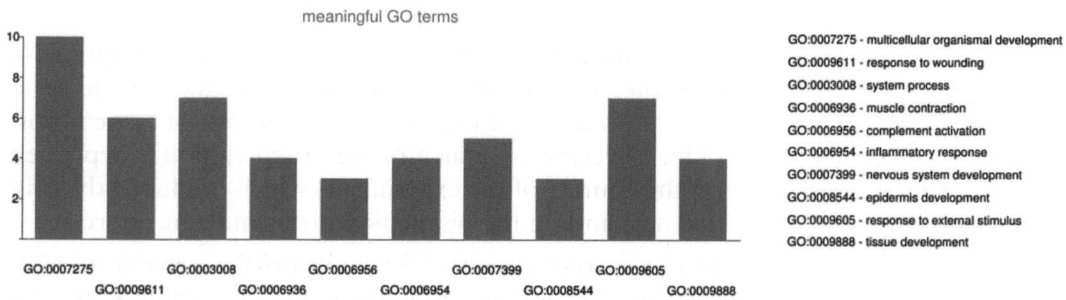

Fig. 9.6. Bar chart of the occurrence of the most representative GO terms within the list of proteins used in the proteomics analysis of cystic fibrosis.

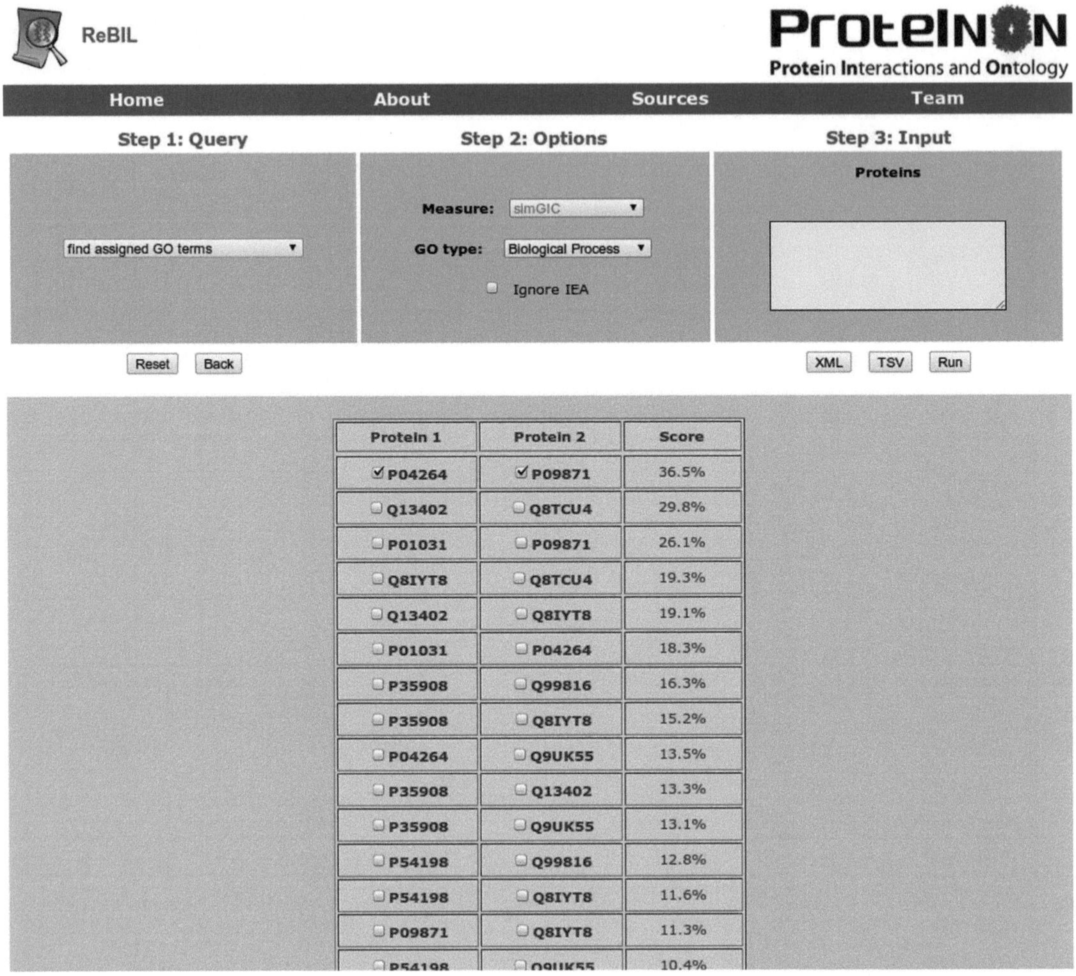

Fig. 9.7. Semantic similarity scores for pairs of representative gene products annotated with the GO term *multicellular organismal development*.

4. Notes

1. Along this chapter, and as example of use and interpretation of ProteInOn results, we present the analysis of the set of gene products used in a proteomics analysis of cystic fibrosis (11). Nevertheless, much of the interpretation is dependent on the context of the experiments which produced the original data and on the biomedical problem being addressed.
2. In our example, a set of 34 UniProtKB accession numbers used in (11) was given as input for ProteInOn's *find GO term representatitvity* option. We chose to analyze the *biological process* ontology, since it is evidently the most interesting for candidate gene identification. However, *molecular*

function terms can also be of interest, and although the *cellular component* ontology is of limited usefulness in this context, it may serve as a means of validating results.

3. The *find GO term representativity* option results in a list of relevant GO terms ranked by e-value, which includes the number and frequency of occurrences of each term in the gene product data set, and the information content of the term to provide a measure of its specificity.
4. This choice can be based on e-value alone; however, users should take occurrence and IC values into consideration as well. For instance, in some cases there maybe some relatively general terms (with information content below 0.3) whose occurrence is very significant because they are highly overrepresented in the data set. This is often due to an inherent experimental bias, for example, in an experiment based on cell membrane proteins, it is expected that *binding* and *protein binding* are overrepresented terms. In these cases, the presence of these terms is useful only as an additional validation of the experimental results and should generally be ignored for the purpose of identifying functional aspects of interest. Another critical aspect in selecting GO terms is the duality between specificity and frequency of occurrence (or representativity). For a given threshold e-value, often there are several related terms with the more general terms occurring in more gene products than the more specific ones. For instance, in our example (**Fig. 9.5**) the term *complement activation* and its ancestor *inflammatory response* have similar e-values because despite being less specific the latter occurs in one protein more than the former. Thus, we have to choose between the specificity of the functional aspect considered and its representativity of the dataset, a choice which naturally depends on the context of the problem. To support this we recommend the utilization of a GO browser (http://www.geneontology.org/GO.tools.browsers.shtml) to investigate the relations between GO terms with similar e-values.
5. In our example, we selected the term *multicellular organismal development,* so ProteInOn could calculate the semantic similarity between the subset of gene products that are annotated with it (**Fig. 9.7**). This enables researchers to analyze the topology of this subset of gene products at the functional level and identify clusters of similar gene products within that subset that merit a more detailed analysis. Most of the semantic similarity values between the gene products annotated to the term *multicellular organismal development* are low, which is not unexpected considering that this term is fairly general. However, by selecting the gene products of

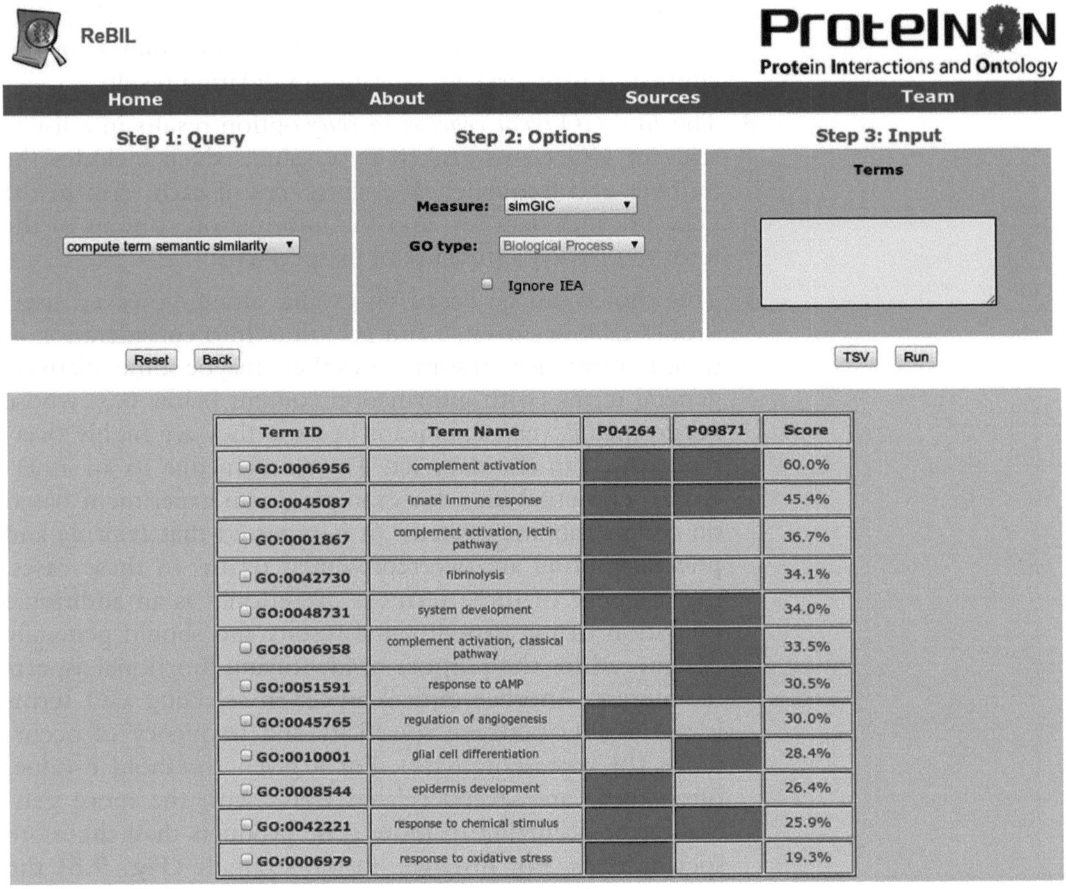

Fig. 9.8. GO terms from the *biological process* ontology that annotate the selected proteins, Complement C1s subcomponent and Keratin type II cytoskeletal.

the highest scoring pair and using them as input for the *find assigned GO terms* option we find that these gene products have an interesting set of annotations. These are shown in **Fig. 9.8** and include terms relevant for cystic fibrosis such as *innate immune response*. In fact one of these proteins, Complement C1s subcomponent, is related to early onset of multiple autoimmune diseases, whereas the other, Keratin, type II cytoskeletal 1, is related to several genetic skin disorders caused by defects in the gene KRT-1. Thus, by applying ProteInOn's gene finding method we were able to identify two relevant candidate genes to cystic fibrosis.

References

1. Tabor, H. K., Risch, N. J., and Meyers, R. M. (2002) Candidate-gene approaches for studying complex genetic traits: practical considerations. *Nat Rev Genet* 3, 391–397.
2. Zhu, M., and Zhao, S. (2010) Candidate gene identification approach: progress and challenges. *Int J Biol Sci* 3, 420–427.

3. Oti, M., and Brunner, H. G. (2007) The modular nature of genetic diseases. *Clin Genet* 71, 1–11.
4. Bodenreider O., and Stevens, R. (2006) Bio-ontologies: current trends and future directions. *Brief Bioinfo* 7, 256–274.
5. Gene Ontology Consortium (2000) The gene ontology tool for the unification of biology. *Nat Genet* 25, 25–29.
6. Bada, M., Stevens, R., Goble, C., et al. (2004) A short study on the success of the Gene Ontology. *Web Semantics: Science, Services and Agents on the World Wide Web, 2003 World Wide Web Conference*, 1, 235–240.
7. Khatri, P. Draghici, S., Ostermeier, G. C., and Krawetz S. A. (2002) Profiling gene expression using onto-express. *Genomics* 79, 266–270.
8. Khatri, P., and Drăghici, S. (2005) Ontological analysis of gene expression data: current tools, limitations, and open problems. *Bioinformatics* 21, 3587–3595.
9. Rivals, I., Personnaz, L., Taing, L., and Potier MC. (2007) Enrichment or depletion of a GO category within a class of genes: which test? *Bioinformatics* 23, 401–407.
10. Xu, T., Gu, J., Zhou, Y., and Du, L. (2009) Improving detection of differentially expressed gene sets by applying cluster enrichment analysis to Gene Ontology. *BMC Bioinformatics* 10, 240.
11. Charro, N., Hood, B. L., Pacheco, P., et al. (2011) Serum proteomics signature of cystic fibrosis patients: a complementary 2-DE and LC-MS/MS approach. *J Proteome Res* 74, 110–126.
12. Barrell, D., Dimmer, E., Huntley, R. P., et al. (2009) The GOA database in 2009 – an integrated Gene Ontology Annotation resource. *Nucleic Acids Res* 37, D396–D403.
13. Pesquita, C., Faria, D., Bastos, H., et al. (2008) Metrics for GO based protein semantic similarity: a systematic evaluation. *BMC Bioinformatics* 9, S4.
14. Rada, R., Mili, H., Bicknell, E., and Blettner, M. (1989) Development and application of a metric on semantic nets. *IEEE Trans Syst Man Cybernet* 19, 17–30.
15. Wu, Z., and Palmer, M. S. (1994) Verb semantics and lexical selection. *Proceedings of the 32nd. Annual Meeting of the Association for Computational Linguistics (ACL 1994)*. pp. 133–138.
16. Resnik, P. (1995) Using information content to evaluate semantic similarity in a taxonomy. *Proceedings of the 14th International Joint Conference on Artificial Intelligence*. Montreal, Quebec: Canada.
17. Couto, F. M., Silva, M. J., and Coutinho, P. M. (2005) Semantic similarity over the gene ontology: Family correlation and selecting disjunctive ancestors. *Proceedings of the ACM Conference in Information and Knowledge Management*. Bremen: Germany.
18. Lin, D. (1998) An information-theoretic definition of similarity. *Proceedings of the 15th International Conference on Machine Learning*. San Francisco, CA: Morgan Kaufmann. pp. 296–304.
19. Jiang, J., and Conrath, D. (1997) Semantic similarity based on corpus statistics and lexical taxonomy. *Proceedings of the 10th International Conference on Research on Computational Linguistics*, Taiwan.
20. Pesquita, C., Faria, D., Falcão, A. O., et al. (2009) Semantic Similarity in Biomedical Ontologies. *PLoS Comput Biol* 5, e1000443.
21. Gentleman, R. (2005) Visualizing and Distances Using GO. URL http://www.bioconductor.org/docs/vignettes.html.
22. Lord, P., Stevens, R., Brass, A., and Goble, C. (2003) Investigating semantic similarity measures across the Gene Ontology: the relationship between sequence and annotation. *Bioinformatics* 19, 1275–1283.
23. Guo, X., Liu, R., Shriver, C. D., Hu, H., and Liebman, M. N. (2006) Assessing semantic similarity measures for the characterization of human regulatory pathways. *Bioinformatics* 22, 967–973.
24. Aranda, B., Achuthan, P., Alam-Faruque, Y., et al. (2010) The IntAct molecular interaction database in 2010. *Nucleic Acids Res* 38(Database issue), D525–D531.
25. UniProt Consortium (2010) The Universal Protein Resource (UniProt) in 2010. *Nucleic Acids Res* 38(Database issue), D142–D148.
26. Faria, D. Pesquita, C., Couto F. M. and Falcão A. (2007) ProteInOn: a web tool for protein semantic similarity. DI/FCUL TR 07-6, Department of Informatics, University of Lisbon.

Chapter 10

Phenotype Mining for Functional Genomics and Gene Discovery

Philip Groth, Ulf Leser, and Bertram Weiss

Abstract

In gene prediction, studying phenotypes is highly valuable for reducing the number of locus candidates in association studies and to aid disease gene candidate prioritization. This is due to the intrinsic nature of phenotypes to visibly reflect genetic activity, making them potentially one of the most useful data types for functional studies. However, systematic use of these data has begun only recently. 'Comparative phenomics' is the analysis of genotype–phenotype associations across species and experimental methods. This is an emerging research field of utmost importance for gene discovery and gene function annotation. In this chapter, we review the use of phenotype data in the biomedical field. We will give an overview of phenotype resources, focusing on PhenomicDB – a cross-species genotype–phenotype database – which is the largest available collection of phenotype descriptions across species and experimental methods. We report on its latest extension by which genotype–phenotype relationships can be viewed as graphical representations of similar phenotypes clustered together ('phenoclusters'), supplemented with information from protein–protein interactions and Gene Ontology terms. We show that such 'phenoclusters' represent a novel approach to group genes functionally and to predict novel gene functions with high precision. We explain how these data and methods can be used to supplement the results of gene discovery approaches. The aim of this chapter is to assist researchers interested in understanding how phenotype data can be used effectively in the gene discovery field.

Key words: Phenotype, comparative phenomics, phenotype clustering, text mining, gene discovery, function prediction, RNA interference

1. Introduction

Phenotypes are traceable changes or variations in behaviour or appearance, differentiating one individual of a species from another on all but the genetic levels. Being more accessible to observation and experimentation than genotypes, they are a highly valuable type of information at the interface of medicine

B. Yu, M. Hinchcliffe (eds.), *In Silico Tools for Gene Discovery*, Methods in Molecular Biology 760, DOI 10.1007/978-1-61779-176-5_10,

and biology. In particular, phenotypes can be used to dissect the relationships between genetic diseases and their responsible genes. In the last few years, a number of new methods have been developed to find more relationships between genotypes and phenotypes in less time. These efforts have culminated in the development of high-throughput phenotype screening methods such as RNA interference (RNAi) (1) and in combination with public databases (2, 3), phenotypes have become an acknowledged and widely used component of functional genomics. Mostly, they are interpreted on a gene-by-gene level for functional annotation, limiting the analysis to each single genotype–phenotype relationship, since it is the most immediate result of such a screen. This simple type of evaluation can already uncover the involvement of genes in processes or diseases and may lead to novel insights and therapeutic approaches (4). The ever increasing amount of available phenotype screening data has also driven the creation of public phenotype data repositories addressing phenotypes across experimental methods, species and purpose of the original assay [for more details, see the survey on phenotype data resources by Groth and Weiss (5)]. Having such large collections of phenotypes readily available opens the door to new approaches of their analysis. As is the case in other large-scale, whole-genome approaches (such as microarray experiments), data mining algorithms or (hypothesis-free) meta-analyses can be applied to analyze the data systematically and to uncover patterns of similar behaviour (6). Thus, phenotypes have the potential to be even more useful for functional studies than many other types of data. The large-scale integration and the joint analysis of genotype–phenotype data also enable discoveries across species which are especially useful when original data is comparably sparse, as in the case of human diseases (7).

In gene prediction from a defined locus, as it is referred to in this chapter, the task is to predict the gene most likely responsible for the given disease (or phenotype) (8). Here, phenotypes have the potential to deliver the next valuable clues towards ranking or identifying the best candidates. For example, it has been observed that groups of identical or highly similar phenotypes can be caused by mutations in different genes (so-called genotypic heterogeneity) (9, 10). In such cases, the genes responsible for these similar phenotypes are often very likely to be related to members of the same pathway or biological process (10, 11). This fact has been used successfully, e.g., in gene prediction settings where a disease locus has already been defined, i.e. when candidate prioritization becomes the essential next step to predict the gene most likely responsible for a disease (or phenotype) of interest.

Gefen et al. (9) have recently presented 'Syndrome to gene' (S2G), a tool to identify candidate genes for human diseases prioritizing known genes from the same locus whose defects cause phenotypically similar syndromes based on their involvement in pathways, protein–protein interactions (PPIs), common regulation, protein family association and orthology. Similarly, Lage et al. (12) and van Driel et al. (13) described approaches for identifying disease candidates based on phenotype similarity in humans.

However, all the described methods depend on readily available phenotype data in textual form and most of these studies are strictly limited to human diseases and their related phenotype database, e.g. the Online Mendelian Inheritance in Man (OMIM) (14). They thus ignore the wealth of further phenotype information available in other formats that have been derived from other species. In general, the available phenotype *repertoire* ranges from descriptions of the outcome of RNAi knock-down experiments in model organisms such as *Caenorhabditis elegans* with single terms from a controlled vocabulary, like 'lethal' or 'reduced egg size' in WormBase (15), knockout studies in *Mus musculus* described with free-text supplemented with terms from the Mammalian Phenotype (MP) ontology (16) in the Mouse Genome Database (MGD) (17), all the way to clinicians' free-text descriptions of genetic diseases in *Homo sapiens* in OMIM. Unfortunately, there is no common vocabulary to describe these observations and most of the phenotype resources are poorly annotated with common vocabulary (18). When describing phenotypes, researchers tend to use home-grown term lists, highly species-specific vocabularies or simply plain English text. Due to the resulting heterogeneity in descriptions, and in order to maintain the ability to use all the available phenotype data in cross-species and cross-method meta-analyses, the broadest common denominator for describing a phenotype is its plain textual description.

In this chapter, we first present the database PhenomicDB (19, 20) which is an integrated repository of large amounts of genotype–phenotype data across methods and species (*see* **Sections 2.1** and **3.1**). Then, we present a method to group similar phenotypes based on text clustering of textual phenotype descriptions from PhenomicDB (*see* **Sections 2.2**, **2.3**, **3.2** and **3.3**). We have previously shown that the intrinsic similarity of the resulting phenotype clusters reflects their biological coherence and that they can be used to successfully predict gene function (21).

We show here how the tools within PhenomicDB can be used as part of a gene prediction workflow, e.g., to identify all genes associated with a disease of interest, to show the group of most similar diseases and their responsible genes or to present genes with similar diseases and their interaction partners (*see* **Section 3.4**). Although it is too young to have a proven record in gene discovery, we will give valid examples of its usefulness and its ability to present good results in this application (*see* **Section 3.4**).

Our approach provides novel means to group phenotypes by similarity that is complementary to others. We are currently developing other useful features like candidate ranking, which will be deployed with PhenomicDB in the near future. At the same time, we are working on overcoming the main drawback of the method, namely the species-specific clustering when using cross-species phenotypes (*see* **Note 1**) due to the existence of heterogeneous phenotype vocabulary describing essentially the same things (*see* **Note 2**).

2. Materials

2.1. Integration of Genotype–Phenotype Data into PhenomicDB

The large-scale, cross-species, genotype–phenotype data repository (*see* **Section 3.1**) hosts phenotypes from studies as diverse as mutant screens, knockout mice or RNAi, spanning various species (ranging from yeast to human) and deriving from a variety of sources, namely OMIM (14), the Mouse Genome Database (MGD) (17), WormBase (15), FlyBase (22), the Comprehensive Yeast Genome Database (CYGD) (23), the Zebrafish Information Network (ZFIN) (24) and the MIPS *Arabidopsis thaliana* database (MAtDB) (25). Additional RNAi data was also obtained from FlyRNAi, maintained by the *Drosophila* Resource Screening Centre (DRSC) (13,900 targeted genes; available at http://www.flyrnai.org) (26), PhenoBank (24,671 RNAi phenotypes for 20,981 genes; available at http://www.phenobank.org) (3) and RNAiDB (59,991 RNAi phenotypes; available at http://www.rnai.org) (2).

In total, the current database version contains 327,070 unique phenotypes connected to 70,588 genes. Approximately 36% of the phenotypes are associated with genes from either *Drosophila melanogaster* or *C. elegans.* Genes from *Saccharomyces cerevisiae*, *M. musculus* and *H. sapiens* are associated with 12.5, 6 and 1% of the phenotypes, respectively. The remaining 27,800 phenotypes are associated with genes from other species.

Furthermore, genotypes were grouped by orthology information taken from the NCBI's HomoloGene (27).

PhenomicDB specifically has been built to enable analysis across techniques and species. Comparison of phenotypes from orthologous genes can help gain insight into the function of a gene, especially if there is no phenotypic information available for the primary gene of interest. Therefore, PhenomicDB incorporates 43,998 eukaryotic orthology groups from the NCBI's HomoloGene database (27) (using the file homologene.data available from ftp://ftp.ncbi.nih.gov/pub/HomoloGene/current). Through orthology, 98,543 genes having no phenotype *directly* associated with them become connected to the phenotypic annotation of orthologs. For example, only 2,405 human genes are *directly* linked to a human phenotype, but another 8,389 human genes can be associated with a phenotype by orthology, raising the percentage of human genes with at least some associated phenotypic information from 5.8 to 26.3% based on the Entrez Gene index (see also (19)). Transferred phenotype information across species even for orthologous genes should of course always be considered with care to ensure its biological validity.

2.2. From Phenotypes to Vectors

1. Raw textual phenotype data within PhenomicDB is available from the 'Downloads' section at http://www.phenomicdb.de/downloads.asp
2. To further prepare textual phenotype descriptions for clustering (*see* **Sections 3.2** and **3.3**), the doc2mat program was downloaded from http://glaros.dtc.umn.edu/gkhome/fetch/sw/cluto/doc2mat-1.0.tar.gz
3. 'Stop-words' (i.e. words of high frequency not adding to the distinctiveness of any feature vector) were eliminated using stop word lists integrated in doc2mat.
4. All remaining words were stemmed using the stemming algorithm from the doc2mat program which implements Porter's stemming algorithm (28).
5. The resulting documents, named 'phenodocs', were transformed into a numeric vector using the doc2mat package.

2.3. From Vectors to Phenoclusters

1. We used the open-source software CLUTO for clustering textual phenotype descriptions (*see* **Section 3.3**) (Clustering Toolkit, version 2.1.1, 9.3 MB, file cluto-2.1.1.tar.gz). CLUTO is available at http://glaros.dtc.umn.edu/gkhome/cluto/cluto/download (29).
2. Specifically, the scalable implementation of the bisecting *k*-means algorithm from the CLUTO package, called *vcluster*, was used (*see* **Note 3**).

3. Methods

3.1. Integration of Genotype–Phenotype Data into PhenomicDB

Systematic data integration is an essential first step when dealing with such diverse data from multiple sources of phenotypes (5). Usually, and as is the case here, large-scale data integration is only a semi-automated process, where mappings of fields between databases have to be defined manually and custom software programs need to be written to transform formats, term lists or database identifiers. Furthermore, there are cases where data download is not supported by a data source, leaving 'screen scraping' (i.e. data download by programming a script against the interface of the data source) as the only method for data retrieval. In order to build a common database of cross-species phenotypes, data (*see* **Section 2.1**) was downloaded, reorganized and eventually semantically integrated as described by Kahraman et al. (20). This included the physical (i.e. materialized) integration of phenotype data from various sources, where each data field from each data source was mapped manually (by coarse-grained semantic mapping) to the data fields of the target database. Furthermore, the genotypes directly associated with each phenotype were mapped to a common gene index, namely the NCBI's Entrez gene index. By application of these methods, PhenomicDB was created.

3.2. From Phenotypes to Vectors

PhenomicDB version 2 offered 428,150 phenotype entries which were downloaded (*see* **Section 2.2**). Those 411,102 entries directly associated with at least one gene were considered for further analysis. For each entry, its corresponding Entrez gene identifier and the available texts of all associated phenotypes using the PhenomicDB fields 'names', 'descriptions', 'keywords' and 'references' were compiled. Phenotypes with less than 200 characters were skipped. They were deemed to be too short to deliver reasonable results in text clustering (*see* **Note 4**). A further 511 ambiguous phenotypes (i.e. linked to more than one gene) were also removed. Next, so-called 'stop-words' (i.e. words of high frequency not adding to the distinctiveness of any feature vector) were eliminated (*see* **Section 2.2**). All remaining words were stemmed (*see* **Section 2.2**). The resulting documents, named 'phenodocs', were transformed into a numeric vector using the doc2mat package (on Unix command line '*doc2mat -mystoplist=<PubMed list of stopwords> -skipnumeric -nlskip=1 -tokfile <PhenoDocs.txt downloadable from PhenomicDB> <Name of resulting matrix file>*'). This resulted in a data set of 39,610 'phenodocs' associated with 15,426 genes from seven species: 1.7% *Danio rerio* (zebrafish), 19.9% *C. elegans* (earth worm), 1.7% *Dictyostelium discoideum* (slime mold), 24.1% *D. melanogaster* (fruit fly), 15.6% *H. sapiens* (human), 28.7% *M. musculus* (mouse) and 8.3% *S. cerevisiae* (yeast). In total, the numeric vectors consist of 73,188 unique features (derived from 113,283 unique words) with an average of 67.87 features per vector (min., 12 features; max., 364 features).

3.3. From Vectors to Phenoclusters

We used the open-source software CLUTO for clustering textual phenotype descriptions (*see* **Section 2.3** and **Note 3**). Three main parameters determine the *k*-means algorithm behaviour: the number of clusters *k* (here the command-line parameter *nclusters*), the similarity (or distance) measure (the command-line parameter *colmodel*, e.g. 'idf' when the input features' values are given as term frequencies and the TFIDF scoring scheme should be calculated, or 'none' when the given values should be accepted as they are) and the criterion function (the command-line parameter *crfun*, typically I_2 – *see* **Note 5**).

Clustering was done using *vcluster* (*see* **Section 2.3**). Prior to clustering, the phenotypes had to be converted into vectors using the doc2mat package (*see* **Section 2.2**). The resulting *matrix* file was stored and given as the command-line parameter *filename.mat*. Two other very useful optional files can be created using doc2mat, namely the *rlabel* file (giving the phenodocs' identifiers in order of appearance in the *matrix* file) and the *clabel* file (containing all unique words as represented by feature identifiers in the *matrix* file). The clustering program was called using '*vcluster -colmodel=<string> -crfun=<string> <filename.mat> <nclusters>*' on a Unix command line.

3.4. Using Phenotype Similarity for Gene Prediction

As outlined in **Section 1**, several ways for using phenotypes for gene function prediction exist. The search interface of PhenomicDB (*see* **Fig. 10.1**) is a good starting point, as it is based on the largest phenotype database worldwide, which also offers a set of associated tools. A user can search the database using keywords or identifiers, and searches can be refined by limiting them to a specific data field (e.g. 'phenotype keyword') or to a specific species. Also, one can manipulate the format of the result, for instance, by adding new columns such as chromosome number. The result of a query is a list of genes and their associated phenotypes matching the search terms (*see* **Fig. 10.2**).

Usage of this feature is best explained by a real use case. Cirelli et al. (30) had screened for *D. melanogaster* mutations affecting the daily amount of sleep, finding 15 strains with a mean daily amount of sleep at least two standard deviations less than the average for both male and female fruit flies. They found that likely gene candidates must affect sleep duration rather than sleep rhythm and that they must be located on the X chromosome. Furthermore, they noticed that all affected animals 'exhibited a transient shaking of the legs and scissoring of the wings when recovering from diethyl ether anaesthesia' (31). With these indications, they painstakingly screened the literature manually to eventually designate four genes as the most likely candidates: *shaker*, *ether a go-go*, *hyperkinetic* and *shaking b*. Indeed they experimentally confirmed that short sleepers can be rescued with a *shaker*$^+$ transgene. They do not elaborate in detail on how they came up with these candidates, but such a task nowadays could easily be solved using PhenomicDB. Searching for 'shak* and (leg* or wing*) and

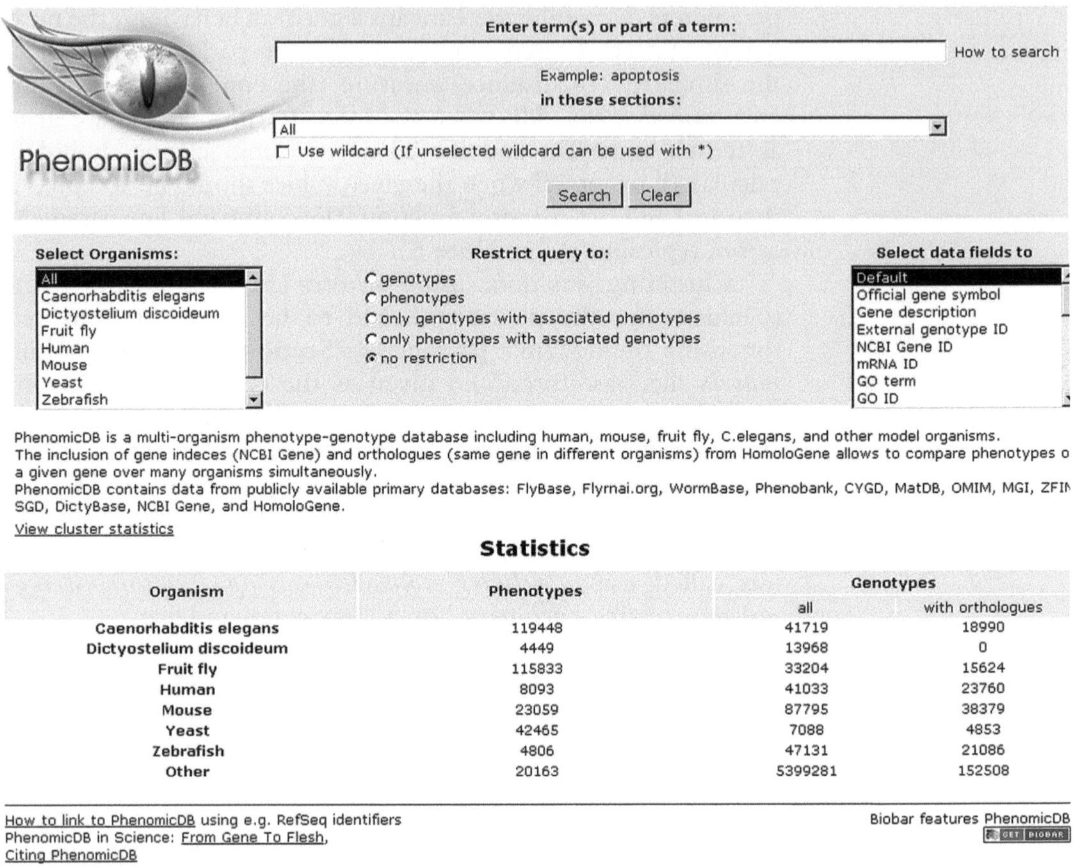

Fig. 10.1. Search interface of PhenomicDB (at http://www.phenomicdb.de). Any term or identifier can be entered in the search field at the top. Below, the search can be limited to specific data fields, e.g. Entrez Gene identifier and phenotype description. The query can be further restricted to an organism of interest (left selection box), or genotypes only, phenotypes only or only when a genotype is associated with at least one phenotype (or vice versa). Finally, the result list can be customized, showing either a default set of data fields or selected fields of interest. Also, the page shows the number of genotypes and phenotypes within PhenomicDB as well as the current database version and data freeze for reference.

ether*' in phenotype descriptions limited to fruit fly phenotypes and configuring the output to report also chromosome numbers, PhenomicDB delivers *hyperkinetic*, *ether a go-go*, *shaker*, *shaking B*, *flutter*, *shaking A* and *section* 2 as genes on chromosome X.

This exemplifies the benefit of integrated phenotype resources; however, PhenomicDB can also be used for more complex searches. Once an interesting phenotype has been identified inside the database, one can use phenoclusters to find the most similar phenotypes and their associated genes. Advanced visualization is a key feature to handle the resulting amount of information effectively. To do so, each phenotype has a 'Show Cluster' button, opening PhenomicDB's phenocluster visualization software in a new window (**Fig. 10.3**). A new window appears, divided into a centre screen, an 'actions and information' pane at the side and

shak* and (leg* or wing*) and ether*: **10** genotypes and **216** phenotypessection 'All', organisms 'Fruit fly'

☐ Toggle all		Organism name	Official gene symbol	Official gene name	NCBI Gene ID	Chromosome
☐ Orthologies	Show Entry	Drosophila melanogaster	Hk	Hyperkinetic	31955	X

	External phenotype ID	Phenotype description	Phenotype name	Phenotype symbol
Show Entry Show Cluster	FlyBase: FBal0005497	**Mutant phenotype:** RK1 Following etherisation legs vibrate rapidly. Non-etherised flies respond to hand moving above the vial by falling about as if completely uncoordinated. **Mutant phenotype:** RK1 Non-etherised flies respond to hand moving above the vial by falling about as if uncoordinated. **Mutagen:** ethyl methanesulfonate	Hk[2]	Hk^{2T}
Show Entry	FlyBase: FBal0005498	**Mutagen:** spontaneous	Hk[3]	Hk^{73}
Show Entry Show Cluster	FlyBase: FBal0083425	**Mutant phenotype:** Flies are significantly more sensitive to acrolein than wild-type flies. **Mutagen:** ethyl methanesulfonate	Hk[101]	Hk^{101}
Show Entry	FlyBase: FBal0160332	**Mutagen:** P-element activity	Hk[EY10029]	$Hk^{EY10029}$
Show Entry	FlyBase: FBal0207295	**Mutagen:** in vitro construct - regulatory fusion **Mutagen:** in vitro construct - RNAi **Nature of the lesion:** Scer\UAS regulatory sequences drive expression of an inverted repeat.	Hk[GD15937]	$Hk^{GD15937}$

Fig. 10.2. Resulting list (abridged) when searching PhenomicDB with query 'shak* and (leg* or wing*) and ether*' limited to hits in *D. melanogaster*. The default view has been expanded showing also the chromosome location of the gene. Here, the first gene on the result list is the fly gene *hyperkinetic* (Entrez Gene ID 31955). Below, phenotypes associated with that gene are shown, e.g. the phenotype HK^{2T}. In total, 10 genes have been found, to which 216 phenotypes are associated. Functional buttons are 'Show Entry', leading to the full entry for genes and phenotypes, including links to the original data sources, 'Orthologies', leading to the list of orthologs and associated phenotypes (if applicable), and 'Show Cluster', opening the phenocluster tool in a new window.

six tabs at the top. The centre screen always shows the phenotypes (or genes) of the current cluster as a graph (or alternatively as a tabular list – *see* **Note 6**). Nodes are coloured according to taxonomy and cluster membership. Mouse-click tooltips give detailed node information. Graphs can be downloaded in 'xdot' and 'png' format from the 'actions and information' pane.

Using the tabs will change the view on the cluster members. The 'overview' tab displays all phenotypes within a cluster as either unconnected nodes ('graph') or a table. The three similarity tabs ('cosine similarity', 'GO similarity' and 'AA sequence similarity') will connect the cluster members (or their associated genes) labelled with their mutual similarity (if surpassing a given similarity threshold), i.e., textual similarity of phenotype descriptions, functional similarity of GO annotations or amino acid sequence similarity. The orthology tab displays only those clustered genes for which there is an orthology relation. The protein–protein interaction ('PPI') tab adds protein interactions to the graph by means of an 'expansion' feature: Genes of a phenocluster are

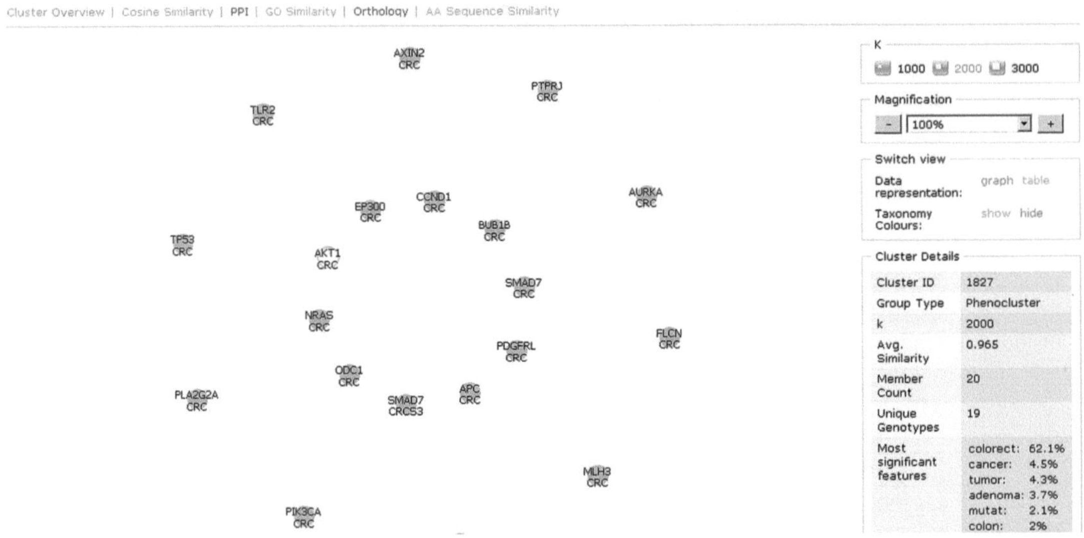

Fig. 10.3. Example of the Cluster Overview for the phenocluster ($k = 2{,}000$) of the human phenotype named 'Colorectal Cancer' (CRC) associated with the gene *AKT1* (v-akt murine thymoma viral oncogene homolog 1) found in PhenomicDB by searching for Entrez Gene ID 207. The 'actions and information' pane on the right provides statistics, e.g. it can be seen that the phenotype terms 'colorect' and 'cancer' are the most important features that have led to this cluster. The top section shows the six tabs, enabling a change to the presentation of similarity scores and other views.

connected based on cosine similarity, and the network will be enriched with those genes that are PPI partners of a gene in the cluster. Thus, even nodes without a similar phenotype, but a certain chance of being functionally related, are seamlessly included in the analysis.

Phenoclusters allow for a multitude of discoveries unavailable with other methods (32). For instance, users may query PhenomicDB for genes annotated with a certain disease name or phenotypic feature, and explore their phenoclusters for genes showing similar phenotypes which have not been associated with this disease or biological process so far. Along that line, if a biological pathway is to be inhibited pharmacologically but contains no known druggable targets, phenoclusters may now allow a search for as yet undiscovered members of that pathway which may be modulated by drugs. The value of these approaches has also been reported by others (33).

Following up on the above example, **Fig. 10.4** shows the PPI view of the phenocluster for $k = 1{,}000$ of the phenotype named HK^{2T}, being the first on the result list when searching PhenomicDB's *D. melanogaster* phenotype description with 'shak* and (leg* or wing*) and ether*'. The gene *hyperkinetic*, which is responsible for this phenotype, appears in the networks. The closest genes in that cluster that are also located on chromosome X are *hyperkinetic*, *paralytic*, *ether-a-go-go and shaker*. In combination with the candidate list named above, this leaves a very feasible

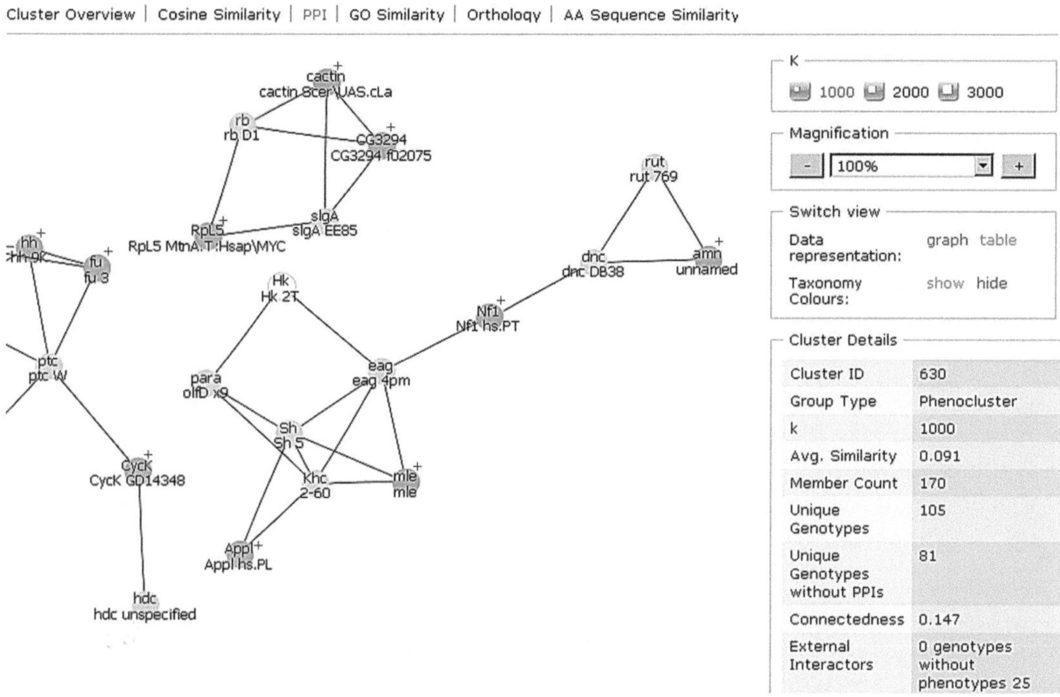

Fig. 10.4. Phenocluster of the hyperkinetic phenotype HK2T associated with the *D. melanogaster* gene *hyperkinetic* (Hk) visualized with $k = 1{,}000$. This cluster was found searching for 'shak* and (leg* or wing*) and ether*' in PhenomicDB limited to phenotypes from fruit fly and clicking on the 'Show Cluster' button of the first phenotype associated with the first gene on the list. It can be seen that the genes para (*paralytic*) and eag (*ether-a-go-go*) are directly connected to Hk (*hyperkinetic*) and that Sh (*shaker*) and Khc (*kinesin heavy chain*) are also in close relation by protein interactions. Furthermore, all of these genes have an associated phenotype from the same phenocluster (shown as unmarked nodes, blue in PhenomicDB). Genes associated with phenotypes from the cluster connected by protein interactions are shown as unmarked nodes (blue in PhenomicDB). Connected genes with phenotypes that are not within the cluster are shown as *darker* nodes (marked with '+', green in PhenomicDB). There are no genes without associated phenotypes, which would otherwise be shown in PhenomicDB as red nodes.

list of only three likely candidates (*hyperkinetic*, *ether-a-go-go* and *shaker*) that can now be analyzed with laboratory methods, leading ultimately, as shown (30), to the successful identification of the responsible gene.

In another example, shown in **Fig. 10.5**, human DAG1 has no phenotype described in PhenomicDB. However, the 'PPI' view of the rippling muscle disease (RMD) phenotype, which is known to be caused by caveolin-3 (CAV3), is composed of genes of similar phenotypes associated with 'dystrophy' (23.3%) and 'muscular' (22.6%) as the most significant similarity features. Human DAG1 through its protein–protein interaction with CAV3 becomes connected to the mouse ortholog of DAG1 which indeed is associated with a 'muscular dystrophy' phenotype, giving in combination a strong indication also that human DAG1 may be involved in such a phenotype.

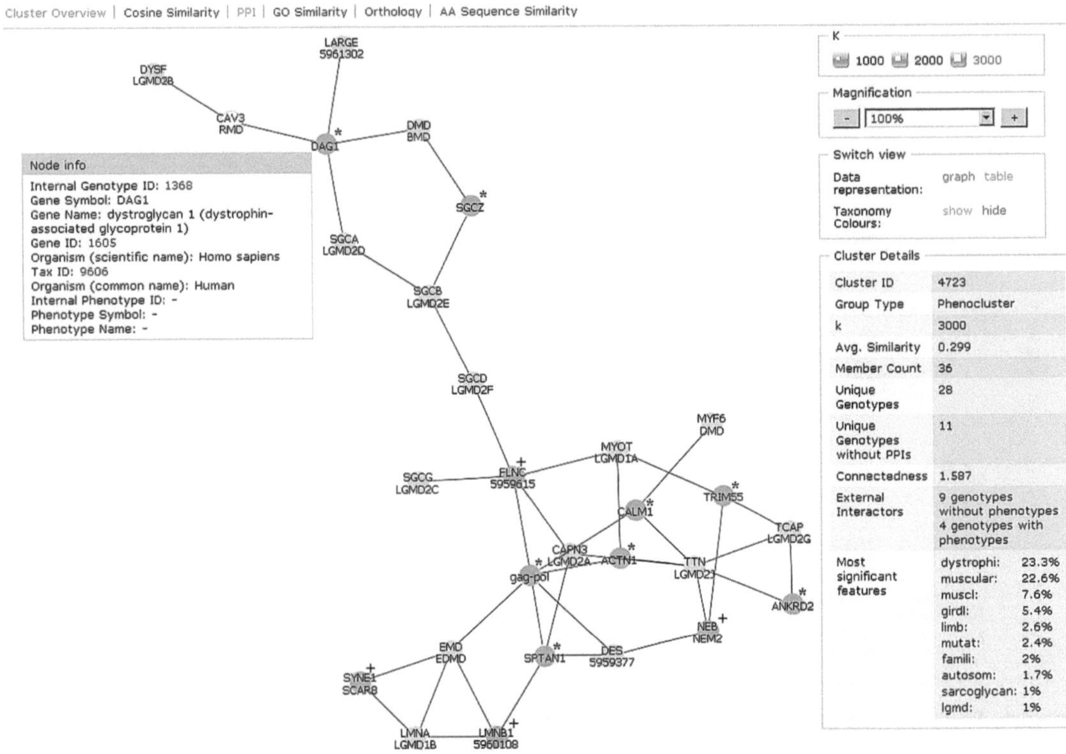

Fig. 10.5. Phenocluster of the rippling muscle disease (RMD) phenotype associated with caveolin-3 (CAV3) visualized with $k = 3{,}000$ for an optimal view. The cluster was found searching for 'rippling muscle disease' in phenotype descriptions. Genes associated with phenotypes from the cluster connected by protein interactions are shown (unmarked nodes, blue in PhenomicDB). Connected genes with phenotypes that are not within the cluster (nodes marked with '+', green in PhenomicDB) and genes with no phenotypes associated (nodes marked with '*', red in PhenomicDB) are also shown. The 'actions and information' pane on the right provides statistics, a legend and enables altering of the view. The top section enables changing the presentation of similarity scores.

4. Notes

1. A further issue in cross-species phenotype analyses is the semantic heterogeneity of the phenotype descriptions due to species- or domain-specific terminology. In a recent study (21), we showed that text clustering inherently overcomes this diversity at least partially and that a clustering of phenotype descriptions (phenoclustering) can be used to predict gene function from the groups of associated genes with high precision. Still, despite our cross-species setting, almost 90% of the phenotypes were grouped into single-species clusters due to the usage of highly species-specific terminology.
2. This currently predominant use of such species-specific terminology can only be partly justified scientifically. Many phenotypic observations are common across species, e.g. in

regard to survival, fertility, motility and growth, and could be described easily using a common vocabulary (probably with species-specific extensions). The multitude of synonyms for essentially the same phenotype currently in use leads to clustering artefacts, i.e. phenotypes being clustered separately which in fact describe a very similar observation albeit in a different organism – or laboratory. Such discrepancies can be resolved by using well-curated ontologies (34). Recently, Washington et al. (33) have shown that rigorous application of ontology-based phenotype descriptions to 11 gene-linked human diseases from OMIM (14) can be used as a means to identify gene candidates of human diseases by utilizing similarities to phenotypes from animal models. We have already started making more use of phenotype ontologies to, e.g., weight such terms higher and see significant improvement (35).

3. From the available clustering algorithms in the public domain, CLUTO has been chosen here for its reliability, availability and because it has been proven to perform well on textual data sets from the life science domain on several occasions (29, 31, 36, 37). In any case, quality and coherence of a clustering depend more on the correct choice of parameters than on the algorithm's implementation.
4. One of the obstacles when clustering phenotypes by their textual description is the variance in description length. In our first approach implemented in PhenomicDB, we disregard phenotype descriptions shorter than 200 characters, as clustering textual descriptions with hundreds of words to descriptions with only one or two words is not useful. Unfortunately, this excludes quite a large number of phenotypes, especially those being created by high-throughput RNAi screens (e.g. 'embryonic lethality'). This loss of data is a sacrifice to feasibility and we have tackled it partially in the most recent release of PhenomicDB (in April 2010) by reducing this cut-off to 50 characters. An alternative method for dealing with short feature vectors is the transformation of descriptions into Boolean 'absence' or 'presence' calls which can be clustered using vector similarity, as described by Piano et al. (38).
5. The choice for the criterion function, i.e. the function that uses the similarity measure in order to assign samples to their best (i.e. nearest) centroid, is highly dependent on the choice of similarity measure, which in turn is dependent on the clustered data (39). The cosine similarity measure is the best choice for document clustering for which CLUTO's criterion function I_2 has been suggested (37).

6. The list can be browsed or, for a more detailed analysis, exported into tabular or XML format (e.g. as input to a gene candidate ranking method). To also include 'orthologous phenotype information', we recommend initially not limiting the search to a particular species; information from orthologous genes can be instrumental to expand the candidate list even if no direct information for the gene of interest is available. Examples are human genes with no associated phenotypes but an ortholog in mice which has been used for the creation of a mouse knockout. Users can use the 'Orthologies' button (*see* **Fig. 10.2**) to find out whether a gene with a particular phenotype has orthologs in other species.

References

1. Tuschl, T., and Borkhardt, A. (2002) Small interfering RNAs: a revolutionary tool for the analysis of gene function and gene therapy. *Mol Interv 2*, 158–167.
2. Gunsalus, K. C., Yueh, W. C., MacMenamin, P., and Piano, F. (2004) RNAiDB and PhenoBlast: web tools for genome-wide phenotypic mapping projects. *Nucleic Acids Res 32*, D406–D410.
3. Sonnichsen, B., Koski, L. B., Walsh, A., et al. (2005) Full-genome RNAi profiling of early embryogenesis in *Caenorhabditis elegans. Nature 434*, 462–469.
4. Kittler, R., Surendranath, V., Heninger, A. K., et al. (2007) Genome-wide resources of endoribonuclease-prepared short interfering RNAs for specific loss-of-function studies. *Nat Methods 4*, 337–344.
5. Groth, P., and Weiss, B. (2006) Phenotype data: a neglected resource in biomedical research? *Curr Bioinform 1*, 347–358.
6. Kent, J. W., Jr. (2009) Analysis of multiple phenotypes. *Genet Epidemiol 33(Suppl 1)*, S33–39.
7. Prosdocimi, F., Chisham, B., Pontelli, E., Thompson, J. D., and Stoltzfus, A. (2009) Initial implementation of a comparative data analysis ontology. *Evol Bioinform Online 5*, 47–66.
8. Yu, B. (2009) Role of in silico tools in gene discovery. *Mol Biotechnol 41*, 296–306.
9. Gefen, A., Cohen, R., and Birk, O. S. (2009) Syndrome to gene (S2G): in-silico identification of candidate genes for human diseases. *Hum Mutat 31*, 229–236.
10. Robinson, P. N., Kohler, S., Bauer, S., et al. (2008) The Human Phenotype Ontology: a tool for annotating and analyzing human hereditary disease. *Am J Hum Genet 83*, 610–615.
11. Oti, M., Snel, B., Huynen, M. A., and Brunner, H. G. (2006) Predicting disease genes using protein–protein interactions. *J Med Genet 43*, 691–698.
12. Lage, K., Karlberg, E. O., Storling, Z. M., et al. (2007) A human phenome–interactome network of protein complexes implicated in genetic disorders. *Nat Biotechnol 25*, 309–316.
13. van Driel, M. A., Bruggeman, J., Vriend, G., et al. (2006) A text-mining analysis of the human phenome. *Eur J Hum Genet 14*, 535–542.
14. McKusick, V. A. (2007) Mendelian Inheritance in Man and its online version, OMIM. *Am J Hum Genet 80*, 588–604.
15. Rogers, A., Antoshechkin, I., Bieri, T., et al. (2008) WormBase 2007. *Nucleic Acids Res 36*, D612–D617.
16. Smith, C. L., Goldsmith, C. A., and Eppig, J. T. (2005) The Mammalian phenotype ontology as a tool for annotating, analyzing and comparing phenotypic information. *Genome Biol 6*, R7.
17. Bult, C. J., Eppig, J. T., Kadin, J. A., et al. (2008) The Mouse Genome Database (MGD): mouse biology and model systems. *Nucleic Acids Res 36*, D724–D728.
18. Oti, M., Huynen, M. A., and Brunner, H. G. (2009) The biological coherence of human phenome databases. *Am J Hum Genet 85*, 801–808.
19. Groth, P., Pavlova, N., Kalev, I., et al. (2007) PhenomicDB: a new cross-species genotype/phenotype resource. *Nucleic Acids Res 35*, D696–D699.
20. Kahraman, A., Avramov, A., Nashev, L. G., et al. (2005) PhenomicDB: a multi-species genotype/phenotype database for comparative phenomics. *Bioinformatics 21*, 418–420.

21. Groth, P., Weiss, B., Pohlenz, H. D., and Leser, U. (2008) Mining phenotypes for gene function prediction. *BMC Bioinformatics* *9*, 136.
22. Drysdale, R. (2008) FlyBase: a database for the *Drosophila* research community. *Methods Mol Biol* *420*, 45–59.
23. Guldener, U., Munsterkotter, M., Kastenmuller, G., et al. (2005) CYGD: the Comprehensive Yeast Genome Database. *Nucleic Acids Res* *33*, D364–D368.
24. Sprague, J., Bayraktaroglu, L., Bradford, Y., et al. (2008) The Zebrafish Information Network: the zebrafish model organism database provides expanded support for genotypes and phenotypes. *Nucleic Acids Res* *36*, D768–D772.
25. Schoof, H., Ernst, R., Nazarov, V., et al. (2004) MIPS *Arabidopsis thaliana* Database (MAtDB): an integrated biological knowledge resource for plant genomics. *Nucleic Acids Res* *32*, D373–D376.
26. Flockhart, I., Booker, M., Kiger, A., et al. (2006) FlyRNAi: the *Drosophila* RNAi screening center database. *Nucleic Acids Res* *34*, D489–494.
27. Sayers, E. W., Barrett, T., Benson, D. A., et al. (2010) Database resources of the National Center for Biotechnology Information. *Nucleic Acids Res* *38*, D5–D16.
28. Porter, M. F. (1980) An algorithm for suffix stripping. *Program* *14*, 130—137.
29. Zhao, Y., and Karypis, G. (2003) Clustering in life sciences. *Methods Mol Biol* *224*, 183–218.
30. Cirelli, C., Bushey, D., Hill, S., et al. (2005) Reduced sleep in Drosophila Shaker mutants. *Nature* *434*, 1087–1092.
31. Zhao, Y., and Karypis, G. (2005) Data clustering in life sciences. *Mol Biotechnol* *31*, 55–80.
32. Groth, P., Kalev, I., Kirov, I., Traikov, B., Leser, U., and Weiss, B. (2010) Phenoclustering: Online mining of cross-species phenotypes. *Bioinformatics* *26*(15), 1924–1925.
33. Washington, N. L., Haendel, M. A., Mungall, C. J., et al. (2009) Linking human diseases to animal models using ontology-based phenotype annotation. *PLoS Biol* *7*, e1000247.
34. Mungall, C. J., Gkoutos, G. V., Smith, C. L., et al. (2010) Integrating phenotype ontologies across multiple species. *Genome Biol* *11*, R2.
35. Groth, P., Weiss, B., and Leser, U. (2010) Ontologies improve cross-species phenotype analysis. In *Special Interest Group on Bio-ontologies: Semantic Applications in Life Sciences* (Shah, N., Ed.). National Center for Biomedical Ontology, Boston, MA. p. 192.
36. Tagarelli, A., and Karypis, G. (2008) A segment-based approach to clustering multi-topic documents. In *Text Mining Workshop, SIAM Datamining Conference*. Atlanta, GA.
37. Steinbach, M., Karypis, G., and Kumar, V. (2000) A Comparison of Document Clustering Techniques. In *KDD Workshop on Text Mining*. Boston, MA.
38. Piano, F., Schetter, A. J., Morton, D. G., et al. (2002) Gene clustering based on RNAi phenotypes of ovary-enriched genes in *C. elegans*. *Curr Biol* **12**, 1959–1964.
39. Zhao, Y., and Karypis, G. (2002) Criterion functions for document clustering, University of Minnesota, Department of Computer Science/Army HPC Research Center, Minneapolis.

Chapter 11

Conceptual Thinking for In Silico Prioritization of Candidate Disease Genes

Nicki Tiffin

Abstract

Prioritization of most likely etiological genes entails predicting and defining a set of characteristics that are most likely to fit the underlying disease gene and scoring candidates according to their fit to this "perfect disease gene" profile. This requires a full understanding of the disease phenotype, characteristics, and any available data on the underlying genetics of the disease. Public databases provide enormous and ever-growing amounts of information that can be relevant to the prioritization of etiological genes. Computational approaches allow this information to be retrieved in an automated and exhaustive way and can therefore facilitate the comprehensive mining of this information, including its combination with sets of empirically generated data, in the process of identifying most likely candidate disease genes.

Key words: Candidate disease genes, disease gene prioritization, disease gene prediction, computational disease gene prioritization.

1. Introduction

Disease gene identification can lead to improved diagnostic, prognostic, and therapeutic applications in the clinic. The identification of genetic factors underlying susceptibility to complex diseases, however, is a significant challenge, and bioinformatic approaches have a fundamental role to play in identification of most likely genetic candidates prior to embarking on empirical research. Such computational approaches can prioritize candidate genes through integration of data on gene characteristics, gene annotation, existing knowledge in the biomedical literature, and experimental data. This in turn can facilitate more effective, economical, and focused research in the laboratory and clinic.

B. Yu, M. Hinchcliffe (eds.), *In Silico Tools for Gene Discovery*, Methods in Molecular Biology 760,
DOI 10.1007/978-1-61779-176-5_11,

Experimental techniques increasingly focus on genome-wide experiments such as linkage (*see* **Chapter 2**), genome-wide association studies (*see* **Chapter 3**), and microarray analysis. These approaches select regions of the genome containing up to several hundred genes or generate large gene lists that contain candidate etiological genes. Consequently, there has been a shift from the historical approach of hypothesis-driven analysis of single candidate disease genes to large-scale experimental analysis that acts as the starting point from which to develop novel hypotheses about disease mechanisms.

In parallel, there is increasing focus on the genetics of complex diseases rather than single gene (Mendelian) diseases (1, 2). This makes it harder to identify the many etiological genes each making small contributions to the disease state, as opposed to a single causative gene. In synergy with this, prioritization of candidate genes relies increasingly on approaches analyzing gene regulatory networks underlying disease, rather than the functions of single genes.

The resources available for disease gene prioritization are rapidly expanding. Publicly available databases contain vast amounts of genetic data, including genomic data, gene sequence data, epigenetic data, variation data, expression data, regulatory network data, and biomedical literature linking genes and phenotypes. Computational approaches allow an objective, ordered and systematic approach to harnessing the enormous amounts of genetic data to allow prioritization of candidate disease genes. This can facilitate identification of the most likely etiological genes and aid in generating hypotheses about disease mechanisms.

Disease gene prioritization requires a process of defining the characteristics of most likely etiological genes and using these characteristics to filter and rank all candidates according to this profile for the most likely disease gene. In this chapter, the approach to disease gene prioritization is described in three stages. The first is to define existing information about the disease in question, its phenotype, and previously identified underlying etiological factors. The second is to use this information to define the characteristics that are likely to belong to genes underlying the disease, based on the known features of the disease and its etiology. The third is to use these characteristics to filter and rank the set of potential candidates according to the likely characteristics of genes underlying the disease.

2. Materials

In silico disease gene prioritization can be conducted with a minimum of equipment. A standard, up-to-date desk-top or laptop computer and a broadband connection to the Internet to facilitate access and datamining of public databases are required. Much of the software that can be used for datamining (e.g., Python or Perl software) and data management (e.g., MySQL for data storage, see **Section 3.3.2**) are open access and can be downloaded free of charge from the Internet.

3. Methods

3.1. Defining Existing Information about the Disease and Its Known Causative Genes

In order to prioritize etiological genes for a particular disease or phenotype, it is imperative to first establish as comprehensive an understanding of this phenotype as possible. This can assist in focusing the gene prioritization process, for example, whether the researcher should aim to prioritize a single good candidate or look for a gene regulatory network; whether there is a particular tissue in which the etiological gene must be active; or whether the disease gene should interact with a particular environmental factor. Each disease phenotype has its own set of characteristics that can be exploited to this end. Examples of these and how they may be exploited are described below.

3.1.1. Range of Symptoms

Some diseases present with a single defining symptom. For example, many cancers are defined by a primary tumor occurring within a particular tissue, or essential hypertension that presents with elevated blood pressure. In other cases, however, the disease presents as a syndrome or composite phenotype that has multiple possible classes of symptoms which do not fall into such neatly separated categories. Examples of these include human malformation syndromes (reviewed in (3)), metabolic syndrome (investigated in (4)), and fetal alcohol syndrome (investigated in (5)). Syndromes present an opportunity to look for overlap in genes selected as good candidates for each of the individual symptoms with which the patient may present. Candidate etiological genes can be prioritized for each of the symptoms, and then the gene lists investigated for commonality to establish genes that have the capacity to underlie multiple facets of the syndrome. In this case, it is also useful to examine upstream regulatory elements, such as signal transduction cascades, that may be common to the candidates prioritized for each of the sets of symptoms. Electronic tools are able to identify common regulatory/promoter motifs in candidate gene lists and predict upstream molecules that bind to these promoter motifs, for example, BioBase ExPlain (http://www.biobase.de) (6).

3.1.2. Mendelian and Complex Diseases

It is useful to note the mode of inheritance or heritability of the disease under investigation and the phenotypic heterogeneity of the disease. Historically, research has focused on Mendelian, or monogenic disorders, in which a familial trend and modes of inheritance have been established. For such diseases, disease gene prioritization can focus on finding a single causative gene with crucial function. Often, linkage or association studies of affected families provide a smaller starting set of candidate genes from a well-defined disease-associated locus. Modes of inheritance can give insights into the type of genes under investigation. In an extreme example, disease inheritance in the offspring of affected mothers but not of affected fathers would suggest involvement of mitochondrial genes, as seen with Leber Optic Atrophy (LHON; OMIM #535000).

For complex diseases, however, multiple etiological genes as well as environmental factors can each contribute a small part toward disease phenotype, and the mode of inheritance and penetrance of disease genes can be unclear (7). In the process of prioritizing disease genes for complex diseases, it becomes necessary to look for multiple contributory genes or gene regulatory networks underlying disease, rather than focusing on single causative genes. Some disease gene prioritization tools, such as Prioritizer (http://www.prioritizer.nl) (8) and the Genetrepid Common Pathway Scanning (CPS) method (http://www.gentrepid.org) (9), are designed specifically to address this issue.

3.1.3. Population Specificity

The distribution of the disease within the general population can provide useful clues toward the type of gene causing the phenotype. In a simple example, for a disease that affects only male or female patients, genes located on the X or Y chromosome make good candidates. A bias in geographical, social, or socioeconomic grouping of patients may also give clues to possible gene–environment interactions underlying complex disease. For example, phenylketonuria (PKU; OMIM #261600) results from a genetic variant that leads to deficient metabolism of the amino acid phenylalanine; in the presence of normal protein intake, phenylalanine accumulates and is neurotoxic. PKU occurs only when both the genetic variant (phenylalanine hydroxylase deficiency) and the environmental exposure (dietary phenylalanine) are present. One could therefore expect lower incidence of the disease in those with a protein-poor diet. Prevalence of disease in a particular ethnic group should be noted, although this tends to be more useful at the level of identifying disease variants within identified disease genes. Differences in disease occurrence between ethnic groups can, however, be used in scoring and ranking potential candidates in some cases, as demonstrated in a study of candidate genes for metabolic syndrome, in (4).

3.1.4. Resources for Defining Disease Phenotype

The existing caucus of biomedical literature is invaluable and can be accessed online through PubMed (http://www.ncbi.nlm.nih.gov/pubmed). Additionally, the Online Mendelian Inheritance in Man database (http://www.ncbi.nlm.nih.gov/omim) provides a wealth of information about genetic phenotypes. Clinical disease phenotype data, however, is rarely captured in databases in a standardized way by clinicians. The Database of Chromosomal Imbalance and Phenotype in Humans using Ensembl Resources (DECIPHER) (10) is a recent development aiming to centralize clinician-sourced phenotype data and their relationship to gene copy number, and is a first step toward databasing clinical phenotype data. Additional phenotype databases are assessed in (11). Ontologies can provide a standardized approach to phenotype description (*see* **Chapter 9**). They are formalized representations of a set of concepts within a domain of knowledge and define terms and relationships between those terms in a standardized way. The MeSH ontology, as reviewed in (12, 13), represents a set of biomedical concepts, and is used to annotate abstracts of the biomedical literature in PubMed and OMIM with phenotype-specific terms relating to the article. PhenoGO is another such ontology that includes information about diseases and clinical phenotypes (14). Such annotation can be used to search and group information in these databases by disease type or symptoms. Clinical case studies in the biomedical literature are also a good source of phenotype information (*see* **Note 1**). An example of this is the disease Ankylosing Spondylitis (AS, OMIM #106300), which is commonly described as an autoimmune disease affecting the cartilage of the spine. An additional symptom for a subset of patients is iritis. This provides an unrelated, discrete tissue type in which the disease gene is also likely to be active (15).

3.1.5. Existing Genetic Information Associated with the Phenotype of Interest

In many cases, there will be some level of existing information about the genetics underlying any particular disease. This information can take many different forms, but most may be used to assist in prioritizing candidate genes. Karyotypes of patients and/or diseased tissue may give an indication of areas of the genome that have undergone gross rearrangements, deletions, or expansions. This information can provide an area of the genome, denoted by chromosomal banding, that is highly likely to contain etiological genes. Candidate genes that fall in these grossly disrupted regions can receive preferential weighting in the search for good candidates. For example, in Angelman syndrome (OMIM #105830), the majority of cases are due to a deletion of segment 15q11-q13 on the maternally derived chromosome 15. Cytogenetic analyses such as fluorescent in situ hybridization (FISH) (16) and comparative genomic hybridization (CGH) (17) are also able to give a higher resolution identification of regions with duplications or deletions. Areas of the genome that have undergone translocation are likewise able to indicate areas of the genome that are likely to contain etiological genes, with preferential weighting of candidate genes lying in these regions of the genome. Finally, linkage analysis and association studies performed on cohorts of affected/unaffected individuals identify loci, often lying scattered across the genome, that are linked to the phenotype under study (*see* **Note 2**). The likelihood of etiological genes lying in these regions is high; and genes falling within the locations thus defined can be used to populate the starting set of candidate genes – usually a significant reduction in gene numbers when compared to the whole genome. Examples of linkage and association studies defining the starting set of candidate genes can be seen for candidate gene prioritization for type 2 diabetes/obesity (18) and metabolic syndrome (4).

Another resource that can be effectively harnessed to prioritize candidate disease genes includes genes that are already identified as underlying a particular disease. There are frequently multiple genes that can underlie a single disease phenotype, and in many cases the functions of the various disease genes are found to be closely related. Therefore candidate genes with very similar functions or properties make likely candidates to similarly underlie the disease when dysregulated. An example of this is Liddle syndrome (OMIM #17720): mutations of the *SCNN1B* or the *SCNN1G* gene both result in dysfunction of the renal epithelial sodium channel for which they encode discrete subunits. Another example is Cardio–facio–cutaneous syndrome (OMIM #115150), which can be caused by mutations in *MEK1*, *MEK2*, *KRAS*, or *BRAF*, all members of the same *RAS/ERK* signal transduction pathway (reviewed in (19)). Therefore it is possible to investigate the role and function of the known genes with the aim of prioritizing candidate genes that have similar characteristics. Some computational tools make use of this likelihood of similarity between disease genes, including G2D (20), POCUS (21), TOM (22), ENDEAVOUR (23), the Gentrepid Common Module Profiling method (9), and SUSPECTS (24). A limitation of this approach, however, is that only a small percentage of known genes have an experimentally verified function (25).

3.1.6. Experimental Models of the Disease

Although there are inevitable limitations of information from animal models when applied to human disease, the ability to collate detailed phenotypic disease information from animal models is not possible in human patients. Large-scale projects are underway to induce targeted knockouts in mice and analyze the corresponding phenotypes thoroughly (26). The data generated by genetic manipulations in animal models can be used to associate human genes with phenotypes according to properties of orthologous genes. This approach is used by such methods as GeneSeeker (27) and ToppGene (28) (mouse data). With increasing evolutionary distance between species, determining orthology becomes more difficult, although not impossible, as shown in the method of Fraser and Plotkin (yeast data) (29).

3.2. Defining the Characteristics of the "Perfect" Disease Gene

With a full understanding of the disease phenotype under study and its existing genetic information, it becomes possible to design a description of the kind of gene most likely to underlie the disease. In order to use this information for computational prioritization of disease genes, it is necessary to define the "perfect gene" profile in a way that is computationally meaningful, and various tools are available to do so. Examples of these are given in the following.

3.2.1. Intrinsic Gene Properties

Some studies have analyzed the intrinsic properties of known disease genes, regardless of their associated disease phenotype, and have identified several properties associated with etiological genes. For example, longer gene length, larger proteins, longer intergenic distance, a higher proportion of promoter CpG islands, and longer regulatory regions (such as 3'-UTR) have all been associated with disease-causing genes. Lower mutation rates, broader phylogenetic breadth, and fewer paralogs are similarly associated with disease-causing genes. These factors can be taken into consideration when defining the properties attributable to a strong candidate disease gene, and some electronic tools already do so, for example, DGP ((30) – now incorporated into ENDEAVOUR (23)) and PROSPECTR (31)). A limitation of these studies that must be taken into consideration, however, is the reliance of the definition of "disease genes" and "non-disease genes"; a boundary which becomes blurred when moving from Mendelian diseases to complex diseases.

3.2.2. Chromosomal Location

With the availability of cytogenetic, linkage, or association data, it is possible to define the area/s of the genome in which the candidate is likely to be located. Chromosomal location may be given in a variety of units and sometimes the area of interest may be defined by markers – in which case the position of the markers in the genome must be determined from their IDs. In order to use this information properly, it is important to collate it in a standardized way, especially where there are multiple sources of data on genomic location; and in the process of standardizing the units of chromosomal location, it is also important to note which strand of DNA the marker coordinates refer (*see* **Note 2**). Most public genomic databases (e.g., Ensembl, http://www.ensembl.org (32); UCSG, http://genome.ucsc.edu/ (33); NCBI, http://www.ncbi.nlm.nih.gov (34)) include information of genetic location of each gene and genetic markers in the database.

3.2.3. Expression Profile of the Disease Gene

A full understanding of the tissues affected in most patients allows the investigator to draw up a list of tissues or cell types in which the etiological gene is likely to be expressed. In this instance, the use of an anatomical- or cell type-specific ontology allows for a standardized way to define the tissues and cell types in which the disease gene is expressed, providing a controlled vocabulary to describe the tissues and cell types of interest, and avoiding ambiguity that can occur with synonyms and interchangeable terminologies. Such an ontology is eVOC (http://www.evocontology.org (35)), which offers anatomical and cell-type terms, which have been linked to cDNA libraries and transcripts at a genome-wide level. eVOC annotation of genes is incorporated in the Ensembl database, and therefore all terms selected to represent the preferred gene expression profile of the etiological gene can be used directly to filter genes from the Ensembl database. A similar source of gene expression data, defined by tissue, is the H-Angel database containing human gene expression data across 40 distinct tissues and 7 different platforms (http://www.h-invitational.jp/hinv/h-angel/ (36)). Additionally, a global map of human gene expression is a recently developed expression data resource developed by the European Bioinformatics Institute (http://www.ebi.ac.uk/gxa/ (37)).

3.2.4. Functional Annotation of the Disease Gene

Given the types of functions that are dysregulated in the disease, it is possible to define gene functions that the candidate gene may fulfill. Again, when describing gene function, ontologies offer a standardized vocabulary that can then be used to filter annotated genes. The Gene Ontology (GO, http://www.geneontology.org (38)) is highly developed and widely used and consists of three ontologies that cover "cellular component," "biological process," and "molecular function" of any given gene product. The annotation of genes with GO terms is widespread and can be accessed in most public genomic databases, including Ensembl, NCBI, and UCSC databases. Genes annotated with specific terms can also be identified using the AmiGO, the official GO browser available through the GO website. In addition, many web-based, publicly available tools use GO for inferring and defining gene function. Within the field of disease gene prioritization, these include G2D (39), POCUS (21), SUSPECTS (24), ENDEAVOUR (23), and TOM (22). In summary, once a particular function has been defined as a characteristic of the proposed etiological gene it can be described in GO terminology as identified using AmiGO. This terminology will be directly applicable in the process of prioritizing candidate genes based on known function (*see* **Note 3** and **Chapter 9** for information on gene ontology).

Given known genes already implicated in the disease, it is possible to select some gene characteristics that are likely to be in common between these and novel disease candidates. Again, ontologies can be used to define the characteristics of the known genes, including functional annotation and expression data. Where there are many genes already associated with the disease, there are tools available to identify predominant functions within the gene list. These include such tools as GoSTAT (http://gostat.wehi.edu.au/ (40)) and DAVID (http://david.abcc.ncifcrf.gov (41, 42)), which compare the prevalence of each GO annotation in the gene list of interest to the prevalence of that annotation across the genome and provide a ranking for overrepresented annotations. The expression profile of known disease genes can be determined by eVOC annotation, which can be found both from the eVOC website and through the Ensembl database. Currently, however, there is no automated data-miner to calculate the significance of the data set enrichment with a particular profile. This should be taken into consideration (for example, the term "blood" is overrepresented in eVOC because blood samples for cDNA libraries can be obtained non-invasively from patients and are therefore more prevalent). Equally, identified genes from related animal models may be used to define gene function of most likely disease gene candidates: human homologous genes can be identified through the public databases and their functional annotation and expression profile analyzed.

3.3. Filtering the Starting Set of Candidate Genes According to the Characteristics of the "Perfect" Disease Gene

3.3.1. Compiling and Scoring Prioritized Genes

There are two main conceptual approaches to the prioritization of candidate genes. The first is to select a list of possible genes in a binary way: either the gene is selected as a good candidate or it is excluded. In this scenario, the genes are not ranked and the user ends up with a set of equally good candidates (an example of this is found in (43)). In the second approach, which is generally favored, genes are ranked according to a variety of criteria resulting in a list of all genes in order of most likely to least likely candidates. This approach relies on the assumption that a gene that fulfills more of the specified criteria is more likely to be a good candidate, and is better suited to selection of candidates for further empirical research as it provides a list that can be worked through within the limitations of available empirical resources. Thus, for example, a gene that has a specified functional annotation and is expressed in an affected tissue will have a higher prioritization than a gene that fulfills the functional requirements but is not expressed in the affected tissue. This approach is demonstrated in (18) and is used by methods such as ENDEAVOUR (23).

It is also possible to combine these approaches; for example, generating a list of unranked genes for each criterion and then assigning a score to each criterion, so that each gene accrues a cumulative score based on which criteria it fulfills. This approach is used in (4), where candidate gene lists are assembled for each phenotype contributing to a particular syndrome, and then a score is assigned to genes in each phenotype list according to the prevalence of that phenotype in the syndrome.

3.3.2. Retrieving Information from Genomic Databases

Most public genomic databases will incorporate extensive annotation of each gene in the database. Ease of extracting this information in an automated way varies according to database. The author recommends accessing data from the Ensembl database, as it offers querying of data in both a web based and a scripting way. For a bioinformaticist competent in scripting data from an SQL database, Ensembl can be mined as a publicly accessible MySQL server (ensembldb.ensembl.org, user = "anonymous"; or martdb.ensembl.org, user = "anonymous") using standard scripting languages such as Python (http://www.python.org/) or Perl (http://www.perl.org/) (*see* **Note 4**). There is also a Perl API provided by Ensembl, which uses an object-oriented approach to model biological objects, making it straightforward to write scripts that retrieve and analyze data. Current information on retrieving data in these ways is available at the Ensembl website (http://www.ensembl.org/info/data/mysql.html).

For a user without scripting ability, much of the information can be retrieved using the web-based querying interface BioMart (44), which is effective but can be a much slower process for longer gene lists and queries on multiple gene characteristics. BioMart can be accessed through the Ensembl website (http://www.ensembl.org) by clicking on the "Biomart" link, which will open a new query. Several steps are required: The first is to select the database and data set that will be used for the query (*see* **Note 5**). The second is to select filters for genes according to a variety of characteristics, including chromosomal location, expression profile, functional annotation, and orthologous genes. Finally, the third step is to define the gene information and format required for the output file.

Tutorials and information on the latest version of BioMart can be found at the Ensembl website (http://www.ensembl.org/info/data/biomart.html and http://www.ensembl.org/info/website/tutorials/index.html).

3.3.3. Incorporating Information from User-Specified Data Sets

Datamining from public databases such as Ensembl, NCBI, and UCSC databases filters the set of all genes in the human genome. Results from these queries, however, can be combined with additional data sets from other analyses or empirical research to further filter the list of candidate etiological genes. Results from each additional resource can be assembled into a gene list, and each list may also be assigned a weight as described in **Section 3.3.1** and used to further inform the prioritization of "most likely" candidate disease genes. A clear illustration of this approach can be seen in the study by Mootha et al. (45), using DNA, mRNA, and protein data sets to identify *LRPPRC* as an etiological gene for Leigh syndrome, French-Canadian type (LSFC, OMIM # 220111). Experimental data sets are also becoming increasingly available in public databases and can be used to inform disease gene prioritization. In particular, data from functional genomics experiments can be freely accessed from databases such as Array Express (http://www.ebi.ac.uk/microarray-as/ae/ (46)) and Gene Expression Omnibus (GEO, http://www.ncbi.nlm.nih.gov/geo/ (47)).

4. Notes

1. An invaluable source of accurate and informative clinical data is direct interaction with clinicians who specialize in the disease of interest: this is also where the researcher is most likely to gather information on the less commonly reported symptoms of disease, and often these can give a window into refining further the candidate gene search.
2. Care must be taken when defining regions of interest in the genome: there is great inconsistency in methods of defining genetic regions, including karyotype banding (for example, "11p13"), base pair coordinates (base pairs or megabase pairs, bp/Mbp), genetic markers that define boundaries of the regions, and recombinant frequency (centimorgans, cM); and it is most convenient to convert these to base pair coordinates in order to accurately select candidate genes. In general, it is advisable to select the outer limits of defined genomic regions to ensure that all possible candidates are selected.
3. It is important to take into consideration that the use of functional annotation such as Gene Ontology results in an inherent bias toward selecting well-characterized genes. Using functional annotation for disease candidate selection decreases the chance of selecting disease genes that have not yet been characterized or well studied.
4. When writing these scripts, the author recommends that multiple simple queries are run on the databases, the gene lists downloaded locally, and then the complex query assembled locally – complex nested queries of the Ensembl databases are generally slow and are often left "hanging."
5. It is important to note which version of the database is used as the database may be updated during the course of the research project, resulting in slightly different results in the prioritization process.

Acknowledgments

This work was funded by the Medical Research Council of South Africa.

References

1. Risch, N. J. (2000) Searching for genetic determinants in the new millennium. *Nature* ***405***, 847–856.
2. Yang, Q., Khoury, M. J., Botto, L., et al. (2003) Improving the prediction of complex diseases by testing for multiple disease-susceptibility genes. *Am J Hum Genet 72*, 636–649.
3. Oti, M., and Brunner, H. G. (2007) The modular nature of genetic diseases. *Clin Genet 71*, 1–11.
4. Tiffin, N., Okpechi, I., Perez-Iratxeta, C., et al. (2008) Prioritization of candidate disease genes for metabolic syndrome by computational analysis of its defining phenotypes. *Physiol Genomics 35*, 55–64.
5. Lombard, Z., Tiffin, N., Hofmann, O., et al. (2007) Computational selection and prioritization of candidate genes for fetal alcohol syndrome. *BMC Genomics 8*, 389.
6. Kel, A., Voss, N., Valeev, T., et al. (2008) ExPlain: finding upstream drug targets in disease gene regulatory networks. *SAR QSAR Environ Res 19*, 481–494.
7. Tabor, H. K., Risch, N. J., and Myers, R. M. (2002) Candidate-gene approaches for studying complex genetic traits: practical considerations. *Nat Rev Genet 3*, 391–397.
8. Franke, L., Bakel, H., Fokkens, L., et al. (2006) Reconstruction of a functional human gene network, with an application for prioritizing positional candidate genes. *Am J Hum Genet 78*, 1011–1025.
9. George, R. A., Liu, J. Y., Feng, L. L., et al. (2006) Analysis of protein sequence and interaction data for candidate disease gene prediction. *Nucleic Acids Res 34*, e130.
10. Firth, H. V., Richards, S. M., Bevan, A. P., et al. (2009) DECIPHER: Database of Chromosomal Imbalance and Phenotype in Humans Using Ensembl Resources. *Am J Hum Genet* 84, 524–533.
11. Oti, M., Huynen, M. A., and Brunner, H. G. (2009) The biological coherence of human phenome databases. *Am J Hum Genet 85*, 801–808.
12. Bodenreider, O. (2004) The Unified Medical Language System (UMLS): integrating biomedical terminology. *Nucleic Acids Res 32*, D267–270.
13. Bodenreider, O. (2008) Biomedical ontologies in action: role in knowledge management, data integration and decision support. *Yearb Med Inform*, 67–79.
14. Sam, L. T., Mendonca, E. A., Li, J., et al. (2009) PhenoGO: an integrated resource for the multiscale mining of clinical and biological data. *BMC Bioinformatics* ***10****(Suppl 2)*, S8.
15. Braun, J., and Sieper, J. (2007) Ankylosing spondylitis. *Lancet* ***369***, 1379–1390.
16. Levsky, J. M., and Singer, R. H. (2003) Fluorescence in situ hybridization: past, present and future. *J Cell Sci 116*, 2833–2838.
17. Gray, J. W., Kallioniemi, A., Kallioniemi, O., et al. (1992) Molecular cytogenetics: diagnosis and prognostic assessment. *Curr Opin Biotechnol 3*, 623–631.
18. Tiffin, N., Adie, E., Turner, F., et al. (2006) Computational disease gene identification: a concert of methods prioritizes type 2 diabetes and obesity candidate genes. *Nucleic Acids Res 34*, 3067–3081.
19. Lahiry, P., Torkamani, A., Schork, N. J., and Hegele, R. A. (2010) Kinase mutations in human disease: interpreting genotype-phenotype relationships. *Nat Rev Genet 11*, 60–74.
20. Perez-Iratxeta, C., Wjst, M., Bork, P., and Andrade, M. A. (2005) G2D: a tool for mining genes associated with disease. *BMC Genet 6*, 45.
21. Turner, F. S., Clutterbuck, D. R., and Semple, C. A. (2003) POCUS: mining genomic sequence annotation to predict disease genes. *Genome Biol 4*, R75.
22. Masotti, D., Nardini, C., Rossi, S., et al. (2008) TOM: enhancement and extension of a tool suite for in silico approaches to multigenic hereditary disorders. *Bioinformatics 24*, 428–429.
23. Tranchevent, L. C., Barriot, R., Yu, S., et al. (2008) ENDEAVOUR update: a web resource for gene prioritization in multiple species. *Nucleic Acids Res 36*, W377–384.

24. Adie, E. A., Adams, R. R., Evans, K. L., et al. (2006) SUSPECTS: enabling fast and effective prioritization of positional candidates. *Bioinformatics 22*, 773–774.
25. Perez-Iratxeta, C., Palidwor, G., and Andrade-Navarro, M. A. (2007) Towards completion of the Earth's proteome. *EMBO Rep 8*, 1135–1141.
26. Auwerx, J., Avner, P., Baldock, R., et al. (2004) The European dimension for the mouse genome mutagenesis program. *Nat Genet 36*, 925–927.
27. van Driel, M. A., Cuelenaere, K., Kemmeren, P. P., et al. (2005) GeneSeeker: extraction and integration of human disease-related information from web-based genetic databases. *Nucleic Acids Res 33*, W758–761.
28. Chen, J., Xu, H., Aronow, B. J., and Jegga, A. G. (2007) Improved human disease candidate gene prioritization using mouse phenotype. *BMC Bioinformatics 8*, 392.
29. Fraser, H. B., and Plotkin, J. B. (2007) Using protein complexes to predict phenotypic effects of gene mutation. *Genome Biol 8*, R252.
30. Lopez-Bigas, N., Blencowe, B. J., and Ouzounis, C. A. (2006) Highly consistent patterns for inherited human diseases at the molecular level. *Bioinformatics 22*, 269–277.
31. Adie, E. A., Adams, R. R., Evans, K. L., et al. (2005) Speeding disease gene discovery by sequence based candidate prioritization. *BMC Bioinformatics 6*, 55.
32. Flicek, P., Aken, B. L., Ballester, B., et al. (2010) Ensembl"s 10th year. *Nucleic Acids Res 38*, D557–D562.
33. Rhead, B., Karolchik, D., Kuhn, R. M., et al. (2010) The UCSC Genome Browser database: update 2010. *Nucleic Acids Res 38*, D613–619.
34. Sayers, E. W., Barrett, T., Benson, D. A., et al. (2010) Database resources of the National Center for Biotechnology Information. *Nucleic Acids Res 38*, D5–16.
35. Kelso, J., Visagie, J., Theiler, G., et al. (2003) eVOC: a controlled vocabulary for unifying gene expression data. *Genome Res 13*, 1222–1230.
36. Tanino, M., Debily, M. A., Tamura, T., et al. (2005) The Human Anatomic Gene Expression Library (H-ANGEL), the H-Inv integrative display of human gene expression across disparate technologies and platforms. *Nucleic Acids Res 33*, D567–572.
37. Lukk, M., Kapushesky, M., Nikkila, J., et al. (2010) A global map of human gene expression. *Nat Biotechnol 28*, 322–324.
38. The Gene Ontology Consortium (2010) The Gene Ontology in 2010: extensions and refinements. *Nucleic Acids Res 38*, D331–335.
39. Perez-Iratxeta, C., Bork, P., and Andrade-Navarro, M. A. (2007) Update of the G2D tool for prioritization of gene candidates to inherited diseases. *Nucleic Acids Res 35* (Web Server issue), W212–216.
40. Beissbarth, T., and Speed, T. P. (2004) GOstat: find statistically overrepresented Gene Ontologies within a group of genes. *Bioinformatics 20*, 1464–1465.
41. Dennis, G., Jr., Sherman, B. T., Hosack, D. A., et al. (2003) DAVID: Database for Annotation, Visualization, and Integrated Discovery. *Genome Biol 4*, P3.
42. Huang da, W., Sherman, B. T., and Lempicki, R. A. (2009) Systematic and integrative analysis of large gene lists using DAVID bioinformatics resources. *Nat Protoc 4*, 44–57.
43. Tiffin, N., Kelso, J. F., Powell, A. R., et al. (2005) Integration of text- and data-mining using ontologies successfully selects disease gene candidates. *Nucleic Acids Res 33*, 1544–1552.
44. Smedley, D., Haider, S., Ballester, B., et al. (2009) BioMart – biological queries made easy. *BMC Genomics 10*, 22.
45. Mootha, V. K., Lepage, P., Miller, K., et al. (2003) Identification of a gene causing human cytochrome c oxidase deficiency by integrative genomics. *Proc Natl Acad Sci USA 100*, 605–610.
46. Parkinson, H., Kapushesky, M., Kolesnikov, N., et al. (2009) ArrayExpress update – from an archive of functional genomics experiments to the atlas of gene expression. *Nucleic Acids Res 37*, D868–D872.
47. Barrett, T., Troup, D. B., Wilhite, S. E., et al. (2009) NCBI GEO: archive for high-throughput functional genomic data. *Nucleic Acids Res 37*, D885–D890.

Chapter 12

Web Tools for the Prioritization of Candidate Disease Genes

Martin Oti, Sara Ballouz, and Merridee A. Wouters

Abstract

Despite increasing sequencing capacity, genetic disease investigation still frequently results in the identification of loci containing multiple candidate disease genes that need to be tested for involvement in the disease. This process can be expedited by prioritizing the candidates prior to testing. Over the last decade, a large number of computational methods and tools have been developed to assist the clinical geneticist in prioritizing candidate disease genes. In this chapter, we give an overview of computational tools that can be used for this purpose, all of which are freely available over the web.

Key words: Disease gene prediction, disease gene prioritization, bioinformatics, genetic diseases, genome, phenotype.

1. Introduction

Historically, linkage mapping and candidate gene-based association studies have been used to investigate the genetic basis of inherited diseases (1). However, linkage mapping frequently results in large loci containing many genes, and the candidate gene-based approach to association studies met with limited success due to limitations in statistical power and knowledge of disease biology (1). More recent genome-wide association studies (GWAS) have proven more successful at detecting associations between SNPs and complex diseases (1) but have also made it more difficult to determine which are genuine and which are false positives. Therefore, both linkage and GWAS analyses would benefit greatly from the ability to computationally sift through large numbers of candidate disease genes to identify which are the most likely to be involved in the disease in question. Happily,

B. Yu, M. Hinchcliffe (eds.), *In Silico Tools for Gene Discovery*, Methods in Molecular Biology 760,
DOI 10.1007/978-1-61779-176-5_12, © Springer Science+Business Media, LLC 2011

the genomic era heralded in by the sequencing of the complete human genome has resulted in the generation of large amounts of biological data which can be used for just such a purpose. Consequently, the past decade has seen the development of a large number of computational candidate disease gene prioritization tools.

Chapter 11 provides a practical overview of general approaches to prioritizing candidate disease genes in disease genetic research. It also mentions several computational resources and tools that can be applied to this purpose. The present chapter delves further into computational tools that can be used to predict, prioritize, or explore candidate disease genes, describing their underlying approaches and the circumstances of their applicability. It is directed toward users of online candidate gene prioritization systems and is intended to complement existing reviews which focus more on the conceptual basis of such approaches than on their practical usage (e.g., (2–5)). All tools have also been published in peer reviewed journals and have been subjected to some form of validation such as benchmarking. The large number of tools precludes their in-depth treatment, but links are provided to online help pages or tutorials describing their use in more detail. Instead, this chapter focuses on giving the reader an overview of available tools, along with practical guidelines on which tools to use under which circumstances, and what pitfalls to bear in mind when using them.

Although the list of tools described here is comprehensive, it may not be exhaustive. Recent years have seen the introduction of a large number of such tools and more are undoubtedly in development. To keep up with the latest progress, the Gene Prioritization Portal website (http://www.esat.kuleuven.be/gpp) was created (6). This web portal summarizes web-based candidate disease gene prediction and prioritization tools and, as it is actively maintained, should continue to reflect available web tools into the future. The associated paper describing the portal (6) is similar in spirit to this chapter, but is styled more as a review than a handbook and does not feature easy lookup of tool-specific information (although such information is available on the portal website).

Only freely available web-accessible candidate disease gene prediction and prioritization tools are included in this chapter. Approaches without end user web tools, such as ACGR (7), CAESAR (8), CFA (9), DRS (10), PDG-ACE (11), POCUS (12), PRINCE (13), and the methods described by Ala et al. (14), Care et al. (15), Freudenberg and Propping (16), Karni et al. (17), Lage et al. (18), Li and Agarwal 2009 (19), Linghu et al. (20), Oti et al. (21–22), and Tiffin et al. (23), are not covered. We have also not covered previously available online tools that are no longer available such as DGP (24) and the online version of Prioritizer (25), or tools with mandatory login requirements (e.g., GeneRECQuest (26)). Offline tools such as Endeavour (27) and Prioritizer (25), though very useful and available free of charge to clinical geneticists, are also excluded from treatment here as they require more work to set up and use. These two tools are nevertheless comparatively easy to install if desired, as they are written in the widely supported Java programming language. Instructions are available from their corresponding websites (Endeavour: http://www.esat.kuleuven.be/endeavour; Prioritizer: http://www.prioritizer.nl/).

Most candidate gene prediction tools were designed for use on one or a few genetic loci and were originally intended for use with Mendelian disorders. Due to the weaker associations between genetics and disease phenotype, complex disease gene prioritization is even more difficult to tackle computationally. Nevertheless, several tools – particularly those designed to prioritize genes from the whole genome rather than a defined locus – can be applied to this problem. Some tools and approaches, such as the above-mentioned CAESAR (8) approach and the CANDID web tool (28), have even been designed specifically with complex diseases in mind. Pathway analyses of genome-wide association study (GWAS) data have demonstrated the tractability as well as the difficulties of candidate disease gene identification for complex diseases (29–34). This area of research is set to expand in the near future due to the current high interest in research into this type of disease, so more complex disease-oriented candidate gene prediction tools can be expected in the coming years.

We start by providing a brief conceptual overview of the different research requirements addressed by these tools and the kinds of data they provide. We classify the various tools according to these criteria and provide a guide indicating which tools can be used for which purposes. Subsequent to this general overview we summarize the important characteristics of each tool individually, including information such as web URLs for its home and help pages, what it can be used for, what kinds of data it requires, how actively it is maintained, and other tool-specific information.

2. Materials

All tools described here are implemented as online web servers, so all that is needed is a computer with an Internet connection and web browser. The operating system and browser used should not be important. **Table 12.1** provides an overview of the tools described in this chapter.

Table 12.1
Overview of web-based candidate disease gene prioritization/exploration tools described in this chapter

Tool	URL	References
aBandApart, aGeneApart	http://tomcat.esat.kuleuven.be/abandapart/, http://tomcatbackup.esat.kuleuven.be/sanger/	(56)
AlignPI, CIPHER	http://bioinfo.au.tsinghua.edu.cn/alignpi/, http://bioinfo.au.tsinghua.edu.cn/cipher/cipher_search.html	(57–58)
BITOLA	http://ibmi.mf.uni-lj.si/bitola/	(59)
CANDID	https://dsgweb.wustl.edu/hutz/candid.html	(28)
Endeavour	http://homes.esat.kuleuven.be/~bioiuser/endeavour/index.php	(48)
GeneDistiller	http://www.genedistiller.org/	(60)
Gene Prospector	http://www.hugenavigator.net/HuGENavigator/geneProspectorStartPage.do	(61)
Genes2Diseases (G2D)	http://www.ogic.ca/projects/g2d_2/	(62)
GeneSeeker	http://www.cmbi.ru.nl/GeneSeeker/	(63)
GeneWanderer	http://compbio.charite.de/genewanderer/GeneWanderer	(64)
Gentrepid	https://www.gentrepid.org/	(65)
GFINDer	http://www.bioinformatics.polimi.it/gfinder/	(66)
MimMiner	http://www.cmbi.ru.nl/MimMiner/	(67)
PGMapper	http://www.genediscovery.org/pgmapper/index.jsp	(68)
PhenoPred	http://www.phenopred.org/	(69)
PolySearch	http://wishart.biology.ualberta.ca/polysearch/index.htm	(70)
PosMed	http://omicspace.riken.jp/PosMed/	(71)
SNPs3D	http://www.snps3d.org/	(72)
SUSPECTS	http://www.genetics.med.ed.ac.uk/suspects/	(73)
Syndrome To Gene (S2G)	http://fohs.bgu.ac.il/s2g/	(74)
TOM	http://www-micrel.deis.unibo.it/~tom/	(75)
ToppGene	http://toppgene.cchmc.org/	(76)

3. Methods

In this section a brief overview is given for each of the candidate disease gene prioritization web tools covered in this chapter. Here the term *prioritization* may be used to indicate prioritization of an existing user-defined list of genes, for example, the output of a microarray experiment; or it may be used in a hierarchical sense as

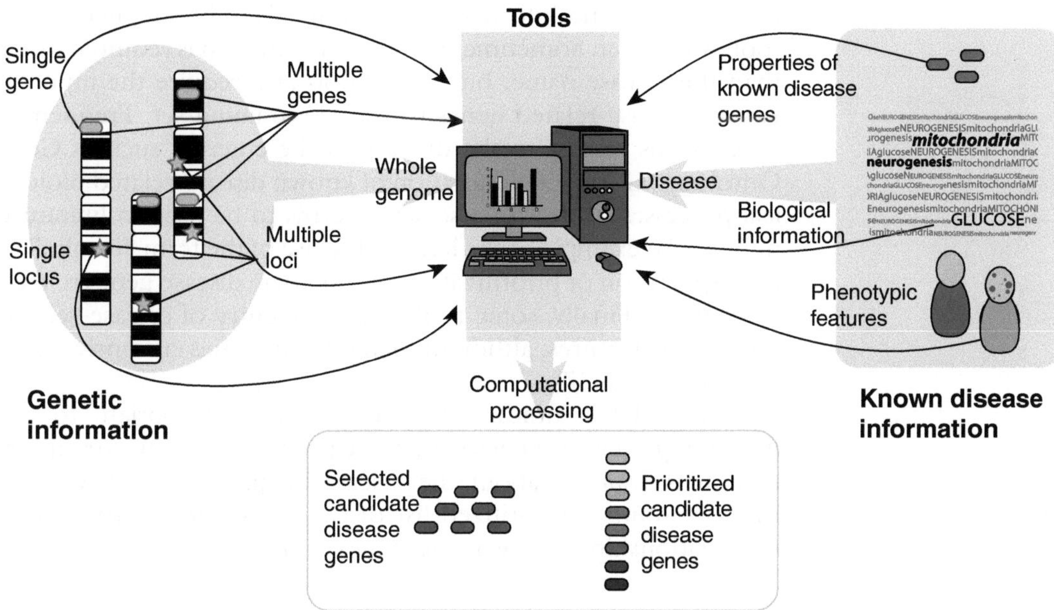

Fig. 12.1. Types of data required by candidate disease gene prioritization web servers. Some web servers provide unranked selections of candidate gene sets, while others provide prioritized lists of candidate genes.

a catchall term to indicate both *prediction* and *prioritization* of candidates. For some tools, no ranking of candidates is attempted, with candidates simply being predicted or not, and in this case *prioritization* simply indicates *prediction*.

The various disease gene prioritization and exploration tools require different kinds of candidate gene data. **Figure 12.1** gives an overview of the various types of input data required by the prioritization tools, grouped into two main categories: sources of candidate disease genes; and known disease-related information. There are tools, such as AlignPI, CIPHER, PhenoPred, and PolySearch, that do not require the entry of any candidate disease genes at all, instead prioritizing the whole genome, or at least those genes in the genome that are amenable to their prioritization approaches. Other tools, such as aGeneApart, BITOLA, and SNPs3D, enable a specific candidate disease gene to be investigated for links to a disease phenotype. Most, however, prioritize candidate genes from one or more genomic loci or from lists of genes which are associated with the disease – for instance, those that are differentially expressed in patients.

In addition to candidate genes, several other kinds of information about the disease are used by different tools in their prioritization processes. Frequently, such information is automatically retrieved based on genes known to be associated with the disease; or what is already known about the disease in the literature, or in databases. As this chapter focuses on practical tool usage, we only consider the extra information which needs to be supplied to the tool by the user. Sometimes no extra information is required other than the disease name, but many tools also require the input of known disease-related genes to use as a training set. Frequently, other terms related to the disease can be entered, such as Gene Ontology (GO) (35) annotation of known disease-related biological processes or disease-associated terms to be used in literature mining. An example of the latter is the use of the term "insulin" in the exploration or prioritization of candidate disease genes related to diabetes. Finally, some tools allow the entry of disease-related phenotypic features, although such information is currently under utilized (3, 36–37).

Table 12.2 indicates which tools are appropriate to use depending on what genes need to be prioritized, what extra information is available about the disease in question, and whether the user wants a prioritized list of candidates or just to explore the relationships between the genes and the disease. This table

Table 12.2
Overview of which tools to use depending on available candidate disease genes and disease-related data. Numbers reference tools designated in the footnote and described in Table 12.3

		Genetic information				
		Single locus	Multiple loci	Single gene	List of genes	No candidates (whole genome)
Disease information	Disease name	3.8, 3.10, 3.19	3.8	3.18		3.2, 3.7, 3.13, 3.15, 3.16, 3.18, 3.19
	Known genes	3.5, 3.6, 3.8, 3.10, 3.11, 3.19, 3.20, 3.21	3.5, 3.8, 3.21		3.5, 3.6, 3.22	3.19, 3.20
	Phenotypic features	3.1, 3.6, 3.9		3.1	3.6	
	Disease-associated keywords	3.1, 3.4, 3.5, 3.6, 3.14, 3.17, 3.19	3.4, 3.5	3.1, 3.3	3.5, 3.6, 3.14	3.4, 3.7, 3.16, 3.17, 3.19
	None				3.12	

3.1, aBandApart and aGeneApart; 3.2, AlignPI and CIPHER; 3.3, BITOLA; 3.4, CANDID; 3.5, Endeavour; 3.6, GeneDistiller; 3.7, Gene Prospector; 3.8, Genes2Diseases (G2D); 3.9, GeneSeeker; 3.10, GeneWanderer; 3.11, Gentrepid; 3.12, GFINDer; 3.13, MimMiner; 3.14, PGMapper; 3.15, PhenoPred; 3.16, PolySearch; 3.17, PosMed; 3.18, SNPs3D; 3.19, SUSPECTS; 3.20, Syndrome To Gene (S2G); 3.21, TOM; 3.22, ToppGene.
Underlined tools are exploratory only, while the remaining tools prioritize candidate genes. Tools that select subsets of likely genes without ranking them are treated as prioritization tools here.

can be used to determine which web servers to consult given the researcher's needs and available data. However, many tools have issues that need to be taken into account when using them. The majority of these tools rely on gene functional annotation data, which are unevenly distributed across genes in the genome, leading to potential bias issues (*see* **Note 1**). Also, for those tools that use training sets, the candidate gene sought may not be adequately represented by the known genes used in the training set (*see* **Note 2**). Given the different strengths and weaknesses of each tool, it is advisable to use several and look for consensus predictions rather than selecting a single one (*see* **Note 3**). Nevertheless, regardless of how many tools predict a given gene, it is wise to bear in mind that these are still just computational predictions and are subject to the associated limitations (*see* **Note 4**). Finally, in addition to these specialized disease gene prediction tools, there are other useful computational tools that the clinical geneticist can use for analyzing candidate genes (*see* **Note 5**) or preprocessing data (*see* **Note 6**) that fall outside the scope of this chapter. In the rest of this section, we give a brief overview of each of these tools (*see* **Table 12.3**).

4. Notes

1. *Effect of annotation bias on predictions*: Annotation bias is an issue that needs to be borne in mind when using these tools, as most predictions rely heavily on annotation (either in the form of literature mining or manual curation). Well-studied genes will be better annotated and therefore more easily prioritized, but the target disease gene might not be well annotated. Indeed, such biased genome coverage is a general phenomenon regardless of data type. And while tools that combine data sources increase their overall coverage, there will still be large differences between the genes in the amount of information available for use in their prioritization. The real disease gene may fail to rank highly due to a lack of data rather than low functional relevance.
2. *Choice of training set genes can affect predictions*: Several tools use sets of known disease genes as training sets for their candidate disease gene prediction. Such training sets determine the kinds of genes that can be detected by the tool, which can be a disadvantage if the unknown disease gene differs substantially from the genes used in the training set (for instance, if it is part of a novel disease pathway). This is something to bear in mind when using tools trained

Table 12.3
Useful computational tools for analyzing candidate genes or preprocessing data

	3.1 aBandApart and aGeneApart	3.2 AlignPI and CIPHER
Home page:	http://tomcat.esat.kuleuven.be/abandapart/, http://tomcatbackup.esat.kuleuven.be/sanger/	http://bioinfo.au.tsinghua.edu.cn/alignpi/, http://bioinfo.au.tsinghua.edu.cn/cipher/cipher_search.html
Help/Tutorial:	Interactive help information in web interface.	http://bioinfo.au.tsinghua.edu.cn/alignpi/help.html, http://bioinfo.au.tsinghua.edu.cn/cipher/help_cipher.html
Summary:	Uses text mining of MEDLINE abstracts and data from other databases to link genes in chromosomal loci (aBandApart), or the whole genome (aGeneApart), to syndrome features.	Both align a phenotype network with a protein–protein interaction network; AlignPI further identifies phenotype modules that map to genetic modules. Disease genes are predicted based on these mappings.
When to use:	Prioritization of genes (aGeneApart) or chromosomal bands (aBandApart) associated with specific phenotypic features, or features associated with specific genes or chromosomal bands.	Prediction of candidate disease genes. If the relevant disease is not in the data set, a phenotypically similar OMIM disease can be used.
Input data:	Genes (Ensembl Gene ID).	Disease (name or OMIM ID), chromosomal locus or gene (HGNC gene symbol).
Updates:	Publication states "regular automated updates". Frequency unclear. aGeneApart is still under development at the time of writing.	Results of specific studies (both in 2008). Not updated.
Comments:	aBandApart was primarily designed for application to inherited chromosomal aberration syndromes. Not applicable to tumors as it maps genes to phenotypic features.	Pre-calculated results for specific sets of OMIM diseases. Approach scales to whole genome, e.g., complex disease GWAS data.
	3.3 BITOLA	3.4 CANDID
Home page:	http://ibmi.mf.uni-lj.si/bitola/	https://dsgweb.wustl.edu/hutz/candid.html
Help/Tutorial:	http://ibmi.mf.uni-lj.si/bitola/	https://dsgweb.wustl.edu/hutz/instructions.html
Summary:	Attempts to link concepts (e.g., diseases and genes) together using literature mining. The intention is to identify previously unrealized links.	Candidate disease gene prioritization tool that utilizes several different data sources.
When to use:	Exploration of candidacy of suspected disease genes.	Prioritization of candidate disease genes for complex diseases.

(continued)

Table 12.3 (continued)

Input data:	Concepts to be linked, e.g., gene and disease names.	GWAS SNPs or linkage loci, genes, literature keywords.
Updates:	Update frequency unclear. Last publication in 2006.	About once or twice per year.
Comments:	Unwieldy to use for large numbers of candidates.	Is specifically designed for complex diseases. Can be used for GWAS data.
	3.5 Endeavour	3.6 GeneDistiller
Home page:	http://homes.esat.kuleuven.be/~bioiuser/endeavour/index.php	http://www.genedistiller.org/
Help/Tutorial:	http://homes.esat.kuleuven.be/~bioiuser/endeavour/help.php	http://www.genedistiller.org/GeneDistiller/manual.html
Summary:	Candidate disease gene prioritization tool that utilizes and combines several different data sources. Scores candidate disease genes based on similarity to known disease genes using these data types.	Integrates gene data from several different data sources, enabling interactive filtering and prioritization based on them.
When to use:	Prioritization of candidate disease genes when known disease genes are available.	Interactive exploration of biological information on candidate disease genes.
Input data:	Known disease genes (training set), candidate loci or genes.	Candidate disease genes.
Updates:	Actively maintained.	Actively maintained.
Comments:	Can be applied to the whole genome as well as to loci or candidate gene lists.	Can be used simply to display various kinds of functional information about candidate genes, or can filter or prioritize them based on user-selected criteria.
	3.7 GeneProspector	3.8 Genes2Diseases (G2D)
Home page:	http://www.hugenavigator.net/HuGENavigator/geneProspectorStartPage.do	http://www.ogic.ca/projects/g2d_2/
Help/Tutorial:	http://www.hugenavigator.net/HuGENavigator/HNDescription/instGenePros.htm	http://www.ogic.ca/projects/g2d_2/info/tutorial.html
Summary:	Uses literature mining of GWA studies to identify links between genes and (complex) diseases.	Prioritizes positional candidate disease genes either by linking candidate genes directly to disease phenotype using literature mining or by using functional links between candidates in one locus and either known disease genes or those in a different candidate locus.
When to use:	Genome-wide prioritization of disease genes based on existing GWAS data.	Prioritization of positional candidate disease genes.

(continued)

Table 12.3 (continued)

Input data:	Disease or risk factor.	Candidate locus/loci, known disease genes or OMIM disease ID.
Updates:	Actively maintained.	Does not appear to be actively updated. Last update March 2007.
Comments:	Is a component of the HuGE Navigator (http://www.hugenavigator.net/), a collection of search and exploration tools for human genetic association and genome epidemiology data.	When using disease phenotype, if the disease is not in G2D's OMIM ID list, an OMIM ID for a similar disease can be used instead. This web tool processes a maximum of two loci at a time.
	3.9 GeneSeeker	3.10 GeneWanderer
Home page:	http://www.cmbi.ru.nl/GeneSeeker/	http://compbio.charite.de/genewanderer/GeneWanderer
Help/Tutorial:	http://www.cmbi.ru.nl/GeneSeeker/help.html	http://compbio.charite.de/genewanderer/tutorial.pdf
Summary:	Predicts positional candidate disease genes by mapping their expression patterns to disease phenotypic features. Also uses mouse data.	Prioritizes candidate disease genes based on their proximity to known disease genes in a gene interaction network. Different proximity measures are available.
When to use:	Prediction of positional candidate disease genes.	Prioritization of positional candidate disease genes when known disease genes are available.
Input data:	Genomic locus, disease phenotypic features.	Chromosomal locus, known disease genes.
Updates:	Website maintained. Dynamically queries external databases, so update frequency is dependent on those databases.	Update frequency unclear (published 2008).
Comments:	Selects a subset of candidate disease genes but does not prioritize them.	The authors tested several proximity measures and found that the random walk approach, which is based on the likelihood of reaching a candidate gene from a known disease gene through randomly chosen paths through the network, worked the best.
	3.11 Gentrepid	3.12 GFINDer
Home page:	http://www.gentrepid.org/	http://www.bioinformatics.polimi.it/gfinder/
Help/Tutorial:	https://www.gentrepid.org/scripts/help.html	http://genoma.bioing.polimi.it/GFINDer_new/eng/tutorial.asp
Summary:	Prioritizes positional candidate disease genes based on the sharing of biochemical pathways or protein domains with known disease genes.	Enables lists of genes, e.g., up- or down-regulated microarray genes, to be explored toward finding which pathways/functional annotation/disease phenotypic features are overrepresented within them.

(continued)

Table 12.3 (continued)

When to use:	Prioritization of positional candidate disease genes when known disease genes are available.	Exploration of functional biology and phenotypic features associated with candidate gene list.
Input data:	Chromosomal locus, known disease genes.	List of genes.
Updates:	Actively maintained.	Actively maintained. Update frequency unclear.
Comments:	Will be able to alternatively use multiple candidate loci and/or known disease genes in the future.	Similar to more general gene functional analysis tools, but includes disease phenotype information as well. Usage scenario similar to that of aBandApart; identifies which genes in a list affect which features.
	3.13 MimMiner	3.14 PGMapper
Home page:	http://www.cmbi.ru.nl/MimMiner/	http://www.genediscovery.org/pgmapper/index.jsp
Help/Tutorial:	http://www.cmbi.ru.nl/MimMiner/help.html	http://www.genediscovery.org/pgmapper/tutorial.html
Summary:	Determines phenotypic similarity between diseases based on shared features.	Maps candidate genes to phenotype-related terms in OMIM or PubMed databases.
When to use:	When identifying which genes are known to cause similar diseases to query disease.	Exploration of phenotypic terms associated with candidate gene list.
Input data:	Disease OMIM ID.	Genomic region or gene list.
Updates:	Maintained, but not regularly updated. Last publication in 2006.	Dynamically queries external databases (Ensembl, OMIM, and PubMed).
Comments:	If relevant disease is not in OMIM, an OMIM ID of a similar disease can be used.	Conceptually somewhat similar to aGeneApart/aBandApart in that it links genes to phenotypes through keyword searches. However, the user can define search terms to use in querying databases and so can explore different term combinations.
	3.15 PhenoPred	3.16 PolySearch
Home page:	http://www.phenopred.org/	http://wishart.biology.ualberta.ca/polysearch/index.htm
Help/Tutorial:	Help information integrated with web interface.	http://wishart.biology.ualberta.ca/polysearch/cgi-bin/help.cgi
Summary:	Predicts gene-disease associations based on several different data types, using the Support Vector Machine algorithm.	Uses text mining to find relationships between genes, diseases, and various other biomedical concepts such as drugs and metabolites.

(continued)

Table 12.3 (continued)

When to use:	Predicting genes that may be involved in a disease, or diseases that may be affected by a gene.	Identifying candidate disease genes associated with a given disease or identifying which diseases may be associated with a given gene.
Input data:	Gene or disease.	Gene or disease (among others).
Updates:	Data sets apparently not being updated. The most recent paper was in 2008.	Some external databases queried dynamically. In-house database update frequency unclear.
Comments:	Uses Disease Ontology instead of OMIM diseases.	Similar to BITOLA.
	3.17 PosMed	3.18 SNPs3D
Home page:	http://omicspace.riken.jp/PosMed/	http://www.snps3d.org/
Help/Tutorial:	http://omicspace.riken.jp/tutorial/HowToUsePosMed_Eng.pdf, http://omicspace.riken.jp/tutorial/HowToUseGPS_Eng.pdf	Help information in web interface (only limited help available).
Summary:	Prioritizes genes in a genomic interval based on their links to phenotypic keywords in MEDLINE literature and other databases. These links are encoded in a neural network-like structure.	Uses literature mining to link genes to diseases or to other genes, and also analyses possible effects of non-synonymous SNPs on protein functions. Gene-gene networks can be browsed.
When to use:	Prioritization of disease candidate genes.	Genome-wide candidate disease gene prioritization. Identifies genes that might be involved in a given disease, or diseases that are associated with a given gene.
Input data:	Genomic region or gene list.	Gene or disease.
Updates:	Website actively maintained. Data update frequency unclear.	Does not appear to be updated anymore. Last update was with dbSNP 128 data in 2008.
Comments:	Uses the GRASE (38) semantic web statistical search engine. A lot of information is provided with the results.	Pre-computed results available for many diseases. The Java runtime environment is required for gene network browsing.
	3.19 SUSPECTS	3.20 Syndrome To Gene (S2G)
Home page:	http://www.genetics.med.ed.ac.uk/suspects/	http://fohs.bgu.ac.il/s2g/index.html
Help/Tutorial:	http://www.genetics.med.ed.ac.uk/suspects/help.shtml	http://fohs.bgu.ac.il/s2g/howto.php
Summary:	Prioritizes candidate disease genes based on similarity to known disease genes using several different data types.	Prioritizes candidate disease genes based on similarity to known disease genes underlying both the query disease and phenotypically similar diseases, using data from 18 databases.

(continued)

Table 12.3 (continued)

When to use:	Prioritization of disease candidate genes.	Prioritization of candidate disease genes, either from specific genomic loci or from the whole genome.
Input data:	Genomic region, or annotation criteria that candidate genes should fulfill.	Known disease genes and (optionally) genomic locus.
Updates:	Not actively updated. It is based on Ensembl version 28 from 2005.	Actively maintained. Update frequency unclear. Latest paper published in 2010.
Comments:	Supersedes PROSPECTR (http://www.genetics.med.ed.ac.uk/prospectr/), which uses fewer data types.	Can also be used to identify phenotypically similar diseases in the OMIM disease database, or functionally related genes using their gene similarity network.
	3.21 TOM	3.22 ToppGene
Home page:	http://www-micrel.deis.unibo.it/~tom/	http://toppgene.cchmc.org/
Help/Tutorial:	http://www-micrel.deis.unibo.it/~tom/modules/tom/manual/index.htm	http://toppgene.cchmc.org/help/help.jsp
Summary:	Uses microarray co-expression and gene function annotation to prioritize positional candidate disease genes based on similarity either between candidate genes from one locus and known disease genes or between candidate genes from two loci.	Prioritizes candidate disease genes based on functional similarity to known disease genes using many different data types, including mouse data.
When to use:	Prioritization of positional candidate disease genes.	Prioritization of candidate disease genes. Candidate disease genes need not necessarily be positional, they could also be, for instance, differentially expressed in patients.
Input data:	Genomic loci and known disease genes.	List of candidate disease genes and of known disease genes.
Updates:	Update frequency unclear. Last publication in 2006.	Actively maintained and frequently updated.
Comments:	Maximally handles two loci at a time. If more loci are available, use different pair combinations.	Suite of related tools which can also be used for prioritization of candidate genes in protein–protein interaction networks (ToppNet) or detection of functional enrichment in gene sets (ToppFun).

on Mendelian disease genes (as these tools generally are) to predict genes for complex diseases.

3. *Use multiple tools, but weigh results appropriately*: It is advisable to use multiple tools and identify which candidate genes are commonly reported by several of them (39–43).

However, bear in mind that there is substantial overlap between many of the tools including which data sources are used, so try to choose complementary tools that use different data types. It is also important to bear in mind that there may be differences between tools in prioritization performance, which can also vary between disease types. Results from tools shown to have higher performance, or those that are more appropriate for the disease at hand, should be given more credence. The Gene Prioritization Portal website (http://www.esat.kuleuven.be/gpp) contains tables that can be used to identify the degree of data type overlap between different tools, as well as providing validation information for several of them.

4. *Consider predictions as suggestions*: Overall, take the output of these tools as suggestions rather than assurances, regardless of what *P*-values the tools assign to the predictions. All tools are benchmarked on known disease genes, and these results may not be representative for novel ones. Furthermore, this could vary from disease to disease. Some tools, e.g., GeneSeeker (44) and Gentrepid (45), have been successfully applied to clinical disease research or association studies (Genes2Diseases (46)), and Endeavour has been successfully applied to candidate gene prioritization in *Drosophila* (47) as well as being retrospectively applied to recently identified disease genes with encouraging results (48). Nevertheless, your mileage may vary. There is no panacea for computational disease gene prediction, and these web servers are simply extra tools in the disease geneticist's toolbox.
5. *Other useful tools for candidate disease gene investigation*: In addition to these specialized candidate disease gene investigation tools, there are other useful but more broadly oriented tools that can be used to gain more insight into disease gene candidacy. Such tools include Ensembl BioMart (http://www.ensembl.org/biomart/martview/), which can be used to filter positional or non-positional candidate genes according to various criteria such as gene function annotation or expression pattern (49). The UCSC table browser (http://genome.ucsc.edu/cgi-bin/hgTables) and Galaxy website (http://main.g2.bx.psu.edu/) also facilitate genome-oriented gene investigation (50). Tools for more general gene function analysis and exploration such as DAVID (http://david.abcc.ncifcrf.gov/) (51), STRING (http://string-db.org/) (52), and iHOP (http://www.ihop-net.org/) (53) can also be used to explore candidate disease gene biology. Finally, non-web server tools which are run locally on the user's computer, such as the candidate

disease gene prioritization tool Prioritizer (25) and the general purpose computational workflow tool Taverna (54), can also be used to investigate candidate genes (55).

6. *Pre-processing input data with Ensembl BioMart*: Tools that require a gene list but which do not accept genomic loci can still be used to prioritize positional candidate genes. Genes located in the disease-associated locus can be retrieved using Ensembl BioMart (http://www.ensembl.org/biomart/martview/) (49), and this gene list can subsequently be used as input for those tools. Furthermore, Ensembl BioMart can also be used to convert gene IDs from one format to another which is useful if a candidate gene prediction tool requires gene IDs in a different format than they already are. For instance, RefSeq mRNA IDs can be converted to Entrez Gene IDs or HGNC gene symbols, and so on. Finally, it can also be applied to retrieve orthologous human genes from model species such as mouse, or vice versa.

Acknowledgments

The authors would like to acknowledge the support of the St. Vincent's Clinic Foundation to M.A.W. and the Australian National Health and Medical Research Council Project Grant 635512 to M.A.W. and M.O.

References

1. Altshuler, D., Daly, M. J., Lander, E. S. (2008) Genetic mapping in human disease. *Science* 322, 881–888.
2. Kann, M. G. (2010) Advances in translational bioinformatics: computational approaches for the hunting of disease genes. *Brief Bioinform* 11, 96–110.
3. Oti, M., Brunner, H. G. (2007) The modular nature of genetic diseases. *Clin Genet* 71, 1–11.
4. Tiffin, N., Andrade-Navarro, M. A., Perez-Iratxeta, C. (2009) Linking genes to diseases: it's all in the data. *Genome Med* 1, 77.
5. van Driel, M. A., Brunner, H. G. (2006) Bioinformatics methods for identifying candidate disease genes. *Hum Genomics* 2, 429–432.
6. Tranchevent, L., Capdevila, F. B., Nitsch, D., De Moor, B., De Causmaecker, P., Moreau, Y. (2010) A guide to web tools to prioritize candidate genes. *Brief Bioinform* 11, 1–11.
7. Yilmaz, S., Jonveaux, P., Bicep, C., et al. (2009) Gene-disease relationship discovery based on model-driven data integration and database view definition. *Bioinformatics* 25, 230–236.
8. Gaulton, K. J., Mohlke, K. L., Vision, T. J. (2007) A computational system to select candidate genes for complex human traits. *Bioinformatics* 23, 1132–1140.
9. Shriner, D., Baye, T. M., Padilla, M. A., et al. (2008) Commonality of functional annotation: a method for prioritization of candidate genes from genome-wide linkage studies. *Nucleic Acids Res* 36, e26.
10. Li, Y., Patra, J. C. (2010) Integration of multiple data sources to prioritize candidate genes using discounted rating system. *BMC Bioinformatics* 11(*Suppl 1*), S20.
11. McEachin, R. C., Keller, B. J. (2009) Identifying hypothetical genetic influences on complex disease phenotypes. *BMC Bioinformatics* 10(*Suppl 2*), S13.

12. Turner, F. S., Clutterbuck, D. R., Semple, C. A. (2003) POCUS: mining genomic sequence annotation to predict disease genes. *Genome Biol* 4, R75.
13. Vanunu, O., Magger, O., Ruppin, E., et al. (2010) Associating genes and protein complexes with disease via network propagation. *PLoS Comput Biol* 6, e1000641.
14. Ala, U., Piro, R. M., Grassi, E., et al. (2008) Prediction of human disease genes by human-mouse conserved coexpression analysis. *PLoS Comput Biol* 4, e1000043.
15. Care, M. A., Bradford, J. R., Needham, C. J., et al. (2009) Combining the interactome and deleterious SNP predictions to improve disease gene identification. *Hum Mutat* 30, 485–492.
16. Freudenberg, J., Propping, P. (2002) A similarity-based method for genome-wide prediction of disease-relevant human genes. *Bioinformatics 18*(*Suppl* 2), S110–115.
17. Karni, S., Soreq, H., Sharan, R. (2009) A network-based method for predicting disease-causing genes. *J Comput Biol* 16, 181–189.
18. Lage, K., Karlberg, E. O., Storling, Z. M., et al. (2007) A human phenome-interactome network of protein complexes implicated in genetic disorders. *Nat Biotechnol* 25, 309–316.
19. Li, Y., Agarwal, P. (2009) A pathway-based view of human diseases and disease relationships. *PLoS One* 4, e4346.
20. Linghu, B., Snitkin, E. S., Hu, Z., et al. (2009) Genome-wide prioritization of disease genes and identification of disease-disease associations from an integrated human functional linkage network. *Genome Biol* 10, R91.
21. Oti, M., Snel, B., Huynen, M. A., Brunner, H. G. (2006) Predicting disease genes using protein-protein interactions. *J Med Genet* 43, 691–698.
22. Oti, M., van Reeuwijk, J., Huynen, M. A., Brunner, H. G. (2008) Conserved co-expression for candidate disease gene prioritization. *BMC Bioinformatics* 9, 208.
23. Tiffin, N., Kelso, J. F., Powell, A. R., et al. (2005) Integration of text- and data-mining using ontologies successfully selects disease gene candidates. *Nucleic Acids Res* 33, 1544–1552.
24. Lopez-Bigas, N., Ouzounis, C. A. (2004) Genome-wide identification of genes likely to be involved in human genetic disease. *Nucleic Acids Res* 32, 3108–3114.
25. Franke, L., van Bakel, H., Fokkens, L., et al. (2006) Reconstruction of a functional human gene network, with an application for prioritizing positional candidate genes. *Am J Hum Genet* 78, 1011–1025.
26. Sadasivam, R. S., Sundar, G., Vaughan, L. K., et al. (2009) Genetic region characterization (Gene RECQuest) – software to assist in identification and selection of candidate genes from genomic regions. *BMC Res Notes* 2, 201.
27. Aerts, S., Lambrechts, D., Maity, S., et al. (2006) Gene prioritization through genomic data fusion. *Nat Biotechnol* 24, 537–544.
28. Hutz, J. E., Kraja, A. T., McLeod, H. L., Province, M. A. (2008) CANDID: a flexible method for prioritizing candidate genes for complex human traits. *Genet Epidemiol* 32, 779–790.
29. Elbers, C. C., van Eijk, K. R., Franke, L., et al. (2009) Using genome-wide pathway analysis to unravel the etiology of complex diseases. *Genet Epidemiol* 33, 419–431.
30. Pan, W. (2008) Network-based model weighting to detect multiple loci influencing complex diseases. *Hum Genet* 124, 225–234.
31. Perry, J. R., McCarthy, M. I., Hattersley, A. T., et al. (2009) Interrogating type 2 diabetes genome-wide association data using a biological pathway-based approach. *Diabetes* 58, 1463–1467.
32. Torkamani, A., Schork, N. J. (2009) Pathway and network analysis with high-density allelic association data. *Methods Mol Biol* 563, 289–301.
33. Torkamani, A., Topol, E. J., Schork, N. J. (2008) Pathway analysis of seven common diseases assessed by genome-wide association. *Genomics* 92, 265–272.
34. Wang, K., Li, M., Bucan, M. (2007) Pathway-Based Approaches for Analysis of Genomewide Association Studies. *Am J Hum Genet* 81, 1278–1283.
35. Ashburner, M., Ball, C. A., Blake, J. A., et al. (2000) Gene ontology: tool for the unification of biology. The Gene Ontology Consortium. *Nat Genet* 25, 25–29.
36. Oti, M., Huynen, M. A., Brunner, H. G. (2008) Phenome connections. *Trends Genet* 24, 103–106.
37. Oti, M., Huynen, M. A., Brunner, H. G. (2009) The biological coherence of human phenome databases. *Am J Hum Genet* 85, 801–808.
38. Kobayashi, N., Toyoda, T. (2008) Statistical search on the Semantic Web. *Bioinformatics* 24, 1002–1010.
39. Elbers, C. C., Onland-Moret, N. C., Franke, L., et al. (2007) A strategy to search for common obesity and type 2 diabetes genes. *Trends Endocrinol Metab* 18, 19–26.

40. Teber, E. T., Liu, J. Y., Ballouz, S., et al. (2009) Comparison of automated candidate gene prediction systems using genes implicated in type 2 diabetes by genome-wide association studies. *BMC Bioinfo* 10(*Suppl 1*), S69.
41. Thornblad, T. A., Elliott, K. S., Jowett, J., Visscher, P. M. (2007) Prioritization of positional candidate genes using multiple web-based software tools. *Twin Res Hum Genet* 10, 861–870.
42. Tiffin, N., Adie, E., Turner, F., et al. (2006) Computational disease gene identification: a concert of methods prioritizes type 2 diabetes and obesity candidate genes. *Nucleic Acids Res* 34, 3067–3081.
43. Tiffin, N., Okpechi, I., Perez-Iratxeta, C., et al. (2008) Prioritization of candidate disease genes for metabolic syndrome by computational analysis of its defining phenotypes. *Physiol Genomics* 35, 55–64.
44. Thiel, C. T., Horn, D., Zabel, B., et al. (2005) Severely incapacitating mutations in patients with extreme short stature identify RNA-processing endoribonuclease RMRP as an essential cell growth regulator. *Am J Hum Genet 77*, 795–806.
45. Sparrow, D. B., Guillen-Navarro, E., Fatkin, D., Dunwoodie, S. L. (2008) Mutation of Hairy-and-Enhancer-of-Split-7 in humans causes spondylocostal dysostosis. *Hum Mol Genet* 17, 3761–3766.
46. Tremblay, K., Lemire, M., Potvin, C., et al. (2008) Genes to diseases (G2D) computational method to identify asthma candidate genes, *PLoS One* 3, e2907.
47. Aerts, S., Vilain, S., Hu, S., et al. (2009) Integrating computational biology and forward genetics in Drosophila. *PLoS Genet* 5, e1000351.
48. Tranchevent, L. C., Barriot, R., Yu, S., et al. (2008) ENDEAVOUR update: a web resource for gene prioritization in multiple species. *Nucleic Acids Res* 36, W377–384.
49. Smedley, D., Haider, S., Ballester, B., et al. (2009) BioMart – biological queries made easy. *BMC Genomics* 10, 22.
50. Woollard, P. M. (2010) Asking complex questions of the genome without programming. *Methods Mol Biol* 628, 39–52.
51. Huang da, W., Sherman, B. T., Lempicki, R. A. (2009) Systematic and integrative analysis of large gene lists using DAVID bioinformatics resources. *Nat Protoc* 4, 44–57.
52. Jensen, L. J., Kuhn, M., Stark, M., et al. (2009) STRING 8 – a global view on proteins and their functional interactions in 630 organisms. *Nucleic Acids Res* 37, D412–416.
53. Hoffmann, R., Valencia, A. (2004) A gene network for navigating the literature. *Nat Genet* 36, 664.
54. Halling-Brown, M., Shepherd, A. J. (2008) Constructing computational pipelines. *Methods Mol Biol* 453, 451–470.
55. Fisher, P., Noyes, H., Kemp, S., et al. (2009) A systematic strategy for the discovery of candidate genes responsible for phenotypic variation. *Methods Mol Biol* 573, 329–345.
56. Van Vooren, S., Thienpont, B., Menten, B., et al. (2007) Mapping biomedical concepts onto the human genome by mining literature on chromosomal aberrations. *Nucleic Acids Res* 35, 2533–2543.
57. Wu, X., Jiang, R., Zhang, M. Q., Li, S. (2008) Network-based global inference of human disease genes. *Mol Syst Biol* 4, 189.
58. Wu, X., Liu, Q., Jiang, R. (2009) Align human interactome with phenome to identify causative genes and networks underlying disease families. *Bioinformatics* 25, 98–104.
59. Hristovski, D., Peterlin, B., Mitchell, J. A., Humphrey, S. M. (2005) Using literature-based discovery to identify disease candidate genes. *Int J Med Inform* 74, 289–298.
60. Seelow, D., Schwarz, J. M., Schuelke, M. (2008) GeneDistiller--distilling candidate genes from linkage intervals. *PLoS One* 3, e3874.
61. Yu, W., Wulf, A., Liu, T., et al. (2008) Gene Prospector: an evidence gateway for evaluating potential susceptibility genes and interacting risk factors for human diseases. *BMC Bioinformatics* 9, 528.
62. Perez-Iratxeta, C., Bork, P., Andrade, M. A. (2002) Association of genes to genetically inherited diseases using data mining. *Nat Genet* 31, 316–319.
63. van Driel, M. A., Cuelenaere, K., Kemmeren, P. P., et al. (2003) A new web-based data mining tool for the identification of candidate genes for human genetic disorders. *Eur J Hum Genet* 11, 57–63.
64. Kohler, S., Bauer, S., Horn, D., Robinson, P. N. (2008) Walking the interactome for prioritization of candidate disease genes. *Am J Hum Genet* 82, 949–958.
65. George, R. A., Liu, J. Y., Feng, L. L., et al. (2006) Analysis of protein sequence and interaction data for candidate disease gene prediction. *Nucleic Acids Res* 34, e130.
66. Masseroli, M., Martucci, D., Pinciroli, F. (2004) GFINDer: Genome Function INtegrated Discoverer through dynamic annotation, statistical analysis, and mining. *Nucleic Acids Res* 32, W293–300.
67. van Driel, M. A., Bruggeman, J., Vriend, G., et al. (2006) A text-mining analysis of the

human phenome. *Eur J Hum Genet* 14, 535–542.

68. Xiong, Q., Qiu, Y., Gu, W. (2008) PGMapper: a web-based tool linking phenotype to genes. *Bioinformatics* 24, 1011–1013.
69. Radivojac, P., Peng, K., Clark, W. T., et al. (2008) An integrated approach to inferring gene-disease associations in humans. *Proteins* 72, 1030–1037.
70. Cheng, D., Knox, C., Young, N., et al. (2008) PolySearch: a web-based text mining system for extracting relationships between human diseases, genes, mutations, drugs and metabolites. *Nucleic Acids Res* 36, W399–405.
71. Yoshida, Y., Makita, Y., Heida, N., et al. (2009) PosMed (Positional Medline): prioritizing genes with an artificial neural network comprising medical documents to accelerate positional cloning. *Nucleic Acids Res* 37, W147–W152.
72. Yue, P., Melamud, E., Moult, J. (2006) SNPs3D: candidate gene and SNP selection for association studies. *BMC Bioinformatics* 7, 166.
73. Adie, E. A., Adams, R. R., Evans, K. L., et al. (2006) SUSPECTS: enabling fast and effective prioritization of positional candidates. *Bioinformatics* 22, 773–774.
74. Gefen, A., Cohen, R., Birk, O. S. (2010) Syndrome to gene (S2G): in-silico identification of candidate genes for human diseases. *Hum Mutat* 31, 229–236.
75. Rossi, S., Masotti, D., Nardini, C., et al. (2006) TOM: a web-based integrated approach for identification of candidate disease genes. *Nucleic Acids Res* 34, W285–292.
76. Chen, J., Bardes, E. E., Aronow, B. J., Jegga, A. G. (2009) ToppGene Suite for gene list enrichment analysis and candidate gene prioritization. *Nucleic Acids Res* 37, W305–W311.

Chapter 13

Comparative View of In Silico DNA Sequencing Analysis Tools

Sissades Tongsima, Anunchai Assawamakin, Jittima Piriyapongsa, and Philip J. Shaw

Abstract

DNA sequencing is an important tool for discovery of genetic variants. The task of detecting single-nucleotide variants is complicated by noise and sequencing artifacts in sequencing data. Several in silico tools have been developed to assist this process. These tools interpret the raw chromatogram data and perform a specialized base-calling and quality-control assessment procedure to identify variants. The approach used to identify variants differs between the tools, with some specific to SNPs and other for Indels. The choice of a tool is guided by the design of the sequencing project and the nature of the variant to be discovered. In this chapter, these tools are compared to facilitate the choice of a tool used for variant discovery.

Key words: DNA sequencing, resequencing, variation, single-nucleotide polymorphism (SNP), Indel, base calling.

1. Introduction

Before the advances in molecular biology, genes were merely abstract units of hereditary known only from the phenotypic expressions of genetic variants (alleles). We now define alleles from variations in DNA sequences. The smallest unit of variation is a change of a single base, either as a substitution (single-nucleotide polymorphism, SNP) or as an insertion/deletion of a base (Indel). A number of in silico tools have been developed to assist in SNP and Indel analysis. Whatever method is used for detecting DNA variants, all putative novel variants must be unequivocally verified by DNA sequencing. Much effort is thus

B. Yu, M. Hinchcliffe (eds.), *In Silico Tools for Gene Discovery*, Methods in Molecular Biology 760,
DOI 10.1007/978-1-61779-176-5_13,

focused toward resequencing genomic regions among cohorts of individuals.

The availability of genome sequences has greatly facilitated the process of DNA variant discovery by the resequencing approach. Novel DNA variants within candidate regions may be rare, in which case the same region may have to be analyzed among several individuals. The "shotgun" approach using next-generation sequencing methods is not appropriate for this task, as most variants discovered would not be within the target region and the cost is still too high to be practical for this application. The conventional/Sanger resequencing approach for variant discovery begins with design of overlapping PCR amplicons for the candidate genomic region from the reference genome sequence. The amplicons are limited to a few hundred base pairs each, since the maximum sequence read length is approximately 800 bp. PCR primers must be designed to specifically amplify the target genomic region and avoid repetitive sequence (including pseudogenes), known SNPs in primers, high GC content, and known copy number variation regions. PCR primer design is facilitated by "in silico PCR" tools, which are described in **Chapters 6** and **18**. Optimal PCR conditions for each primer pair also need to be determined empirically. Once the conditions optimal for each amplicon are known, the amplicons are sequenced using the same primers. Sequencing is carried out by the Sanger method (1) using BigDye terminator reaction chemistry, and bases detected with capillary-based sequencing machines (2).

Fluorescence-based sequencers generate two data files for each sample read, a chromatogram trace file (e.g., .abi, .scf, .alf, .ctf, and .ztr) and a FASTA base-called sequence file. The automatic base-calling procedure used to generate the FASTA sequence translates the different fluorescent intensities from the chromatogram trace file. When more than one base signal is detected at a calling position, the International Union of Pure and Applied Chemistry (IUPAC) ambiguous nucleotide codes are assigned to that position. Since heterozygous individuals are more common than homozygotes, variants typically manifest in chromatogram traces as mixed signals. These signals are misinterpreted by the automatic base-calling procedure as "N", or calling error. Therefore, the automatic base-called sequence is not suitable for variant detection because variants cannot be distinguished from common sequencing artifacts, which include the following: (1) polymerase slippage, resulting in peak overlap, (2) loss of resolution at the beginning and the end of the read, (3) mixed amplicon/contamination, and (4) dye blob in which unused BigDye masks the nucleotide peak signal. The efficiency of nucleotide variation detection thus relies on the accuracy of in silico tools used to interpret the chromatogram traces. The variant detection tools discussed in this chapter perform base calling and then assess the quality of each base call to identify true variants.

The information captured in the chromatogram trace file is merely the intensity of four different wavelengths generated by the laser-excited fluorophores that pass through sequencing capillaries. The signal intensities of each of the four base signals are captured within a base-call array, which store the sampling interval in the trace corresponding to each base position. DNA variant discovery tools must extract different types of signals and make decisions on whether the signal information is of high enough quality to distinguish variants from noise in the input file of chromatograms.

2. Materials

We compare publicly available in silico tools used for DNA variant discovery from sequencing data. **Table 13.1** presents more information about where they can be obtained and their primary references. Commercial tools (i.e. Mutation Surveyor (*see* **Chapter 14**) and Sequencher) are widely used and their properties are compared, where possible, with the freely available tools below.

Table 13.1
Selected list of DNA variant discovery tools, including primary references and the links for software download

Tool	Download link	Reference
PolyBayes	http://bioinformatics.bc.edu/marthlab/Software_Release	(3)
Genalys	http://software.cng.fr/	(4)
SNPDetector	http://lpg.nci.nih.gov/	(5)
novoSNP	http://www.molgen.ua.ac.be/bioinfo/novosnp/	(6)
InSNPs	http://www.mucosa.de/insnp/	(7)
SeqDoC	http://research.imb.uq.edu.au/seqdoc/	(8)
PolyPhred	http://droog.gs.washington.edu/polyphred/	(9)
AutoCSA	http://www.sanger.ac.uk/genetics/CGP/Software/AutoCSA/	(10)
PolyScan	http://genome.wustl.edu/tools/genome_center_software/polyscan	(11)
VarDetect	http://www4a.biotec.or.th/GI/tools/vardetect	(12)
PineSAP	http://dendrome.ucdavis.edu/adept2/pinesap.html	(13)
Mutation Surveyor®	http://www.softgenetics.com/mutationSurveyor.html	–
Sequencher®	http://www.genecodes.com/	–

3. Methods

3.1. Standard Procedure for Variant Detection

The discovery of DNA sequence variants comprises a number of common steps which can be broadly separated into two parts – production of raw sequencing data and identification of DNA variants.

To obtain the sequence data, DNA samples are collected from the designated cohort of individuals, target regions are amplified by PCR, and the amplicons usually sequenced at a DNA sequencing facility. Sequencing the same region on both strands is also standard, but not always performed. For large projects, there is a trade-off between the greater accuracy of bidirectional sequencing and the lower cost of single-pass sequencing.

Once the raw sequencing data are obtained, DNA variants are identified through a standard procedure. First, the base-calling process generates sample nucleotide sequences. The chromatogram signal can be affected by several factors, such as the sensitivity of the allele detection method and the quality of DNA samples, and is frequently found to be ambiguous. Therefore, quality validation is regularly integrated into the base-calling process, in which a quality score is calculated for each base called. Most tools, including the commercial ones, use the well-known Phred quality score in the base-calling process (9). To assure the accuracy of sequences included for further analysis, low-quality base calls are identified and excluded. Low-quality calls predominate at both ends of the sequence read, which are trimmed generating a defined length of high-quality base calls (*see* **Note 1**). Most tools trim the sequences automatically, with the trimming controlled by user-defined thresholds based on Phred scores. Commercial tools offer more options for trimming (*see* **Note 1**), the trimming boundaries can be visualized, and common artifacts can be automatically removed, e.g. primer/dye blob removal in Sequencher. The next step is sequence alignment and comparison of sample reads against the reference sequence. The commercial tools have a chief advantage over the academic tools for this part of the process, since they can automatically perform the contiguous sequence (contig) assembly by aligning reads from both forward and reverse orientations simultaneously. Most academic tools do not perform contig assembly and rely on other tools to perform this task. Hence, they are less convenient to use, especially for large projects. The base calls from sample-generated sequences that do not match with the reference sequence are highlighted as putative DNA variants. The commercial tools have built-in patented variant detection algorithms (e.g., Mutation Surveyor's anti-correlation technology) which automatically flag the variants, without the need for user intervention to assess the confidence of prediction.

In the past few years, several computational algorithms have been developed to accelerate SNP discovery by increasing the efficiency and accuracy of raw sequence data analysis. Although these programs share the aforementioned standard analysis procedure, they come with various features and parameters which users can choose to match their specific needs and experimental design. The comparative factors in which users should take into consideration for in silico tool selection include pooling of samples, accuracy, detection of Indels, the reference sequence, database cross-checking, and reporting.

3.2. Pooling of Samples

Depending on the cohort sample size, researchers should decide whether to pool DNA samples or not. DNA pooling is a way to reduce sequencing costs when a large number of individuals and SNPs are analyzed. By this means, equal amounts of genomic DNA from individual samples are pooled together prior to the generation of PCR amplicons. The greater potential for ambiguous signals in pooled DNA samples means that the power to detect variants is lower, particularly for rare variants. Furthermore, allele frequency cannot be calculated except when samples are pooled into pairs. The allele frequency of pooled pairs can be estimated by quantification of peak heights of sequence trace. Reading signals from pooled pairs generates five distinct combinations of chromatogram signals. For a given SNP locus, the five outcomes are as follows: (1) both samples are homozygous wild type; (2) both samples are homozygous variant type; (3) one sample is homozygous wild type and the other is homozygous variant type; (4) one sample is homozygous wild type and the other is heterozygous; and (5) one sample is homozygous variant type and the other is heterozygous. Most SNP detection tools are designed for analysis of non-pooled samples; however, a few programs such as Genalys (4) and VarDetect (12) can analyze the input trace sequences obtained from pooled DNA. The commercial tool Mutation Surveyor has an additional feature for analyzing pooled samples not provided by other tools, e.g., somatic mutation detection, mutation quantification, and methylation analysis. In these examples, the pooled samples are typically pooled tissues or cell types from one individual in which accurate quantification of variant frequencies is the focus.

3.3. Base-Calling Accuracy

To guarantee the success of SNP discovery, the critical part is to obtain accurate sequence information. The base-called sequence data are scrutinized to remove data of unacceptable quality. The accuracy of base calling is usually calculated from several parameters including peak spacing and uncalled/called peak resolution. Ideally, the chromatogram trace should have well-defined, evenly spaced peaks and minimum noise. To correctly detect variants, one must be able to distinguish sequencing artifacts from the true variant signals.

Most SNP discovery tools incorporate a base-calling algorithm into their framework for identifying nucleotide sequence from raw chromatogram data. Phred (14, 15) is the most widely used base-calling program, which is also frequently incorporated into SNP discovery tools such as PolyBayes (3), SNPDetector (5), novoSNP (6), PolyPhred (9, 14), and PineSAP (13). Phred reads trace sequence files and assigns a base-specific quality score, which is a log-transformed error probability. The error probability is calculated by examining the peaks around each base call.

Average peak spacing (base-calling bin adjustment) and peak height are common features that are used by Genalys, PolyScan (11), and VarDetect for variant detection. Heuristics are employed by these tools to differentiate variants from sequence artifact mixed peak signals. Furthermore, instead of using Phred quality, these tools (except PolyScan) introduce a quality estimation scheme to be used along with their variant detection heuristics. Genalys strives to generalize SNP variant bases by taking into account the average nucleotide peak height from all samples and the influence of the preceding base on peak height. To detect a variant, the observed peak height is compared with the average peak height of the previous three nucleotides (of the same type). SNPs are called when the peak height drops significantly.

VarDetect does not make use of the peak height information but rather focuses on what the peak shape of a true variant should look like. It also focuses on adjusting the interval in which a base call is to be made. Slippage can increase nucleotide signal at the base-call position, thus leading to potential ambiguity in the peak signal. This artifact is automatically detected and disregarded as a variant by VarDetect. This strategy enables VarDetect to properly adjust base-call spacing (bin adjustment) at positions for which standard base calling algorithms may have marked as unreadable, i.e., reported as "N". While the majority of tools employ a modified base-calling procedure accompanied by a quality score assessment, a few tools such as InSNPs (7) and SeqDoC (8) do not include this module. InSNPs uses the automatic sequencer base-call results and prompts the user to identify SNPs from a candidate list. SeqDoC does not make base calls but rather highlights putative variants by direct comparison of the chromatogram traces between sample and designated reference data.

3.4. Detecting Indel Variations

Insertions or deletions (Indels) are common variations, although it is not yet clear how common, since methods to detect them are not as accurate as for SNPs. A heterozygous sample with an Indel variant generates a mixed-trace chromatogram pattern immediately 3′ to the Indel (*see* **Note 2**). It is difficult to distinguish this pattern from sequence artifact, in particular low-quality read regions at the end of the trace. Indels can be detected reliably by allele-specific amplification, but this solution is expensive and not practical. Computational approaches have been introduced for discovery of Indels from mixed-trace patterns. To identify Indel variants from the mixed trace, the trace corresponding to the reference sequence is subtracted from the continuous mixed trace. The commercial tool CodonCode Aligner uses this approach, whereas the commercial Mutation Surveyor detects Indels using the patented anti-correlation technology. Similar reference subtraction approaches have been adopted by academic variant detection tools including PolyPhred, STADEN (16), novoSNP, InSNP (7), PolyScan, and AutoCSA (10). The accuracy of the sequence subtraction heuristic relies heavily on the reference sequence used. The reference sequence is a consensus of several sequences, which may not be representative of the cohort under investigation. If the reference sequence differs from both alleles, reconstruction (extraction) of the mixed sequence is not possible. Newer in silico tools try to reconstruct continuous mixed sequences without using a reference sequence but rather perform the extraction directly from the mixed traces. These tools include Shift-Detector (17), the newer version of CodonCode Aligner, and Indelligent (18).

3.5. The Reference Sequence (RefSeq)

The detection of DNA sequence variation relies on sequence alignment and identification of base differences from a reference. Poor initial alignments can greatly increase the error rate of DNA variant prediction. Therefore, local alignment methods, e.g. Smith–Waterman algorithm (19) or BLAST (20), are used for this task because they avoid misalignment due to low quality of some sequence regions. Sample sequences are aligned with the genomic reference sequence, which is obtained from a public database for well-annotated genomes. Most variant detection tools require the existing genome reference sequence for identifying putative DNA variants, for example, PolyBayes, SNPDetector, novoSNP, InSNPs, PolyPhred, AutoCSA, PolyScan, VarDetect, and PineSAP. The advantage of using the genomic reference is that the homozygous variant form can be detected. However, the drawback of using the genomic reference is that it may not be representative of the population under investigation. Some nucleotide positions containing the same base in all cohort individuals may be misinterpreted as DNA variants in comparison with the genomic reference. In this case, the nucleotide is not a variant for the sample population. Instead of using a reference, a few tools, e.g. SeqDoC, avoid this problem by automatically selecting a chromatogram trace from the cohort to be the reference. The commercial Mutation Surveyor tool has a special reference sequence feature, in which a synthetic trace is generated from the nucleotide sequence using a proprietary algorithm. This synthetic reference trace is used for quantification of variant frequency, a feature not offered by other tools.

Table 13.2
The feature comparison of DNA variant detection tools

	1999	2002	2005				2006	2007		2008	2009
	PolyBayes	**Genalys**	**SNPDetector**	**novoSNP**	**InSNPs**	**SeqDoC**	**PolyPhred**	**AutoCSA**	**PolyScan**	**VarDetect**	**PineSAP**
Sample DNA											
Overlap fragment (Batch)	/	x	/	/	/	X	/	x	/	/	/
Make use of bidirectional trace	x	/	/	/	/	X	/	x	/	/	/
Two-pooled DNA	x	/	x	x	x	X	x		x	/	x
Base calling											
Algorithm	Phred	Local heuristic	Phred	Phred	x	X	Phred	/	Local heuristic	Local heuristic	Phred
Quality score	Phred	x	Phred	Phred	x	X	Phred	/	x	Local heuristic	Phred
Peak correction	x	Local heuristic	x	x	x	X	x	x	x	Local heuristic	x
SNP identification											
Algorithm	Bayesian inference	Signal ratio peak height	Neighborhood quality	Feature score	Cross-reference	Difference profile	Error probabilities	Peak height	Horizontal/ vertical	Codemap	PolyPhred, PolyBayes with ML
Require RefSeq	/	x	/	/	/	X	/	/	/	/	/

Table 13.2
(Continued)

Indel identification											
Indel algorithm	x	x	x	/	/	/	/	/	/	x	/
Require RefSeq	x	x	x	/	/	/	/	/	/	/	/
Data reporting											
Allele calculation	x	/	x	x	x	X	x	x	x	/	x
Automated sequence annotation	x	x	x	/	x	X	x	x	x	x	x
Data editing	CONSED	x	/	/	/	X	/	/	/	/	x
Usage and platform											
Operation system	UNIX	Mac, Windows	UNIX, Linux	Mac, Windows, UNIX	Windows	Web	Mac OS, Windows, UNIX	Mac OS, Windows, UNIX	Mac, Linux, UNIX	Mac, Windows, UNIX	Web
Easy installation	/	/	/	/	/	x	/	x	/	/	x
Graphic interface	/	/	/	/	/	/	/ with CONSED	/	/	/	x
Command line	x	x	/	/	/	x	/	/	/	/	/

x, not available; /, available

3.6. Database Cross-checking

A number of free public archives have been established to deposit genetic variation data, e.g., dbSNP and Database of Genomic Variants (DGV). If several variants are discovered, it can be laborious to manually cross-check the databases to determine if variants are novel. This cross-checking procedure is facilitated by tools such as SNP BLAST (*see* **Note 3**). The VarDetect tool is linked to the ThaiSNP database, allowing download of the SNP-annotated genomic reference sequence. Users can then visualize the positions of putative SNPs from their data and compare them with the known SNPs of the reference sequence.

3.7. Reporting

All genetic variation detection tools provide reports of putative SNPs and Indels, although the information shown varies. The commercial tools have a great advantage over the academic tools since they have graphical cross-linked displays, allowing intuitive navigation through the whole project-analyzed dataset. A number of programs allow data editing, since automatic procedures may fail to detect some ambiguous signals as variants or conversely may report false positives. In addition to the commercial tools, some academic tools offer data editing, i.e., SNPDetector, novoSNP, InSNPs, PolyPhred, AutoCSA, PolyScan, and VarDetect. The feature comparison of different academic variant detection programs is demonstrated in **Table 13.2**.

4. Notes

Detecting sequence variants using in silico tools is quite straightforward. On the other hand, the accuracy of detection is dependent on several factors, such as the quality of input data, the nature of the variant being detected, and the algorithm used to detect the variant. Finally, putative variants must be cross-checked to determine if they are novel.

1. Assessing chromatogram patterns and trimming reads

   High-quality sequencing data are obviously essential for variant detection. It is recommended to divide the region of interest into fragments of 500–800 bp with at least 30 bases of overlap. Overlap is needed to overcome the problem of low-quality signals at the beginning and the end of the trace. Sequencing both strands (bidirectional traces) is also preferred for most in silico tools to minimize the number of false positives. Once the raw data have been collected, the first step is to assess the overall quality of each trace. Shown below are some common chromatogram patterns that the user should be able to recognize from their data. The pattern also guides the choice of an in silico tool to be used for variant detection. Chromatogram trace external viewer programs, such as Phred, 4Peaks (21), BioEdit (22), and FinchTV (23), are excellent tools for assessing trace raw data. Commercial tools have built-in raw data visualization interfaces, which effortlessly link to the variant detection modules. Furthermore, although these commercial tools cannot be used for the entire variant process without payment, they do have free trial evaluation. With this option, the visualization tools in them can be used to assist the raw data processing for variant discovery using another academic tool, e.g., for validation of variant prediction. Raw data viewers can also generate reverse complement patterns, which are very useful for assessing bidirectional data. The first trace example shown below is typical, in which well-resolved peaks are observed throughout the majority of the trace and most automatic base calls have high scores (**Fig. 13.1a**). From this type of data, SNP variants can be detected. In the second trace example, the read length of automatic base calls with high scores is truncated prematurely at the 3′-end (**Fig. 13.1b, c**). In this type of data, Indel variants may exist. However, if the peaks are uniformly low in height and the automatic base calls have low scores

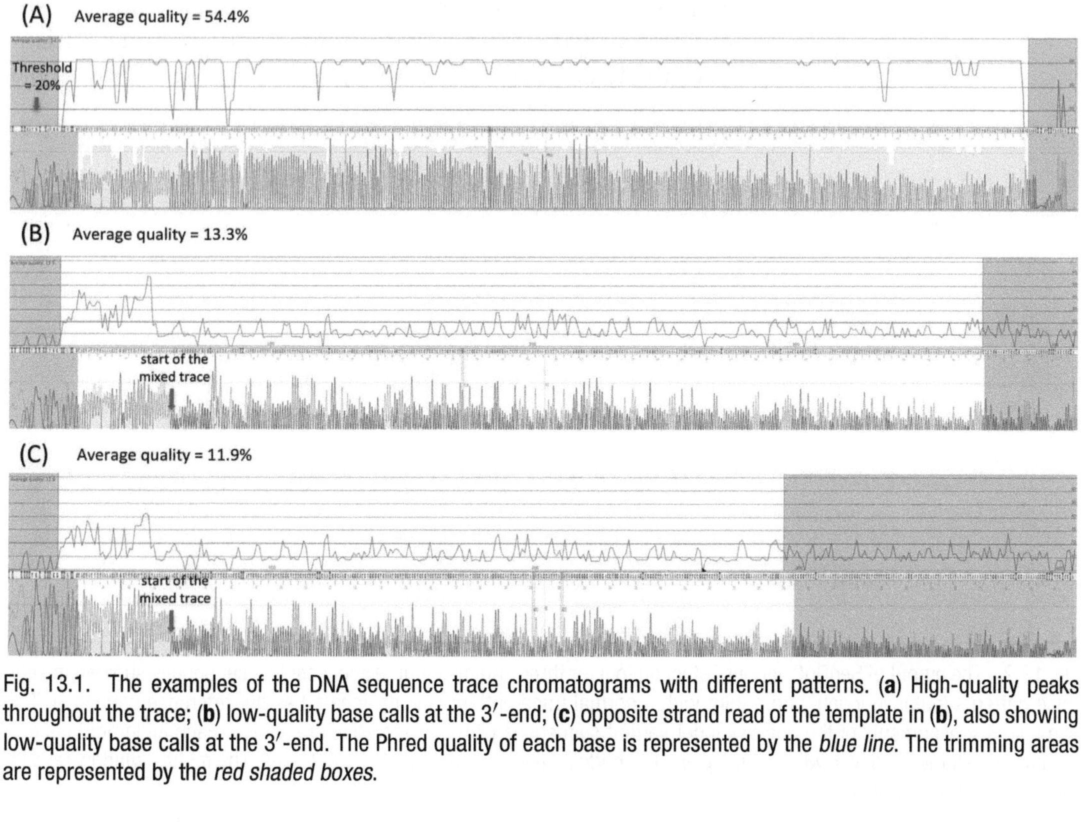

Fig. 13.1. The examples of the DNA sequence trace chromatograms with different patterns. (**a**) High-quality peaks throughout the trace; (**b**) low-quality base calls at the 3′-end; (**c**) opposite strand read of the template in (**b**), also showing low-quality base calls at the 3′-end. The Phred quality of each base is represented by the *blue line*. The trimming areas are represented by the *red shaded boxes*.

throughout, the data are probably unacceptable for variant detection and should be discarded.

In silico tools for SNP detection mask or trim the ends of the data before performing SNP detection. A threshold quality score is chosen for trimming. A default score is incorporated into each tool, removing the need for the user to select a score. However, the default score may not be suitable for every experiment; hence, a better way is to acquire an appropriate cutoff from the trace data. By viewing input sequences using sequence viewer programs, users can estimate the threshold to be used in variant detection. **Figure 13.1** shows three sample sequences of the *ESR* (estrogen receptor) gene from 400-bp amplicons, in which the 4Peaks program was used to visualize the traces. The first trace has an average Phred quality of 54.4% (**Fig. 13.1a**). 4Peaks allows us to visualize the trimming boundaries, which are varied according to the trimming threshold (set to 20% in all sample traces and shown by the red horizontal line).

Close attention should be paid to the traces in **Fig. 13.1b, c**. The overall quality drops to 13.3%. The trimming at the 3′-end appears to be much larger than that of the 5′-end. After observing the trace closely, the trace immediately after the 5′ trimming box has a short stretch with Phred scores well above the 20% threshold (bases 21–58). Immediately 3′ of this region, the Phred scores are below the threshold and a mixed-trace pattern is apparent. An Indel variant may exist, accounting for this pattern. If the bidirectional

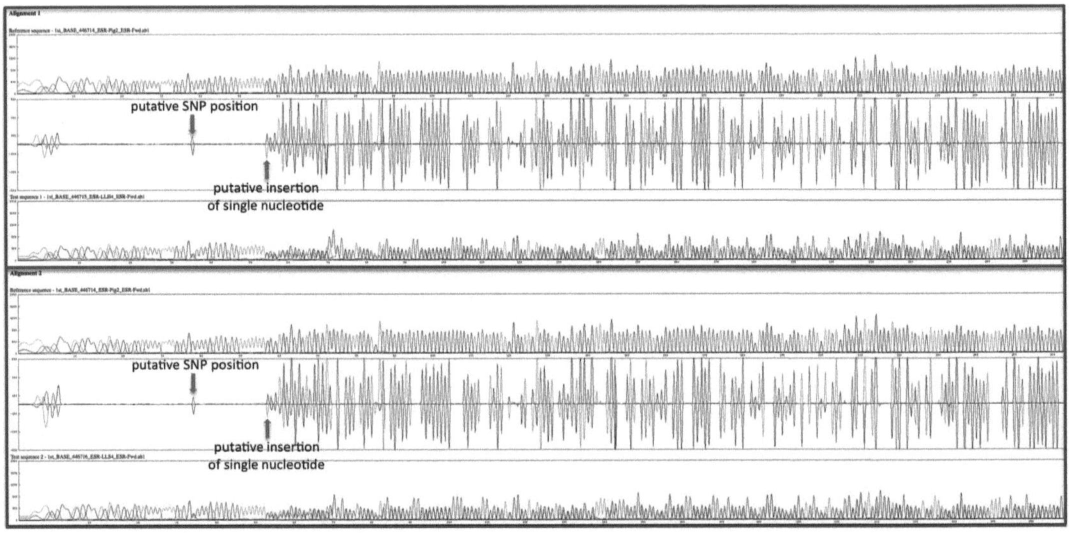

Fig. 13.2. The output of SeqDoC variant detection tool for three sample input sequences: two sequences showed mixed-trace patterns (putative Indel), and a third with a normal trace pattern was designated as the reference sequence. The two pairwise alignments of the putative Indel-variant sequences with the reference are shown. Each alignment pane is structured in three windows, where the *top* and the *bottom* windows present the input traces. The middle window reveals the trace subtraction result.

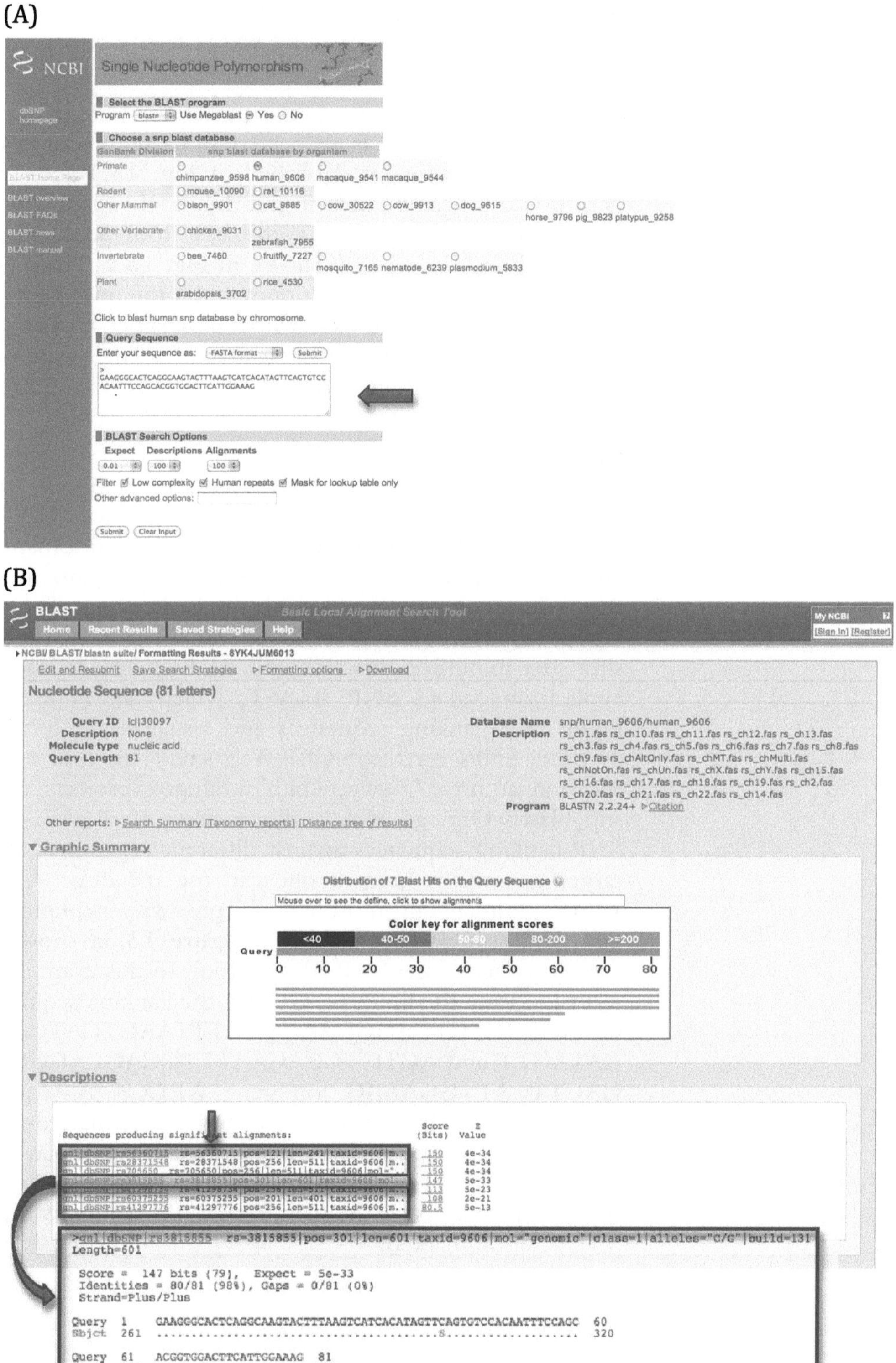

Fig. 13.3. Similarity search for known SNPs deposited in the SNP database using the SNP BLAST tool. (**a**) Snapshot of the SNP BLAST main page. SNP flanking sequences are requested as input. (**b**) The output of SNP BLAST showing the list of SNP rs IDs with high-scoring matches to the input.

sequence of this trace is available (as is the case shown in **Fig. 13.1c**), the same mixed-trace pattern is observed on the other strand.

2. Indel detection from mixed-trace patterns

   If an Indel variant is suspected from the characteristic mixed-trace patterns as described in **Fig. 13.1b, c**, Indel detection tools can be used to test the Indel-variant hypothesis. In this example, the Web-based tool SeqDoC was employed and the result is shown in **Fig. 13.2**. From position 57 onward, the subtraction extracts the mixed trace of the two overlapping traces, whose intensities mirror each other. This result is highly suggestive of a single base deletion at position 56. Furthermore, an SNP at position 38 was also detected.

3. Cross-checking against known variants

   SNP detection tools report putative SNPs in their genomic sequence context by showing the SNP and flanking sequence. Currently, no tool can automatically cross-check against SNP databases to determine if discovered variants are novel. This cross-checking process is laborious, since users must search multiple database Web sites. To minimize this task, NCBI has provided a Web application, called SNP BLAST, which allows users to input SNP flanking sequences and visualize the locations of these SNPs on the NCBI Web site. This tool can be accessed at http://www.ncbi.nlm.nih.gov/projects/SNP/snp_blastByOrg.cgi, which allows users to BLAST their SNP flanking sequences against different organisms. If the target genome is human, one can use the direct link to BLAST human chromosomes (http://www.ncbi.nlm.nih.gov/SNP/snpblastByChr.html). **Figure 13.3a** shows the Web interface of the SNP BLAST tool. In this example, we want to locate the SNP (C/G) with the flanking sequences: GAAGGGCACTCAGGCAAGTACTTTAAGTCATCA-CATAGTT and AGTGTCCACAATTTCCAGCACGGTG-GACTTCATTGGAAAG, on gene *XRCC5*. A sequence comprising of SNP allele C with 5′ and 3′ flanking sequences is used as an input. The BLAST result is displayed in **Fig. 13.3b**. rs3815855 is identified as a known SNP in the query sequence, as can be seen from the alignment with the SNP position marked.

References

1. Sanger, F., Nicklen, S., Coulson, A. R. (1992) DNA sequencing with chain-terminating inhibitors. 1977, *Biotechnology* **24,** 104–108.

2. MacBeath, J. R., Harvey, S. S., Oldroyd, N. J. (2001) Automated fluorescent DNA sequencing on the ABI PRISM 377, *Methods Mol Biol* **167**, 119–152.

3. Marth, G. T., Korf, I., Yandell, M. D., Yeh, R. T., Gu, Z., Zakeri, H., Stitziel, N. O., Hillier, L., Kwok, P. Y., Gish, W. R. (1999) A general approach to single-nucleotide polymorphism discovery, *Nat Genet* **23**, 452–456.
4. Takahashi, M., Matsuda, F., Margetic, N., Lathrop, M. (2003) Automated identification of single nucleotide polymorphisms from sequencing data, *J Bioinform Comput Biol* **1**, 253–265.
5. Zhang, J., Wheeler, D. A., Yakub, I., Wei, S., Sood, R., Rowe, W., Liu, P. P., Gibbs, R. A., Buetow, K. H. (2005) SNPdetector: a software tool for sensitive and accurate SNP detection, *PLoS Comput Biol* **1**, e53.
6. Weckx, S., Del-Favero, J., Rademakers, R., Claes, L., Cruts, M., De Jonghe, P., Van Broeckhoven, C., De Rijk, P. (2005) novoSNP, a novel computational tool for sequence variation discovery, *Genome Res* **15**, 436–442.
7. Manaster, C., Zheng, W., Teuber, M., Wachter, S., Doring, F., Schreiber, S., Hampe, J. (2005) InSNP: a tool for automated detection and visualization of SNPs and InDels, *Hum Mutat* **26**, 11–19.
8. Crowe, M. L. (2005) SeqDoC: rapid SNP and mutation detection by direct comparison of DNA sequence chromatograms, *BMC Bioinformatics* **6**, 133.
9. Ewing, B., Green, P. (1998) Base-calling of automated sequencer traces using Phred. II. Error probabilities, *Genome Res* **8**, 186–194.
10. Dicks, E., Teague, J. W., Stephens, P., Raine, K., Yates, A., Mattocks, C., Tarpey, P., Butler, A., Menzies, A., Richardson, D., Jenkinson, A., Davies, H., Edkins, S., Forbes, S., Gray, K., Greenman, C., Shepherd, R., Stratton, M. R., Futreal, P. A., Wooster, R. (2007) AutoCSA, an algorithm for high throughput DNA sequence variant detection in cancer genomes, *Bioinformatics* **23**, 1689–1691.
11. Chen, K., McLellan, M. D., Ding, L., Wendl, M. C., Kasai, Y., Wilson, R. K., Mardis, E. R. (2007) PolyScan: an automatic indel and SNP detection approach to the analysis of human resequencing data, *Genome Res* **17**, 659–666.
12. Ngamphiw, C., Kulawonganunchai, S., Assawamakin, A., Jenwitheesuk, E., Tongsima, S. (2008) VarDetect: a nucleotide sequence variation exploratory tool, *BMC Bioinformatics* **9** *Suppl 12*, S9.
13. Wegrzyn, J. L., Lee, J. M., Liechty, J., Neale, D. B. (2009) PineSAP – sequence alignment and SNP identification pipeline, *Bioinformatics* **25**, 2609–2610.
14. Bhangale, T. R., Stephens, M., Nickerson, D. A. (2006) Automating resequencing-based detection of insertion-deletion polymorphisms, *Nat Genet* **38**, 1457–1462.
15. Nickerson, D. A., Tobe, V. O., Taylor, S. L. (1997) PolyPhred: automating the detection and genotyping of single nucleotide substitutions using fluorescence-based resequencing, *Nucleic Acids Res* **25**, 2745–2751.
16. Staden, R. (1996) The Staden sequence analysis package, *Mol Biotechnol* **5**, 233–241.
17. Seroussi, E., Ron, M., Kedra, D. (2002) ShiftDetector: detection of shift mutations, *Bioinformatics* **18**, 1137–1138.
18. Dmitriev, D. A., Rakitov, R. A. (2008) Decoding of superimposed traces produced by direct sequencing of heterozygous indels, *PLoS Comput Biol* **4**, e1000113.
19. Smith, T. F., Waterman, M. S. (1981) Identification of common molecular subsequences, *J Mol Biol* **147**, 195–197.
20. Altschul, S. F., Gish, W., Miller, W., Myers, E. W., Lipman, D. J. (1990) Basic local alignment search tool, *J Mol Biol* **215**, 403–410.
21. http://mekentosj.com/science/4peaks/
22. http://www.mbio.ncsu.edu/bioedit/bioedit.html
23. http://www.geospiza.com/Products/finchtv.shtml

Chapter 14

Mutation Surveyor: An In Silico Tool for Sequencing Analysis

Chongmei Dong and Bing Yu

Abstract

DNA sequencing is widely used for DNA diagnostics and functional studies of genes of interest. With significantly increased sequencing outputs, manual reading of sequence results can impede an efficient and accurate analysis. Mutation Surveyor is a useful in silico tool developed by SoftGenetics that assists the detection of sequence variations within Sanger sequencing traces. This tool can process up to 400 lanes of data at a time with high accuracy and sensitivity. It can effectively detect SNPs and indels in their homozygous or heterozygous states as well as mosaicism. In this chapter, we describe the general application of Mutation Surveyor for DNA sequencing analysis and its unique features.

Key words: DNA sequence, in silico variant detection, single nucleotide polymorphism (SNP), indel, mosaicism.

1. Introduction

Since the completion of the human genome sequence and other genome sequences, functional characterisation of genes has become an important challenge. The study of sequence variations and their associated functional changes or disease phenotypes is an effective way of examining the wider fields of functional genomics and clinical genetics. To date, disease-causing alleles and susceptibility SNPs have been identified in 2106 different diseases (1). DNA testing is therefore widely used for clinical diagnosis and carrier screening. Similarly in plants, the completion of *Arabidopsis* and rice genome sequences allowed the rapid development of reverse genetic strategies for gene functional analysis. Targeting-induced local lesions in genomes (so-called TILLING) is a reverse genetic method which allows large-scale screening of chemically

B. Yu, M. Hinchcliffe (eds.), *In Silico Tools for Gene Discovery*, Methods in Molecular Biology 760, DOI 10.1007/978-1-61779-176-5_14,

induced mutations in plants (2). A series of different mutations in a gene of interest can be mined for their functions through phenotypic correlations. DNA sequencing is a gold standard for determining the exact nature of a mutation and has become increasingly important in diagnostic and research applications. Manual analysis of DNA sequence traces (i.e. electropherograms) is labour intensive, time consuming and error prone, especially when a large-scale experiment is performed. There is a need for accurate and rapid analysis tools for assistance in variant detection.

A number of commercial software packages (e.g. Mutation Surveyor, SeqScape, VarDetect, PolyPhred and Sequencher) have been developed for computer-assisted detection of heterozygous and homozygous mutations. However, a comparison of these software programs is beyond the scope of this chapter and interested readers can find the relevant information in **Chapter 13** and references (3–7). In this chapter, we focus on the application of Mutation Surveyor v3.20 (SoftGenetics, Philadelphia, PA, USA) for Sanger sequencing analysis and demonstrate its useful features by using the human low-density lipoprotein receptor (*LDLR*) gene and wheat starch synthase II (*SSII*) gene as examples.

2. Features of Mutation Surveyor Software

A prominent feature of Mutation Surveyor is that it does not rely on base calling from other third-party algorithms. Instead, it compares every physical trace using its own patented anti-correlation technology to perform sequence analysis on both bi-directional and uni-directional sequence data (8). This comparison technology can rapidly locate all differences between the wild-type sequence (reference sequence) and sample traces with excellent accuracy and sensitivity (*see* **Note 1**). More than 99.59% sensitivity (with 95% confidence) has been reported for uni-directional analysis of heterozygous base substitutions (3).

Mutation Surveyor can automatically align and assemble contigs and perform mutation analysis on up to 400 lanes of sequencing data simultaneously in approximately 2 min. It has variant detection sensitivity down to 5% of the primary peak with accuracy greater than 99% in the bi-directional analysis mode. This software has enhanced indel detection at the size range of 1–100 bp with automatic de-convolution of heterozygous indel traces into two clean traces. It can analyse methylation results and detect mosaicism or somatic mutations at cellular levels as low as 20%. Mutation Surveyor is compatible with different formats of sequencing results including [.scf], [.ab1]/[.abi] and [.gz] that are generated from most available DNA sequencers (*see* **Note 2**) and is capable of aligning sequences regardless of sequence quality or text call accuracy. This in silico tool can also provide variant description that is accurate and compliant with nomenclature recommendations from the Human Genome Variation Society (HGVS, http://www.hgvs.org). Other features include GenBank/sequence file editor; automatic GenBank search; sequence data file format conversion; sequence data quality assessment; base call edit; mutation confidence level indication (mutation score) and various report formats including a custom report builder.

3. Methods

3.1. Application Overview

The general application procedure of Mutation Surveyor is summarised in a flowchart (**Fig. 14.1**). Mutation Surveyor starts with a graphic page with information including the version and type (stand alone or network) of the software and a simple menu bar. A new project can simply be established using the "Open Files" function from the "File" menu (**Fig. 14.2a**) and then the GenBank, reference and sample files can be imported into the new project (more details in **Section 3.2**) by clicking the "Add". The imported files will appear on the left pane and the original trace(s) associated with the samples can be called up by double-clicking on a file name.

After the files are imported, one can click on "Options..." from the "Process" menu to select or change the default settings (more details in **Section 3.3**) and then analyse the imported files by clicking the "Run" on the "Process" menu or the "Run"

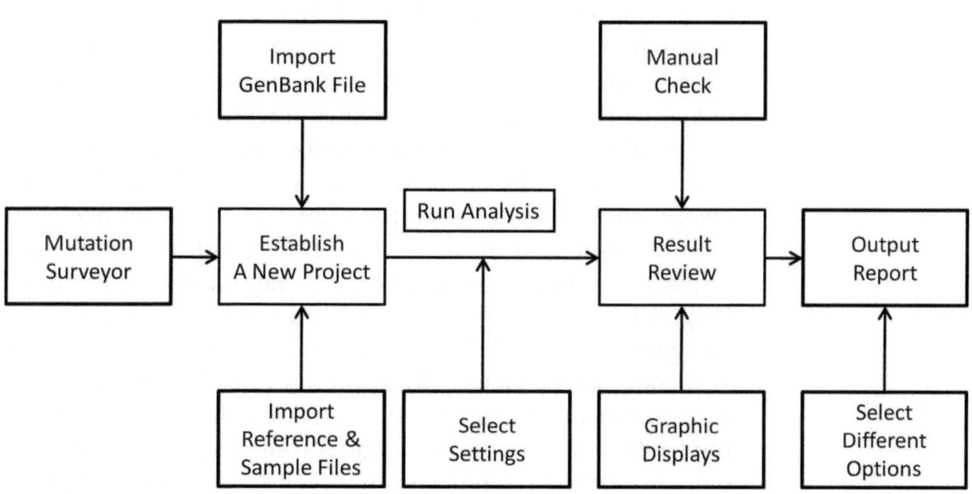

Fig. 14.1. A flowchart showing the general procedures for DNA variant analysis in Sanger sequence traces using Mutation Surveyor.

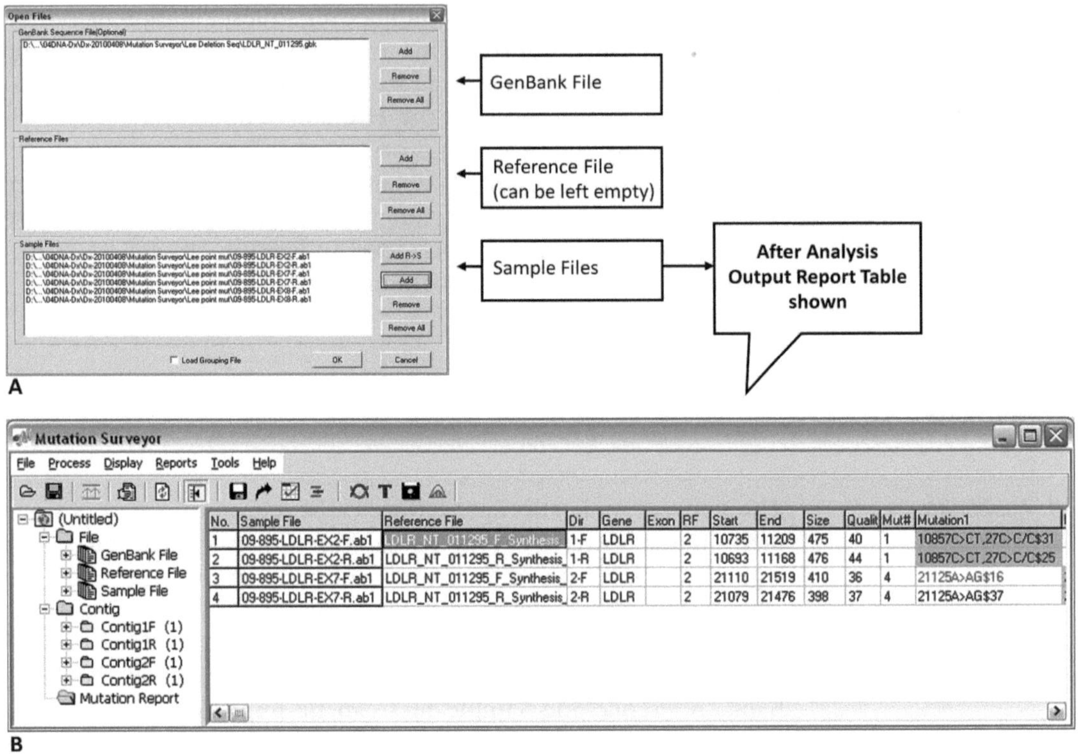

Fig. 14.2. The "Open File" window for file import from GenBank, reference and test samples (**a**). The main project window after the data analysis (**b**). The *left pane* shows all the imported files in a directory/folder structure (File Tree Frame). The mutation report (Output Report Table) on the *right pane* presents the main results with hyperlinks to the analysed sequence trace data in a graphical form, which can be viewed by clicking on any mutations or files.

icon on the tool bar. The results will be arranged into a file tree frame on the left pane and a mutation report (output report table, ORT) on the right pane (**Fig. 14.2b**). Various ORTs can be generated by selecting from the "Reports" menu. An ORT shows all the mutations found during the analysis and they are hyperlinked to their respective sequence traces. One can easily review the graphical analysis display window by clicking any mutations of interest and edit a base or a mutation (*see* **Note 3**). Graphical display shows traces of sample sequence and reference sequence with the mutation in the centre of the window. The mutation is displayed by a peak rising above a threshold in the mutation trace (**Fig. 14.3**). Other parts of analysed sequence can be viewed by navigating the scroll bar above the sequence traces. The whole sequence can be viewed by zooming out (**Fig. 14.4**). Sequence text output can be displayed by clicking the text output icon on the tool bar so that all the fragments are aligned to the GenBank sequence or the reference sequence, and the identified mutations are highlighted with a different colour (**Fig. 14.5**). The project can be saved as a [*.sgp] file.

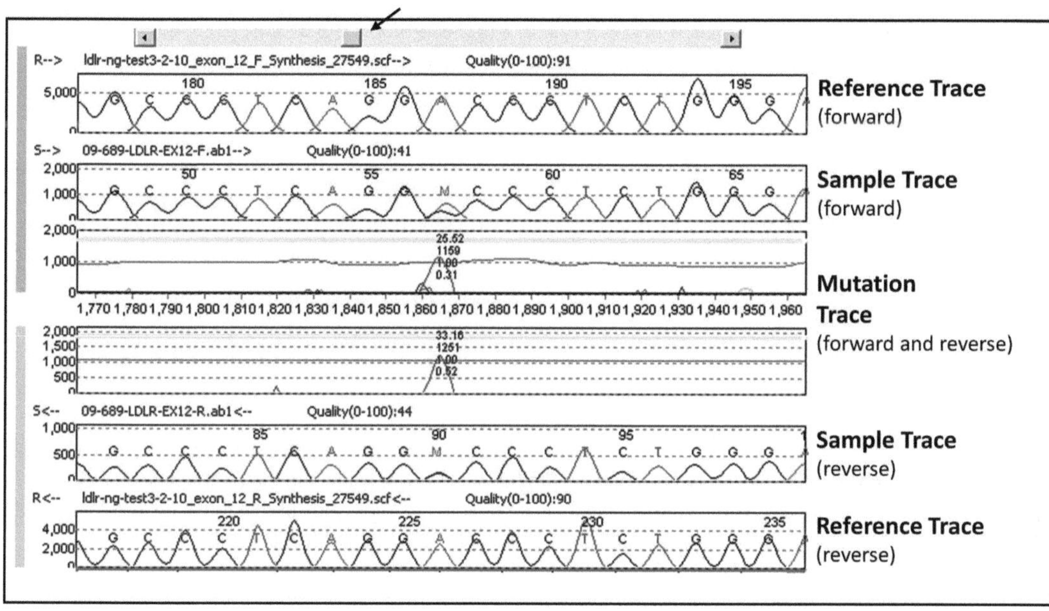

Fig. 14.3. Graphical display of an identified mutation. The mutation is shown in the centre with a peak and mutation score above it. The *arrow* shows the scroll bar which is used for moving the traces to view the other parts of the sequence.

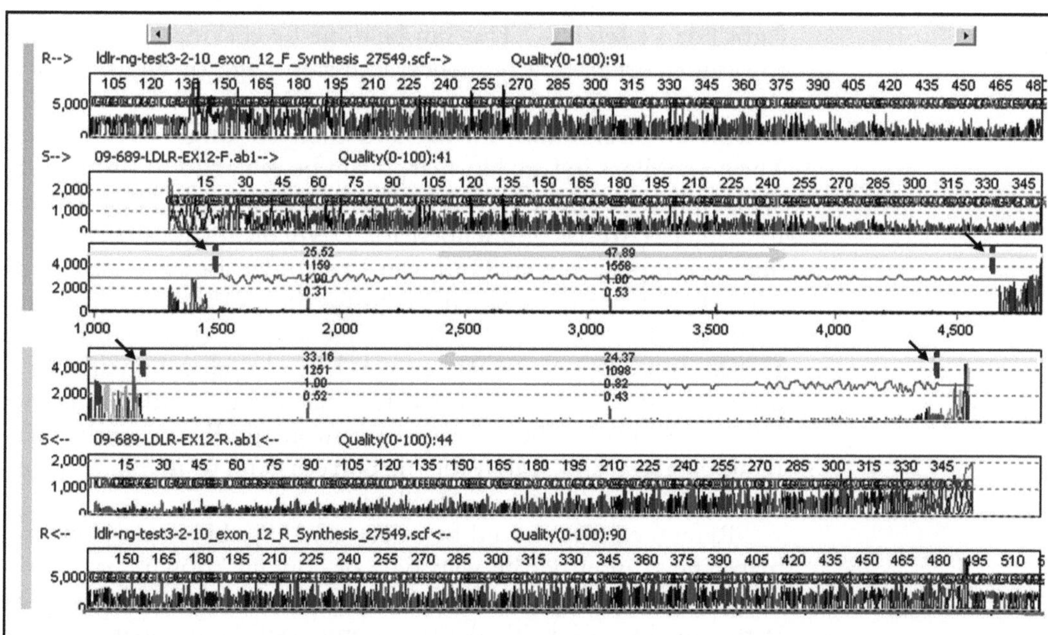

Fig. 14.4. Zoomed out graphical display with the whole analysed sequence. *Arrows* show the thick vertical bars which indicate the cut-off positions of the start and end of the sequence. Mutations are shown in *vertical spikes* with mutation score and other mutation data such as intensity, overlapping and dropping factors above. The *light horizontal bar* (yellow bar) indicates the exon region.

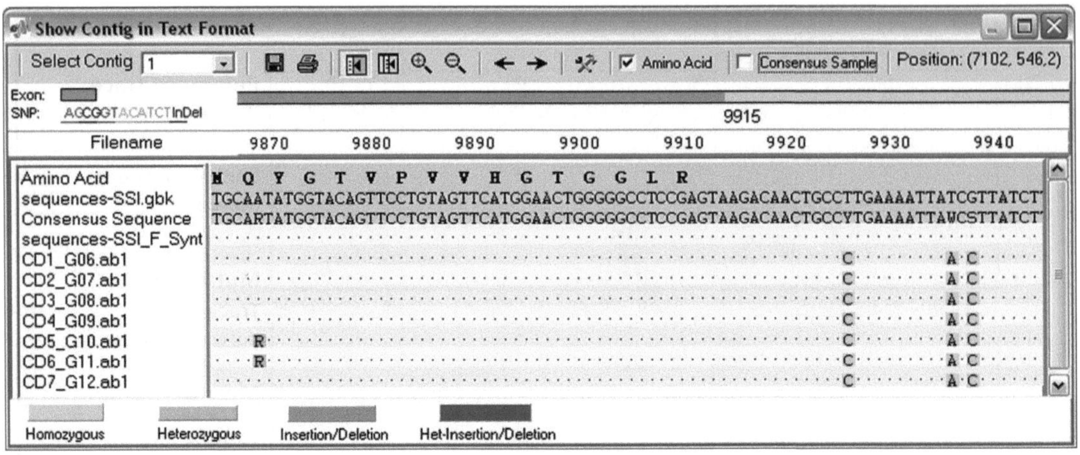

Fig. 14.5. Sequence text output display. All the fragments in the analysis are aligned to the GenBank sequence and the identified mutations are highlighted with different colours according to different types of mutations (*yellow* for homozygous; *blue* for heterozygous; *green* for insertion/deletion and magenta for het-insertion/deletion).

3.2. Importing GenBank and Sample Files

An important feature of Mutation Surveyor is that it can read GenBank files (in a [.seq] or a [.gbk] file format) and create a synthetic reference sequence trace while retaining other information such as exon/intron position, amino acid translation and previously reported SNPs. For any known gene, a GenBank file can be saved from the NCBI website to one's local computer as a [.gbk] or a [.seq] file. This can be done by clicking "send" at the top right corner of a sequence accession page of NCBI, and in the dropdown box, by selecting "Complete Record", "file" and download "GenBank" format and then clicking "Create File". The saved file is in [.gb] format. It can be renamed to [.gbk]. The file can then be added into the "Open File" window (**Fig. 14.2a**). RefSeq files are recommended for DNA diagnostics so that the nucleotide positions in ORT can be standardised for easy comparison. For example, when analysing the *LDLR* gene, it is recommended to use NG_009060 rather than other sequences such as NM_000527 or NT_011295. When analysing human DNA, users have the option to leave the "GenBank" and "Reference File" fields blank. The software can automatically access the GenBank database and search for the correct gene to match the sample files if Internet access is available.

Reference files should be in an [.ab1]/[.abi] or an [.scf] format. They can either be wild type or contain known characteristics. They are used as a control to compare with the test samples. If this section is left blank, the samples will be compared with a GenBank file.

The sample file is a sequence file to be surveyed by the software. It can be in an [.ab1]/[.abi] or an [.scf] format or other sequence trace formats such as [.gz].

When the two-direction analysis mode is used, the forward and reverse file names should be similar except for _F_ in the forward sequence and _R_ in the reverse sequence so that the software can pair the files. The default setting in the software is "Loose Match". This is useful when the filenames have information like capillary number or plate number. For example, in the case of CD15F_F04.ab1 and CD15R_F05.ab1, the software will automatically identify them as a forward and a reverse pair.

3.3. Settings and Analysis

Based on a comparison of a test sample trace to a reference control trace or a GenBank sequence, mutations are called by the software on the satisfaction of the following parameters: mutation height, overlapping factor, dropping factor, signal-to-noise ratio (SnRatio) and mutation score:

- *Mutation height* is the threshold height of a registered mutation peak. In the default setting, mutation height is set at 500. A mutation will be called if its trace peak height is greater than 500 and other parameters are satisfied.
- *Overlapping factor* is a measure of the degree of overlap of the two peaks at the mutation position in horizontal direction. It calculates the horizontal overlapping percentage of a reference peak to the mutation peak. The overlapping factor for a mutation is usually less than its ideal value of 1.0. For example, if the two bases AG overlap by 80%, their overlapping factor is 0.80. In the default setting, the overlapping factor is only set to 0.20, which is the cut-off point for a mutation to be registered.
- *Dropping factor* is the relative intensity drop (height of a peak) of the mutation relative to the neighbouring peaks. It is determined from the relative intensities of the four neighbouring peaks between sample traces and reference traces, two peaks on each side of the potential mutation. Ideally the dropping factor should be 1 (100%) for a homozygous mutation and about 0.5 (50%) for a heterozygous mutation. The default (i.e. minimum detection) setting is 0.20.
- *SnRatio* determines how large the signal has to be relative to neighbouring noise in order for a mutation to be registered. Signal is defined as the mutation peak intensity, and noise is defined as the median peak height of all the minor peaks around the mutation in the mutation trace. The signal-to-noise ratio is used to determine the confidence of the mutation peak; it is calculated based on statistical theory. The default setting is 1.00.
- *Mutation score* is used to call a mutation and rank its confidence level. It is a measure of the probability of error and is derived from signal-to-noise ratio, overlapping factor and dropping factor. Accuracy is defined as 100% minus the error

percentage. The highest possible confidence, 99.9%, corresponds to a mutation score of 30. Scores of 20 and 10 correspond to 99 and 90% accuracy, respectively. Its default setting is 5.00 corresponding to accuracy of around 70%.

Although mutation calling parameters can be specified by a user, it is recommended to use the default settings for a first-time user. The settings can be found in the "Options" window, which can be accessed by selecting "Options…" from the "Process" menu bar. A number of different function bars are presented in this "Options" window (**Fig. 14.6**). In the "Raw" window, "Load Processed Data" is selected in the default setting as most trace files uploaded will include base call information. The "Raw Data" means that sequence trace files do not contain base call information. Default settings of "Contig", "Mutation" and "Display" are shown in **Fig. 14.6**. In the "Display" window, "Check 2D Small Peaks (Mosaic)" should be selected if one wants to detect mosaic mutations (see **Section 3.5**). The "Output" window shows standard output table fields and the "Lane Quality Thresholds" is set to ≥ 0. In the "2 Directions" window, "2 Directions" should be selected if paired forward and reverse sequence data have been entered; while "1 Direction" should be

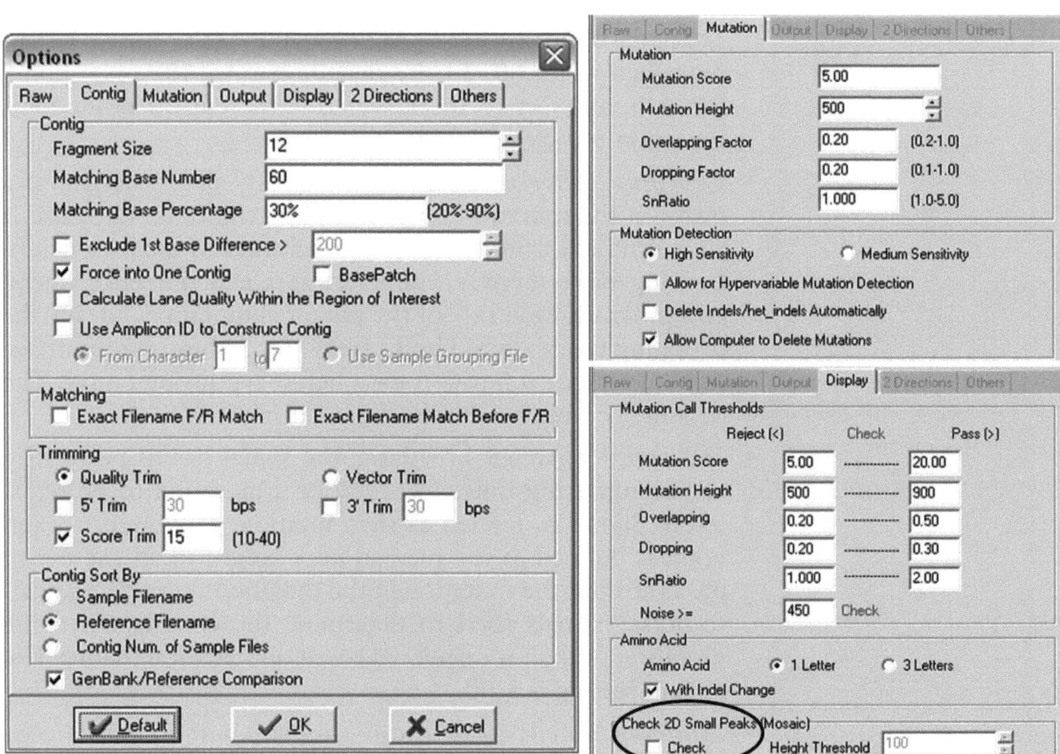

Fig. 14.6. Default settings of "Contig", "Mutation" and "Display" (partial). The *circled* "Check 2D Small Peaks (Mosaic)" in "Display" should be ticked if mosaicism is being surveyed.

used for data in only one direction. The "Others" window contains database URL information that allows an automated search for GenBank files when users leave the GenBank and reference file empty.

After the software finishes its analysis, the main window will contain an ORT (see **Section 3.4**) listing all the mutations detected. These are hyperlinked to an analysed graphical output. ORT and the graphic window are exchangeable by clicking either the "mutation report" on the left-hand pane (in File Tree Window) or a file name or mutation in the ORT.

For heterozygous indels, the graphical display will show a main trace which is aligned to the reference trace and a deconvoluted trace as shown in **Fig. 14.7**.

3.4. Reporting

If running on the default settings, the columns displayed in the basic one-direction ORT are illustrated in **Fig. 14.2b**. The "Gene Name", the "Exon Name" and the "Reading Frame" are automatically extracted from the imported GenBank file, and the "Reading Frame (RF)" will indicate the reading frame number of the first base in a given exon. "Start" and "End" base positions, "Size" and "Lane Quality" are the results from processed sequence. Mutation Surveyor automatically trims off the start and end sequences which have poor quality. The "Lane Quality" score is the average quality score of all the nucleotide physical traces

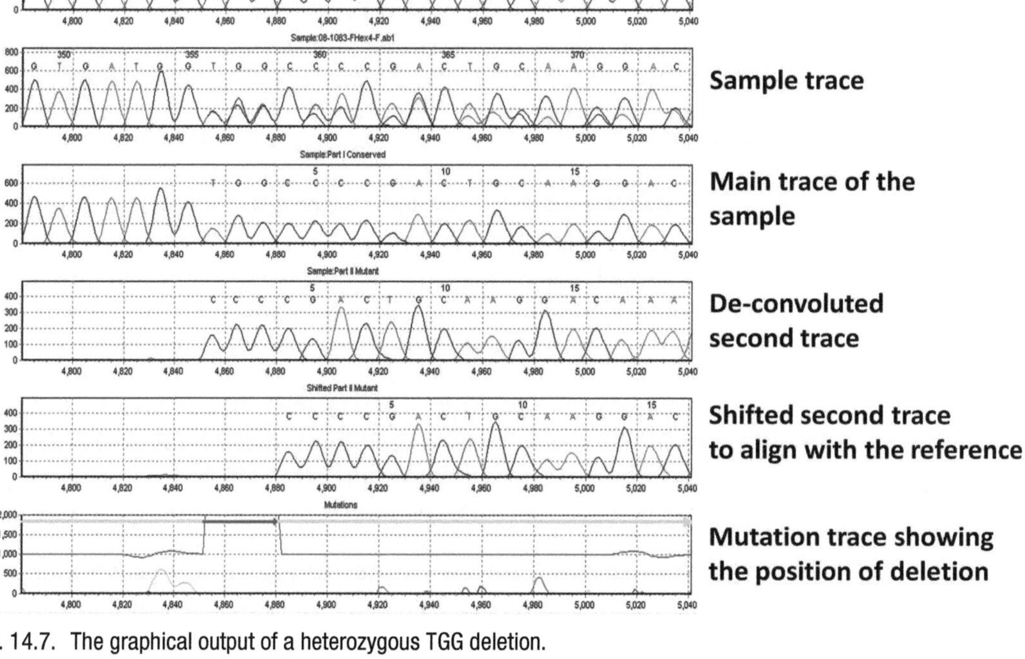

Fig. 14.7. The graphical output of a heterozygous TGG deletion.

measured. The value of a Lane Quality is between 0 and 100 with 100 being the best. If "–1" is presented in "Mutation Number", it means the quality is low. In the "Mutation" column, each mutation has a unique description presented as a base number, reference nucleotide, mutation nucleotide and mutation score. Where appropriate, the amino acid change is also included after the mutation change.

There is also a colour code in the mutation table. Blue text indicates a mutation with a high confidence; red text indicates low confidence and black text signifies that a mutation has been confirmed. Purple background means that the mutation has been recorded in GenBank and a pink background indicates that the mutation results in an amino acid change (either missense or nonsense mutations). No background colour means the mutation does not change any amino acid residue (also called a silent mutation or a synonymous change).

The description of a mutation in Mutation Surveyor includes 1, base number; 2, base identity before and after mutation; 3, type of mutation; and 4, mutation confidence score. The base number refers to the location in the reference sequence that has changed in the sample. If a GenBank file is entered and the mutation is within the region of this GenBank sequence, the base number of the mutation will correspond with the GenBank sequence. The mutation itself is written as G>A, where G is in the reference file and A is the variant base in the sample file. A heterozygous mutation will be G>GA. If the mutation falls in the coding region of the GenBank file, the amino acid changes will be shown after the base letter changes (i.e. 372A>C, 75 N>H). The number following the "$" indicates the mutation confidence score.

For example, "245G>C$34" means the mutation is at the 245th base, which has changed from G to C (homozygously), and the mutation score is 34. "229C>CT, 28R>RC$48" indicates a heterozygous base change at base 229th of the GenBank trace, with a base change from C to CT and a heterozygous amino acid change from R (Arg or arginine) to C (Cys or cysteine), and the mutation score is 48.

For small insertions and deletions, the software monitors the mobility of a fragment relative to the reference. When the sequences no longer align, the program will continue to attempt realignment until it occurs, gapping the sample trace (for a deletion) or the reference (for an insertion). To illustrate an indel, Mutation Surveyor gives a graphical display (**Fig. 14.7**) and provides the text information in ORT as well. For example, "56_57insTAC" indicates the insertion of TAC between bases 56 and 57. "65_67delTGC indicates a deletion of three nucleotides TGC from 65 to 67 bases. "123_127het_delCCTGA" indicates a heterozygous deletion of CCTGA between (and including) bases 123 and 127. The software will automatically de-convolute the mixed trace into two clean traces. However, when the two-direction analysis mode is used, the base number for an indel identified is often slightly different between the forward and reverse sequences. The base number from the forward sequence is usually correct as it names the most 3′ position based on our experience and is also indicated by SoftGenetics (*see* **Note 4**). HGVS' nomenclature rule for naming a deletion of a simple sequence repeat suggests it should use the most 3′ position for naming the deletion (http://www.hgvs.org/mutnomen/).

The basic one-direction ORT can be switched to two-direction ORT and advanced two-direction output by clicking the "2 Dir Output" icon or by selecting the "2 Dir Output" or "2 Dir Advanced" in the "Reports" menu bar. In "2D ORT", yellow and blue highlighting is used to group the forward and reverse samples and the allele frequency is shown as a percentage on the bottom row of each contig. The "2 Dir Advanced" output table allows the user to set display options, such as "reject mutations only in one direction" and "display mosaic mutation". This function is very important in the analysis of mosaic mutations (see **Section 3.5**).

A useful feature in Mutation Surveyor is the HGVS ORT which can be selected from the "Reports" menu. It has similar function as in the "2 Dir Advanced" report. The nomenclature for the mutation calls is displayed following the HGVS guidelines. A homozygous substitution would, for example, be displayed as "c.[76A>C]+[76A>C]", whereas a heterozygous substitution is displayed as "c.[76A>C]+[=]". If a region of interest (ROI) is not specified in the GenBank file (which needs to be done in the GenBank file editor), the "ROI coverage" will be highlighted in red, although the sequences "Read Start" and "End" are clearly indicated.

All forms of the report table can be saved as either a [.txt], an [.xls], a [.htm], or an [.xml] file. An individual cell in the report can also be saved by right clicking on the item; it will then activate a menu with options: "Shrink", "Unshrink", "Copy", "Sort", "Confirmed" and "Deconfirm".

The "Clinical Report" is a custom-formatted report which includes a user-defined header and snapshots of the trace information for all mutations in a sample. By clicking the "Print Clinical Report" icon, the "Print Display Option" box will open. One can then choose customised "Header file" or just use the default SoftGenetics file header, then click OK. The Print Preview window will appear; it can be printed or saved as a PDF file. It is useful to use Screenshot (Print Screen) or Partial Screen Shot (Ctrl+Shift+Hold left click and draw a box, right click and select copy) to copy the graphical display of a mutation and to paste to another document if desired.

3.5. Mosaic Mutation Detection

Due to the nature of sequencing, an artefact peak may appear as real data. However, artefact peaks rarely occur at the same position in both forward and reverse directions. Mosaic mutations appear as a small buried peak under the main sequence peak. They look like a sequence artefact in one direction. To analyse this type of mutation, it is very important to use the two-direction analyse mode. After importing the files for analysis, the setting needs to be changed to mosaic mutation detection. From the "Process" menu, "Option…" is selected and then in the "Display" window, the "check" option under "Check 2D Small Peaks (Mosaic)" is selected. After the analysis, the mosaic mutation which is buried within the baseline is indicated by a short green bar in the graphical display. The normal one-directional report and two-directional report will not show these mosaic mutations. However, they will only be listed in "2 Dir Advanced" report if the option of "display mosaic mutation" is selected. We found that this in silico tool can detect down to 10% of somatic mutations based on a

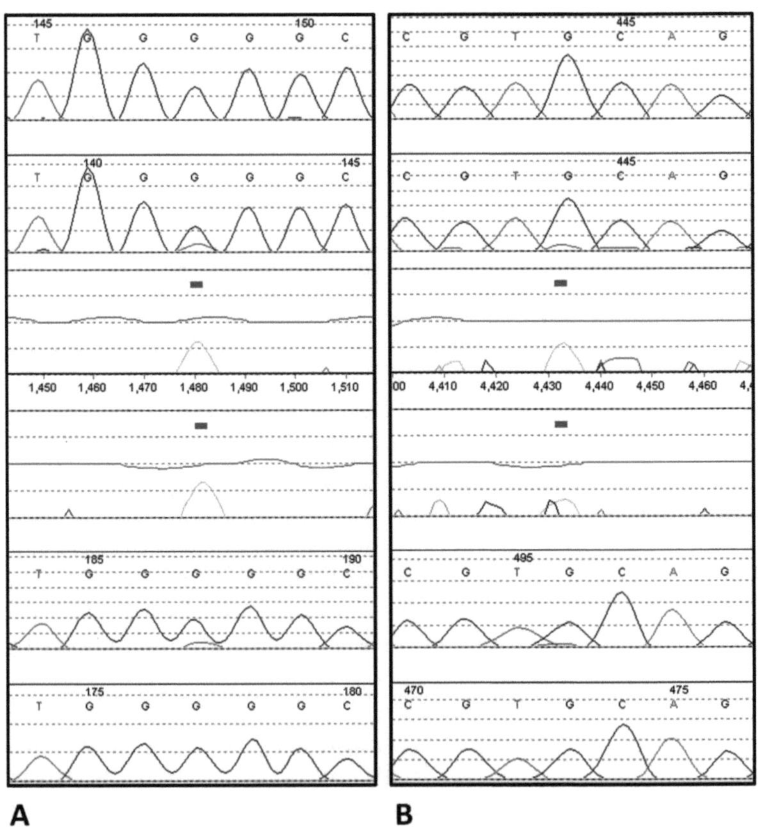

Fig. 14.8. Examples of mosaic mutations indicated by *short horizontal bars*. (**a**) It has higher confidence than the mutation in (**b**). (**b**) There are multiple small mutation peaks (in mutation trace) around the *green bar* indicating mutation peak, which suggest the detected mosaic mutation may actually be the sequencing noise.

detailed study using different ratios of wild-type DNA and mutant DNA (9). Caution must be taken as some baseline noises are often indicated as potential mosaic mutations in this setting. The trace data are recommended to be manually reviewed to confirm those highlighted mutations (*see* **Note 3**). Only those clearly shown in both forward and reverse data should be considered as a genuine mosaic mutation. **Figure 14.8** shows two mosaic mutations with one having higher confidence (a) than the other (b). Further study by high-resolution melting (HRM) analysis of these two samples confirmed that sample a is a genuine mosaic mutation, while b is not (9). The best practice is to confirm these mutations using a second method, such as HRM analysis or DHPLC (9, 10). Detection of mosaic mutations by this in silico tool is useful for not only somatic mutation detection in cancer research but also mutation detection in polyploidy plants.

4. Notes

1. False positive and false negative
   In general, Mutation Surveyor has high accuracy and sensitivity in the identification of sequence variations when sequence quality is good. However, false positives and false negatives (to less an extent) can occur from time to time, especially when the sequence quality is low, for example, in the start and end regions of a sequence. False positives are usually due to noise, low signal intensity, loss of resolution or a sequencing artefact (e.g. a dye blob or spike) in either the test sample or the normal control trace. SoftGenetics does not recommend using a heterozygote as a reference file. A good quality reference file gives better results. False negatives can also be due to poor quality sequence data. The software is able to indicate the mutation in the graphical display by a red dot above the missed mutation but may fail to report the mutation. Therefore, it is highly recommended to do a manual check in the graphical display after an automated analysis (3, 11).
2. File editors
   Mutation Surveyor has comprehensive file editing features, as the software was designed to be extremely flexible with base call analysis. Sample and reference files derived from multiple sources and labelled with user-defined naming conventions can all be uploaded and analysed with Mutation Surveyor. Main file types used in Mutation Surveyor are Trace Files and GenBank Files. Trace files include [.ab1]/[.abi] (standard file types generated by Applied

Biosystems), [.scf] (for Standard Chromatography Files used by Phred) and [.gz] (for GZipped). GenBank files include [.seq], [.gbk], [.fa], [.fasta]. A [.gbk] file is used to represent the sequence text of multiple exons, while a [.seq] file is used to represent the sequence text of one exon. There are functions for file format conversions. For example, the file editor function in Mutation Surveyor can create [.scf] with synthetic or pseudo traces from a GenBank text sequence such as [.seq] and [.gbk]. An [.ab1]/[.abi]/[.fasta] file can also be converted to a [.scf] file, thereby saving data space. "File Name Editor", "Seq File Editor" and "Gbk File Editor" functions are available. "Gbk File Editor" allows editing/entering of information such as gene name, CDS, Region of Interest, etc. The "2 D Filename Match Editor" is useful for defining forward and reverse sequences when sample filenames do not contain *_F_ or *_R_ convention.

3. Base edit and mutation edit
   Base calls in a sequence file, either sample or reference, can sometimes have errors. Mutation Surveyor has an "Edit Base" function. Right click on the base in graphic window and select "Edit Base", the base editing window will open. In this window, by left clicking the base that needs to be changed, one can delete or enter the correct base letter. A warning box appears after closing the base editing window and asks if you would like to save the changes. Confirmation with the selection of "yes" will save the change. Alternatively, click the "Save Base Modified Samples" icon in the main toolbar to save the base call change in the trace file. The modified samples will be saved in the folder selected. The software will automatically correct the base call for similar patterns found in other sample traces. Similarly, a mutation call can also be edited. A right click in the mutation trace allows the user to "Add Mutation". Right click in the mutation table, it opens an action window with the following options: "Edit Comments", "Copy", "Edit", "Delete/Undelete a Mutation", "Delete/Undelete Lane", "Confirm a Mutation" and "De-confirm a Mutation". In the option "Edit", it opens the "Add/Edit Mutation" box, either the numbering or base calling can be changed here. For indel mutations, the software may sometimes make mistakes; one needs to use this function to edit it.

4. Indel mutations
   As mentioned previously (**Section 3.4**), the nucleotide position of an indel mutation called from the forward direction is usually right. If a homozygous indel mutation results in frame shifting, its protein changes are interpreted and displayed in the amino acid text frame above the trace graphical

output. For a heterozygous indel, amino acid residues are displayed according to the wild-type/reference allele. Mutations downstream of a heterozygous indel often fail to be detected. For any single nucleotide substitution with a missense or a nonsense change, Mutation Surveyor will interpret corresponding protein changes irrespective of its homozygous or heterozygous status, but it is unable to identify the protein consequence of splice changes.

References

1. http://www.ncbi.nlm.nih.gov/sites/GeneTests/?db=GeneTests. (viewed in July 2010).
2. Henikoff, S., and Comai, L. (2003) Single-nucleotide mutations for plant functional genomics. *Annual Review of Plant Biology* *54*, 375–401.
3. Ellard, S., Shields, B., Tysoe, C., et al. (2009) Semi-automated unidirectional sequence analysis for mutation detection in a clinical diagnostic setting. *Genetic Testing and Molecular Biomarkers 13*, 381–386.
4. http://droog.gs.washington.edu/polyphred/.
5. http://www.genecodes.com/.
6. Le, H., Hinchcliffe, M., Yu, B., and Trent, R. J. (2008) Computer-assisted reading of DNA sequences, in *Clinical Bioinformatics* (RJ, Trent, Ed.) pp 177–197. Totowa, New Jersey, Humana Press.
7. Ngamphiw, C., Kulawonganunchai, S., Assawamakin, A., et al. (2008) VarDetect: a nucleotide sequence variation exploratory tool. *BMC Bioinformatics 9*, S9.
8. http://www.softgenetics.com/.
9. Dong, C. M., Vincent, K., and Sharp, P. (2009) Simultaneous mutation detection of three homoeologous genes in wheat by high resolution melting analysis and Mutation Surveyor (R) – art. no. 143. *BMC Plant Biology 9*, 143–143.
10. Luquin, N., Yu, B., Trent, R. J., and Pamphlett, R. (2008) DHPLC can be used to detect low-level mutations in amyotrophic lateral sclerosis. *Amyotrophic Lateral Sclerosis 11*, 76–82.
11. Patel, Y., and Wallace, A. (2005) DNA sequence data analysis Automated mutation detection using SoftGenetics® Mutation SurveyorTM v2.51. http://www.ngrl.org.uk/Manchester/sites/default/files/publications/Technology-Assessment/Mutation%20Scanning/Mutation_Surveyor_v5.pdf

Chapter 15

In Silico Searching for Disease-Associated Functional DNA Variants

Rao Sethumadhavan, C. George Priya Doss, and R. Rajasekaran

Abstract

Experimental analyses of disease-associated DNA variants have provided significant insights into the functional implications of sequence variation. However, such experiment-based approaches for identifying functional DNA variants from a pool with a large number of neutral variants are challenging. Computational biology has the opportunity to play an important role in the identification of functional DNA variants in large-scale genotyping studies, ultimately yielding new drug targets and biomarkers. This chapter outlines in silico methods to predict disease-associated functional DNA variants so that the number of DNA variants screened for association with disease can be reduced to those that are most likely to alter gene function. To explore possible relationships between genetic mutations and phenotypic variation, different computational methods like Sorting Intolerant from Tolerant (SIFT, an evolutionary-based approach), Polymorphism Phenotyping (PolyPhen, a structure-based approach) and PupaSuite are discussed for prioritization of high-risk DNA variants. The PupaSuite tool aims to predict the phenotypic effect of DNA variants on the structure and function of the affected protein as well as the effect of variants in the non-coding regions of the same genes. To further investigate the possible causes of disease at the molecular level, deleterious nonsynonymous variants can be mapped to 3D protein structures. An analysis of solvent accessibility and secondary structure can also be performed to understand the impact of a mutation on protein function and stability. This chapter demonstrates a 'real-world' application of some existing bioinformatics tools for DNA variant analysis.

Key words: DNA variants, nonsynonymous variants, SIFT, PolyPhen, PupaSuite, solvent accessibility, secondary structure.

1. Introduction

With the advent of high-throughput DNA variant detection techniques, the number of known nonsynonymous variants is growing rapidly, providing an important source of information for

B. Yu, M. Hinchcliffe (eds.), *In Silico Tools for Gene Discovery*, Methods in Molecular Biology 760,
DOI 10.1007/978-1-61779-176-5_15,

studying the relationship between genotypes and phenotypes of human diseases. The large volume of known and undiscovered genetic variations lends itself well to an informatics approach. The recent sequencing of the human genome (1) together with the large number of DNA variants present in the human population (2, 3) has opened the way for the development of a detailed understanding of the mechanisms by which genetic variation results in phenotype variation. This offers new opportunities for identifying the genetic predisposition to and understanding of the causes of common diseases. Two general strategies for selecting DNA variants for use in association studies include haplotype-tagging methods and targeted selection of candidate genes (*see* **Chapters 11** and **12**) and candidate variants. Whole-genome scans will become increasingly technologically efficient and economically feasible in the near future. Meanwhile, scientists using candidate gene, SNP or haplotype approaches face the challenge of choosing among 10 million possible SNPs (4) or smaller numbers of haplotype-tagging DNA variants (5).

In the context of prioritization of candidate DNA variants that are most likely to be phenotypically relevant, numerous criteria are useful. For example, the location of a DNA variant (within or near genes), the coding effect of a DNA variant (nonsynonymous vs. synonymous), coding vs. non-coding as well as its comparison with other species (6) can yield helpful clues towards functional/phenotypic impact. With the exception of variants lying in promoters or splice sites, it is difficult to determine the effect of non-coding DNA variants on gene expression. For this reason, initial attention has been focused on nonsynonymous variants. These types of alterations are believed to be more likely to cause a change in protein structure and hence compromise its function. For example, nonsynonymous variants may affect the functional roles of proteins involved in signal transduction of visual, hormonal and other stimulants (7). Nonsynonymous variants may inactivate functional sites of enzymes, may destabilize proteins or may reduce protein solubility (9). They may also disrupt exonic splicing enhancers or silencers (11).

To understand the mechanism of phenotypic variations due to nonsynonymous variants, it is important to assess the structural consequences of the amino acid substitution. Over the past few years, many studies have attempted to predict the functional consequences of nonsynonymous variants. These studies attempted to determine whether nonsynonymous variants are disease related or neutral, based on sequence information and structural attributes (12) using computational algorithms such as SIFT (Sorting Intolerant from Tolerant) and PolyPhen (Polymorphism Phenotyping) (13). The structure of a protein can change in various ways due to the biochemical differences of the amino acid variant (acidic, basic or hydrophobic) and by the location of the variant in the protein sequence that affects secondary, tertiary or quaternary structure or the active site where substrate binds (14). Several groups have tried to evaluate deleterious nonsynonymous variants based on three-dimensional (3D) structural information of proteins by in silico analysis. They have indicated that residue solvent accessibility, involving buried residues, is a useful predictor of deleterious substitutions (15).

Although experiment-based approaches provide the strongest evidence for the functional role of a genetic variant, these studies are usually labour intensive and time consuming. In contrast, computational algorithms can be employed on a scale that is consistent with the large number of variants being identified. The flowchart outlined here is based on the integration of multiple bioinformatics sources to provide a systematic analysis of the functionality of nonsynonymous variants (**Fig. 15.1**). The existing in silico methods can also be adapted by any investigator to a priori DNA variant selection or post hoc evaluation of variants identified in whole-genome scans or within haplotype blocks associated with disease. Importantly, the applications of these computational algorithms in association studies will greatly strengthen our understanding of the inheritance of complex human phenotypes.

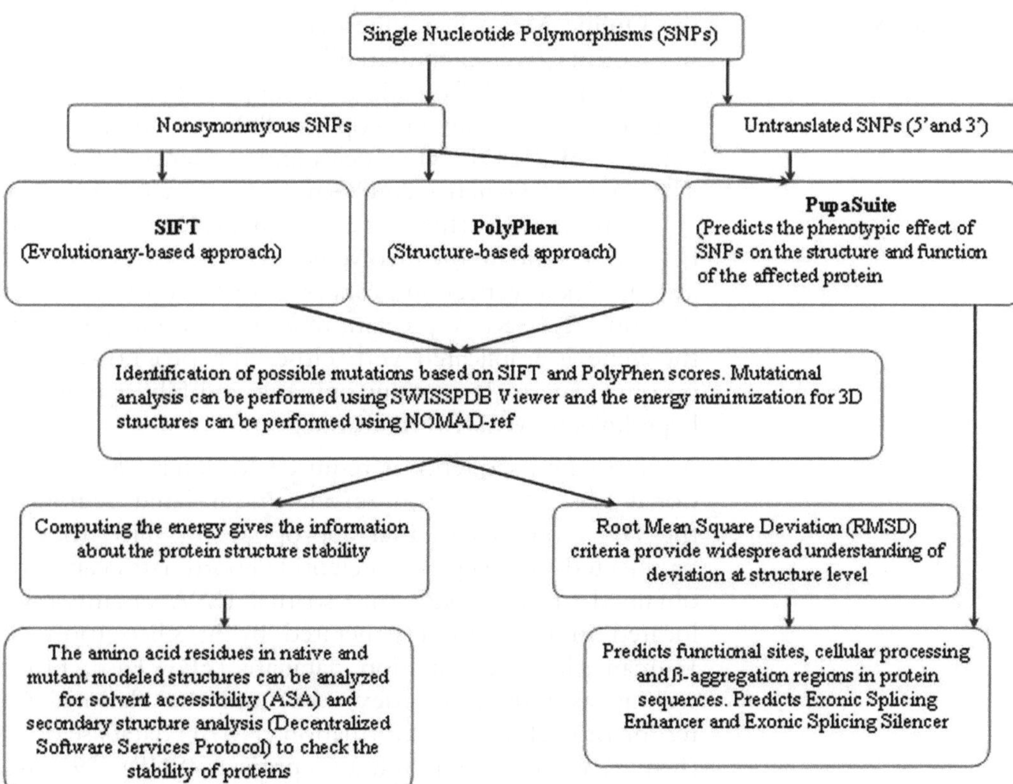

Fig. 15.1. Proposed methodology for disease-associated functional DNA variant analysis.

Therefore, our analysis will provide useful information in selecting DNA variants that are more likely to have potential functional impact and ultimately contribute to an individual's phenotype (*see* **Notes 1** and **2**).

2. Materials

Computational tools will run well on a conventional laptop and desktop with 32-bit Windows 7/Vista/ XP, Linux or Mac OS X 10.5. Internet access is necessary to perform data mining and to use SIFT (version 2.0, http://sift.jcvi.org/), PolyPhen (http://genetics.bwh.harvard.edu/pph/) and Pupa-Suite (http://pupasuite.bioinfo.cipf.es/).

3. Methods

3.1. Database Mining for DNA Variants

1. The genes of interest can be explored and obtained from the Online Mendelian Inheritance in Man (OMIM) website (http://www.ncbi.nlm.nih.gov/omim) (16). OMIM contains textual information, pictures and reference information. It also contains copious links to NCBI's Entrez database of MEDLINE articles and sequence information. The Atlas of Genetics and Cytogenetics in Oncology and Haematology (17) (http://AtlasGeneticsOncology.org) can be used to validate the involvement of a gene in cancer, clinical entities in cancer and cancer- prone disease. It includes data on DNA/RNA, protein, mutations and diseases where the gene is implicated with either the prognosis or data on oncogenesis. It contains only selected bibliography with hyperlinks to MEDLINE abstracts.
2. An annotated sequence is required to determine the functional class (e.g. intron, exon, untranslated regions) of the DNA variants so that appropriate in silico tools can be selected for analyses. Nucleotide coordinates can also be obtained from this sequence so that DNA variants can be located in the output generated by in silico tools. The Human Genome Variation database (HGVBase, http://www.gwascentral.org/index) (18) and the National Center for Biotechnology Information (NCBI) database dbSNP (http://www.ncbi.nlm.nih.gov/projects/SNP) (19) can be used for the retrieval of DNA variants and their related protein for computational analysis. Gene annotations from these

sources may differ. Thus, in silico analyses may produce varied results depending on the source of annotated gene sequences that is utilized.

3. To obtain the annotated sequence, NCBI's Entrez Gene database can be searched by typing a gene name or a symbol into the text box at the top of the page. To restrict searches to human genes, the phrase 'AND human [orgn]' can be added to the end of the query. Once the Entrez Gene web page for a gene is accessed, links to other NCBI resources are provided on the far right-hand side of the page. The 'SNP' link provides lists of all of the SNPs (denoted with a referent sequence number or identifier) that are associated with that gene. 'SNP: GeneView' places the SNPs in the context of the gene, providing functional class information. The NCBI MapViewer can be used to obtain gene and SNP coordinates; from the Gene and Variation maps, the 'Data as Table View' link can be used to obtain gene and SNP genomic coordinates, respectively. FASTA (a standard format of DNA or amino acid sequences with a single line of description followed by lines of sequence data) amino acid sequences can be viewed or downloaded by accessing the NCBI Entrez Protein reports for each gene of interest (through the Entrez Gene 'Links' menu); FASTA must be selected in the report page display menu to obtain the FASTA amino acid sequence for the protein. The amino acid position related to the SNP, which must be submitted to certain in silico tools, is provided in 'GeneView in dbSNP'. For those tools requiring FASTA-formatted nucleotide sequences, the 'dl' link appearing next to the gene name in MapViewer is selected. This opens a sequence download page through which the FASTA sequence of the entire gene can be viewed or downloaded. The correct strand orientation, plus or minus, must be selected. The orientation of the gene sequence is provided in the 'SNP: GeneView' web page. The position of the DNA variants in the nucleotide sequence, which must be noted to utilize the output from the in silico tools, is calculated by subtracting the gene start coordinate from the DNA variant nucleotide coordinate.

3.2. Predictions of Deleterious DNA Variants by Computational Methods

SIFT version 2.0 (http://sift.jcvi.org/) can assist in distinguishing between functional and non-functional coding variants. It predicts whether an amino acid substitution in a protein has a functional effect. SIFT is based on the premise that protein evolution is correlated with protein function. Variants that occur at conserved alignment positions are expected to be tolerated less than those that occur at positions with a diverse list of amino acids through evolution. SIFT takes a query sequence and uses multiple alignment information to predict tolerated and deleterious substitutions for every position of the query sequence. It is a multistep procedure that, given a protein sequence, (1) searches for similar sequences, (2) chooses closely related sequences that may share similar function, (3) obtains the multiple alignment of these chosen sequences and (4) calculates normalized probabilities for all possible substitutions at each position from the alignment. Substitutions at each position with normalized probabilities less than a tolerance index of 0.05 are predicted to be intolerant or deleterious; those greater than or equal to 0.05 are predicted to be tolerated (20). The higher the tolerance index of a particular amino acid substitution, the less likely it is predicted to affect protein function (*see* **Note 3**).

PolyPhen (21) is an automated tool for the prediction of the impact of an amino acid substitution on the structure and function of a human protein. It is available at http://genetics.bwh.harvard.edu/pph/. The predictions are based on straightforward empirical rules which are applied to the sequence including phylogenetic and structural information characterizing the substitution. PolyPhen relies on annotation in the SWALL database (http://srs.ebi.ac.uk) to determine if an amino acid position is involved in metal binding, formation of disulfide bonds or active site catalysis. PolyPhen identifies and aligns homologs of the input sequences via a BLAST search. The alignment is used to calculate a matrix of 'profile scores', which are logarithmic ratios of the likelihood of a given amino acid occurring at a particular position to the likelihood of this amino acid occurring at any position (background frequency). Profile scores of allelic variants are compared to assess whether the substitution is rarely or never observed in the protein family. The amino acid variant is mapped to the known 3D structure to assess whether it is likely to affect the hydrophobic core of a protein, electrostatic interactions, interactions with ligands or other important features of a protein. If the structure of a query protein is unknown, PolyPhen will use homologous proteins with known structure. PolyPhen searches for 3D protein structures using multiple alignments of homologous sequences. It then uses amino acid contact information from several protein structure databases, calculates position-specific independent count (PSIC) scores for each of two variants and then computes the PSIC score difference of two variants. The higher the PSIC score difference, the higher the functional impact a particular amino acid substitution is likely to have. A PSIC score difference of 1.5 and above is considered to be damaging. The query options were left with default values. Results for each variant were classified into 'benign', 'possibly damaging', 'probably damaging' and 'unknown' if not enough information was available. For this study, both 'possibly damaging' and 'probably damaging' were classified as deleterious variants (*see* **Note 4**).

PupaSuite (http://pupasuite.bioinfo.cipf.es/) is now synchronized to deliver annotations for both non-coding and coding variants, as well as annotations for the Swiss-Prot set of human disease mutations (22). PupaSuite retrieves DNA variants that could affect conserved regions that the cellular machinery uses for the correct processing of genes (intron/exon boundaries or exonic splicing enhancers). It uses algorithms like Tango (β-aggregation regions in protein sequences) and FoldX (stability change caused by the single amino acid variation) to predict the effect of nonsynonymous variants on several phenotypic properties such as structure and dynamics, functional sites and cellular processing of human proteins using either sequence-based or structural bioinformatics approaches. It also contains additional methods for predicting DNA variants that are located within transcription factor-binding sites (TFBSs) and splice sites (*see* **Note 5**).

3.3. Structural Effect of DNA Variants

Structural analyses were performed based on the crystal structure of the protein for evaluating the structural stability of native and mutant proteins. The web resources SAAPdb (http://www.bioinf.org.uk/saap/db/) (23) and dbSNP (19) can be used to identify the protein coded by the gene. Then the DNA variant positions and residues were confirmed from this server. The DNA variant positions and residues were in agreement with the results obtained from the SIFT and PolyPhen programs. Each DNA variant was performed using SWISSPDB viewer. Energy minimization for 3D structures was performed using NOMAD-Ref server (http://lorentz.dynstr.pasteur.fr/nomad-ref.php) (24). This last server uses Gromacs as a default force field for energy minimization based on the methods of steepest descent, conjugate gradient and low-memory Broyden–Fletcher–Goldfarb–Shanno quasi-Newtonian minimizer (LBFGS) methods (25). Computing the energy gives the information about the protein structure stability. Then the deviation between the two structures was evaluated by their root mean square deviation (RMSD) values which provide widespread understanding of deviation at the structural level (*see* **Notes 6** and 7).

Solvent accessibility is defined as the ratio between the solvent-accessible surface area of a peptide residue in a three-dimensional structure and that in a Gly-X-Gly extended tripeptide conformation. The solvent accessibility information can be obtained by using NetASAView (26). The entire implementation of ASAView for all PDB proteins, as a whole or for an individual chain, may be accessed at http://www.netasa.org/asaview/. Simply enter the PDB code or the coordinate file for its use. Solvent accessibility was divided into three classes: buried, partially buried and exposed. They indicate low, moderate and high accessibility of the amino acid residues to the solvent, respectively. For a successful analysis of the relation between amino acid sequence and protein structure, an unambiguous and physically meaningful definition of secondary structure is essential. The information about secondary structures of the proteins can be analyzed using the program Decentralized Software Services Protocol (DSSP) (27). The prediction of solvent accessibility and secondary structure has been studied as an intermediate step for predicting the tertiary structure of proteins (*see* **Note 8**).

The vast number of DNA variants now listed challenges biologists and bioinformaticians. Importantly, they can provide information about the relationships between individuals. Stemming from numerous ongoing efforts to identify millions of these DNA variants, there is now also a focus on studying associations between disease risk and these genetic variations using a molecular epidemiological approach. This plethora of DNA variants has created a major difficulty for scientists in planning costly population-based genotyping, including what target DNA variants should be chosen that are most likely to affect phenotypic functions and ultimately contribute to disease development. Many molecular studies are focusing on DNA variants located in coding and regulatory regions, yet many of these studies have been unable to detect significant associations between DNA variants and disease susceptibility. To develop a coherent approach for prioritizing DNA variant selection for genotyping in molecular studies, an evolutionary perspective to DNA variants can be applied for screening. Molecular studies of cancer with respect to nonsynonymous variants can be analyzed using evolutionary conservation levels. The effects of many nonsynonymous variants are predicted to be neutral as natural selection would have removed many deleterious mutations on essential positions. Assessment of non-neutral variants is mainly based on phylogenetic information (i.e. correlation with residue conservation) extended to a certain degree with structural approaches (PolyPhen). Amino acid changes that are evolutionarily conserved might be more likely to be associated with cancer susceptibility. A recent literature survey showed that Universal Mutation Database (UMD) Predictor (http://www.umd.be/) (28) is able to predict functional DNA variants very accurately compared with SIFT and PolyPhen. This tool takes into account the impact of a nucleotide substitution at not only the protein level but also the transcript level. Therefore, it is also able to predict the impact on splicing signals such as acceptor and donor splice sites as well as auxiliary splicing sequences such as exonic splicing enhancers and silencers (ESE and ESS). It is becoming clear that application of the molecular evolutionary approach may be a powerful tool for prioritizing DNA variants to be genotyped in future molecular epidemiological studies (*see* **Note 9**). The prioritization of functional nonsynonymous variants in various forms of cancers including breast cancer (29), leukaemia (30), colon cancer (31), *TP53* (32) and genetic disorders such as cystic fibrosis (33) and the haemoglobinopathies (34) was investigated and was studied by this approach (*see* **Note 10**).

4. Notes

1. Computational biology methods for DNA variant annotations can maximize their contributions to medical genetics research by designing services that are easy for researchers who are not bioinformatics experts to use and understand. These in silico predictions are of great interest in detecting variants for Mendelian and complex diseases, in prioritizing polymorphisms for experimental research in humans and other species, and in analyzing data from genome-wide associations. Using various prediction tools, up to one-quarter of nonsynonymous variants have been diagnosed to be not strictly neutral and are thus thought to harbour signatures of negative or positive selection. The confirmation of pathogenesis may be more straightforward for highly penetrant mutations causing rare Mendelian disorders.
2. Medical geneticists and molecular biologists who are interested in using available DNA variant annotation web servers can select from the following: (i) servers that disseminate original methods to predict biologically important DNA variants (SIFT and PolyPhen); (ii) metaservers (integration of multiple resources), which yield large amounts of heterogeneous bioinformatics information from external servers (PupaSuite) and (iii) hybrids which combine (i) and (ii).
3. In addition to predicting DNA variant functional impact, SIFT builds a multiple sequence alignment of the protein of interest and emails it to the user, allowing alignment analysis with other bioinformatics software.
4. PolyPhen includes additional information about the structure of the protein in the analysis in comparison with SIFT analysis. The structural information includes position within the protein (surface or interior), contribution to well-defined structural elements including helices or sheets, and location within the active site. Although users may perceive DNA variant prediction services as a set of fundamentally different methods, there are major similarities 'underneath the lid'. For example, SIFT and PolyPhen's scores are based on the predictions of multiple sequence alignment between the protein of interest and related

proteins. Although PolyPhen does use protein structural information when it is available, for the majority of queries, its predictions are based on amino acid residue properties and PSIC sequence alignment scores. Like SIFT, the PSIC score measures the probability that a substituted amino acid will be tolerated based on the distribution of amino acids in a multiple sequence alignment column. The measures differ mainly in technical details, such as how pseudocounts and sequence weighting are applied. When SIFT and PolyPhen outputs are substantially different, it is probably because different multiple sequence alignments were used to calculate scores, rather than these details.

5. PupaSuite is an easier alternative than the laborious methodology that we have outlined. Discrepancies between our results and the results from PupaSuite were, in part, due to differences in the annotated sequences used (NBCI vs. Ensembl). For the most part, however, discrepancies were due to differences in the stringency of the analyses.
6. An additional role that can be foreseen for computational analysis is the prediction of the likely site of action of the DNA variant. By modelling the 3D structure of the protein and locating the DNA variant, it should be possible to predict the impact of the DNA variant on the structure and on the protein–protein interactions and regulation.
7. The approaches to analyzing the impact of DNA variants using 3D structures fall along an axis describing the amount of directly relevant structural information used to model the structure of the protein being examined.
8. It is possible to use secondary structure and solvent accessibility prediction to gauge whether a DNA variant might be disruptive of protein structure, although this approach is not informative in many cases. Structure-based approaches are powerful and hold considerable promise for the future.
9. Although it is difficult to determine what criteria or cut-offs are optimal for choosing DNA variants, the strength of our methodology is that individual users can define their own. We presented a methodology born from the necessity to prioritize DNA variant selection in our own studies. Individual investigators may choose to utilize alternative tools or to interpret the output from these tools in an alternative manner.
10. The underlying argument is to use two approaches (SIFT and PolyPhen) that differ in fundamental ways and use the intersection of the results to increase the stringency of the analysis. Interestingly, use of two of these programs to

analyze the DNA variants described in a group of breast cancer or leukaemia-causing genes indicated that a subset of the DNA variants identified appeared in both analyses as likely to have a significant impact (29, 30).

Acknowledgements

The authors thank the Management of Vellore Institute of Technology for providing the facilities to carry out this work.

References

1. Lander, E. S., Linton, L. M., Birren, B. et al. (2001) Initial sequencing and analysis of human genome. *Nature* 409, 860–921.
2. Hinds, D. A., Stuve, L. L., Nilsen, G. B. et al. (2005) Whole-genome patterns of common DNA variation in three human populations. *Science* 307, 1072–1079.
3. The International HapMap Project (2003) The International HapMap Consortium. *Nature* 426, 789–796.
4. Pharoah, P. D., Dunning, A. M., Ponder, B. A., et al. (2004) Association studies for cancer-susceptibility genetic variants. *Nat Rev Cancer* 4, 850–860.
5. Johnson, G. C., Esposito, L., Barratt, B. J., et al. (2001) Haplotype tagging for the identification of common disease genes. *Nat Genet* 29, 233–237.
6. Ferrer-Costa, C., Orozco, M., de la Cruz, X. (2005) Use of bioinformatics tools for the annotation of disease-associated mutations in animal models. *Proteins* 61, 878–887.
7. Smith, E. P., Boyd, J., Frank, G. R. et al. (1994) Estrogen resistance caused by a mutation in the estrogen-receptor gene in a man. *N Engl J Med* 331, 1056–1061.
8. Jaruzelska, J., Abadie, V., Aubenton-Carafa, Y., et al. (1995) In vitro splicing deficiency induced by a C to T mutation at position-3 in the intron 10 acceptor site of the phenylalanine hydroxylase gene in a patient with phenylketonuria. *J Biol Chem* 270, 20370–20375.
9. Proia, R. L., Neufeld, E. F. (1982) Synthesis of betahexosaminidase in cell free translation and in intact fibroblasts: an insoluble precursor alpha chain in a rare form of Tay-Sachs disease. *Proc Natl Acad Sci* 79, 6360–6364.
10. Prokunina, L., Alarcon-Riquelme, M. E. (2002) Regulatory SNPs in complex diseases their identification and functional validation. *Expert Rev Mol Med* 6, 1–15.
11. Cartegni, L., Krainer, A. R. (2002) Disruption of an SF2/ASF-dependent exonic splicing enhancer in SMN2 causes spinal muscular atrophy in the absence of SMN1. *Nature Genet* 30, 377–384.
12. Richard, J. D., Patricia, B. M., Mark, J. C., et al. (2006) Predicting deleterious nsSNPs: an analysis of sequence and structural attributes. *BMC Bioinformatics* 7, 217.
13. Xi, T., Jones, I. M., Mohrenweiser, H. W. (2004) Many amino acid substitution variants identified in DNA repair genes during human population screenings are predicted to impact protein function. *Genomics* 83, 970–979.
14. Melissa, M., Johnson, Houck, J., et al. (2005) Screening for deleterious nonsynonymous single-nucleotide polymorphisms in genes involved in steroid hormone metabolism and response. *Cancer Epidemiol Biomarkers Prev* 14, 1326–1329.
15. Chen, H., Zhou, H. X. (2005) Prediction of solvent accessibility and sites of deleterious mutations from protein sequence. *Nucleic Acids Res* 33, 3193–3199.
16. The Omim database [http://www.ncbi.nlm.nih.gov/entrez/query.fcgi?db=OMIM].
17. Huret, J. L., Dessen, P., Bernheim, A. (2003) Atlas of genetics and cytogenetics in oncology and haematology. *Nucleic Acids Res* 31, 272–274.

18. Fredman, D., Munns, G., Rios, D., et al. (2004) HGVbase: a curated resource describing human DNA variation and phenotype relationships. *Nucleic Acids Res* 32, 516–519.
19. Smigielski, E. M., Sirotkin, K., Ward, M., et al. (2000) dbSNP: a database of single nucleotide polymorphisms. *Nucleic Acids Res* 28, 352–355.
20. Ng, P. C., Henikoff, S. (2001) Predicting Deleterious Amino Acid Substitutions. *Genome Res* 11, 863–874.
21. Ramensky, V., Pork, P., Sunyaev, S. (2002) Human no n-synonymous SNPs: server and survey. *Nucleic Acids Res* 30, 3894–3900.
22. Reumers, J., Conde, L., Medina, I., et al. (2008) Joint annotation of coding and noncoding single nucleotide polymorphisms and mutations in the SNP effect and PupaSuite databases. *Nucleic Acids Res* 36, D825–D829.
23. Cavallo, A., Martin, A. C. (2005) Mapping SNPs to protein sequence and structure data. *Bioinformatics* 8, 443–1450.
24. Lindahl, E., Azuara, C., Koehl, P. et al. (2006) NOMAD-Ref: visualization, deformation and refinement of macromolecular structures based on all-atom normal mode analysis. *Nucleic Acids Res* 34, W52–W56.
25. Delarue, M., Dumas, P. (2004) On the use of low-frequency normal modes to enforce collective movements in refining macromolecular structural models. *Proc Natl Acad Sci* 101, 6957–6962.
26. Ahmad, S., Gromiha, M., Fawareh, H. et al. (2004) ASA view, solvent accessibility graphics for proteins. *BMC Bioinformatics* 51, 51.
27. Kabsch, W., Sander, C. (1983) Dictionary of protein secondary structure: Pattern recognition of hydrogen-bonded and geometrical features. *Biopolymers* 22, 2577–2637.
28. Frederic, M. Y., Lalande, M., Boileau, C. et al. (2009) UMD-predictor, a new prediction tool for nucleotide substitution pathogenicity – application to four genes: FBN1, FBN2, TGFBR1, and TGFBR2. *Hum Mutat* 30, 952–959.
29. Rajasekaran, R., Sudandiradoss, C., George Priya Doss, C. et al. (2007) Identification and in silico analysis of functional SNPs of the BRCA1 gene. *Genomics* 90, 447–452.
30. George Priya Doss, C., Sudandiradoss, C., Rajasekaran, R. et al. (2008) Identification and structural comparison of deleterious mutations in nsSNPs of ABL1 gene in chronic myeloid leukemia: A Bio-informatics study. *J Biomed Info* 41, 607–612.
31. George Priya Doss, C., Sethumadhavan, R. (2009) Investigation on the role of nsSNPs in HNPCC genes-A Bioinformatics approach. *BMC J Biomed Sci* 16(1), 42.
32. George Priya Doss, C., Sudandiradoss, C., Rajasekaran, R. et al. (2008) Application of computational algorithm tools to identify functional SNPs. *Funct Integrat Genomics* 8, 309–316.
33. George Priya Doss, C., Rajasekaran, R., Sudandiradoss, C. et al. (2008) A novel computational and structural analysis of nsSNPs in CFTR gene. *Genomic Med* 2, 23–32.
34. George Priya Doss, C., Sethumadhavan, R. (2009) Impact of Single Nucleotide Polymorphisms in HBB gene causing Haemoglobinopathies: in silico analysis. *New Biotechnol* 25, 214–219.

Chapter 16

In Silico Prediction of Transcriptional Factor-Binding Sites

Dmitry Y. Oshchepkov and Victor G. Levitsky

Abstract

The recognition of transcription factor binding sites (TFBSs) is the first step on the way to deciphering the DNA regulatory code. A large variety of computational approaches and corresponding in silico tools for TFBS recognition are available, each having their own advantages and shortcomings. This chapter provides a brief tutorial to assist end users in the application of these tools for functional characterization of genes.

Key words: Transcription factor-binding sites, in silico, prediction, recognition, transcription regulation

1. Introduction

Specific binding of transcription factors with DNA sequence is one of the key issues in understanding the fundamentals of transcription regulation. Reliable transcription factor binding site (TFBS) recognition methods are essential for computer-assisted annotation of a large amount of genome sequence data. The paramount significance of this problem imposes a great challenge to bioinformaticians, resulting in a constantly increasing variety of approaches (1, 2). Many methods and tools are readily available from the Internet and it is difficult to keep them all in mind. Here we present a limited set of tools, freely available via the Internet, that are helpful for a biologist who is unfamiliar with methods to solve the majority of the tasks that arise when recognition of putative TFBSs is performed for functional characterization of genes (*see* **Note 1**).

B. Yu, M. Hinchcliffe (eds.), *In Silico Tools for Gene Discovery*, Methods in Molecular Biology 760,
DOI 10.1007/978-1-61779-176-5_16,

The basic principle for the development of TFBS recognition methods, based on training samples, is as follows: as a rule, each transcription factor is capable of interacting with DNA sequences differing in their context. Statistical analysis of TFBS samples allows common contextual or context-dependent characteristics useful for recognition of putative sites to be detected. In general, the approaches to TFBS recognition based on training samples differ by the means of detection of these characteristics and their utilization for putative TFBS recognition. The classical approach, involving position weight matrices (PWMs) (3) (*see* **Note 2**), represents a natural development of the search for consensus sequences (4) (*see* **Note 3**). It competes in performance with plenty of alternative approaches (1, 2). TFBS recognition methods based on training samples and appropriate tools can be used if data for training are available including the following: an aligned set of known binding sites for a transcription factor of interest or a frequency matrix or consensus sequence derived from this original set. Large-scale integration of special-purpose databases containing this data has simplified the task of TFBS recognition, thereby offering database-integrated tools for the detection of binding sites for particular transcription factors.

The approach to TFBS recognition described above could be supplemented by using the information on conservation of predicted sites in orthologous sequences from different species (phylogenetic footprinting) to distinguish potentially functional elements from background recognitions (5). The phylogenetic footprinting approach is based on the preferential conservation of functional sequences over the course of evolution by selection pressure, as mutations are more likely to be disruptive if they appear in functional sites, resulting in a measurable difference in evolution rates between functional and non-functional genomic segments.

Therefore, a typical workflow for TFBS recognition is as follows:

1. Retrieve the sequence upstream of the transcription start site (TSS) of a gene of interest or utilize other regulatory sequence(s) of interest.
2. Retrieve the training data for the transcription factor.
3. Utilize the training data for training a preferable TFBS recognition tool for putative TFBS recognition.

A typical workflow for TFBS recognition with database-integrated tools is as follows:

1. Retrieve the sequence upstream of the TSS of the gene of interest or utilize other regulatory sequence(s) of interest.
2. Check available tools for predicting TFBSs for the existence of data for the recognition of a particular transcription factor of interest.

3. Search the potential binding sites of the particular transcription factors of interest, using a set of suitable tools for predicting TFBSs.

A typical workflow for a phylogenetic footprinting approach for TFBS recognition is as follows:

1. Retrieve regulatory sequences of orthologous genes.
2. Utilize them in one of the phylogenetic footprinting approach tools.

2. Materials

A personal computer and an Internet connection are needed. Most of the sequence data used will be in FASTA format, which is quite simple to operate in the text mode. In the FASTA format, the first line begins with the ">" symbol followed by a sequence description, preferably starting with a sequence ID. The nucleotide sequence itself starts from the second line and may contain spaces and numbers. Multiple sequences in the FASTA format are simply placed one after another.

3. Methods

3.1. Retrieving the Regulatory Sequence(s) from Gene(s) of Interest

Sequences, presumed to be regulatory for a gene of interest, are the subject of TFBS searches. Most of these sequences are upstream of an annotated PolII transcription start(s) of the gene(s) of interest, as this region always contains a promoter. One can check the region from –5000... –300 to –1 upstream of the TSS. Also, enhancer regions (if known), 5′- or 3′-untranslated regions (UTRs) and intron sequences of the gene of interest deserve attention. They can be retrieved from the following databases: EPD (6), UCSC Genome Browser (7), DBTSS (8), RefSeq (9), EnsEMBL (10), for example.

3.1.1. Retrieving the Promoter Sequence of the Gene of Interest in EPD

1. Enter *EPD* at http://www.epd.isb-sib.ch/.
2. Choose "Advance search."
3. Enter a query in the boxes on the search page opened. Press "Do query" button below.
4. Find the list of IDs of promoters retrieved at the bottom of the page opened. The details on each are available by clicking the ID.

5. To retrieve promoter(s) in the FASTA format, check the IDs of promoters of interest in the list, check "FASTA" in the "*Promoter Sequence format*" tab, and enter the desired first and last nucleotide positions relative to the transcription start; –499 and 100 are set as default. Click "submit." Find the promoter sequence(s) of the chosen gene(s) in FASTA format on the page opened.

3.1.2. Retrieving Upstream Sequence of the Gene of Interest in EnsEMBL Using RSAT

1. Enter RSAT (11) at http://rsat.ulb.ac.be/rsat/.
2. Choose "Retrieve EnsEMBL sequence" in the "Sequence tools" menu at the left of the page.
3. In the "query organism" menu, choose the organism of interest.
4. Check "Single organism."
5. Specify ID for a gene of interest. These IDs can be EnsEMBL gene, transcript or protein IDs, or IDs from some other databases.
6. For the "Feature type" choose "mRNA". For the "Sequence type," choose upstream/downstream.
7. Specify appropriate 5′- and 3′ boundaries of the requested sequence segments relative to the TSS (e.g., from –500 to –1).
8. The result will be the upstream sequence of the gene of interest in the FASTA format.

3.1.3. Retrieving the Upstream Sequence of the Gene of Interest in UCSC Genome Browser

1. Enter UCSC Genome Browser at http://genome.ucsc.edu/.
2. Choose the "Genomes" tab at the top of the page.
3. Choose the appropriate clade and genome in the menu; the last genome assembly will be chosen by default.
4. Type the gene name in the box marked "position or search term."
5. Press the "Submit" button.
6. The above steps result in a list of known genes listed in the UCSC and RefSeq databases. Choose the desired one.
7. Genome Browser will display gene tracks: Coding exons are shown as bars connected by horizontal lines representing introns. The 5′- and 3′-UTRs are displayed as thinner bars at the leading and trailing ends of the aligned regions. Arrowheads on the connecting intron lines indicate the direction of transcription. In situations where no intron is visible (e.g., single-exon genes, extremely zoomed-in displays), the arrowheads are displayed on the exon block itself. Remember the direction of transcription.

8. Choose the "DNA" tab at the top of the page. The chromosome coordinates of the gene transcript will be displayed at the "Position" window. If the transcription direction for the gene is from left to right (5′ to 3′), choose the lower value in the coordinates of the gene transcript. It will be the transcription start nucleotide. If the transcription direction for the gene is from right to left, choose the greater value. For example, if coordinates were chr8: 2,200–4,400, choose 2,200 in the first case, otherwise choose 4,400.
9. At the "Position" window, enter the chromosome coordinates of the first nucleotide in the transcript. If the transcription direction for the gene is from left to right, change it to the coordinates of the first nucleotide in the transcript (e.g., chr8: 2,200–2,201; the length of the region assignable should be more than 0). In the Sequence Retrieval Region Options, "Add extra bases upstream (5′)" window and "extra downstream" window specify suitable 5′- and 3′ boundaries of the requested sequence segments relative to transcription start site (e.g., –500 and 0). Press the "Get DNA" button.
10. If the transcription direction for the gene is from right to left, change it to the coordinates of the first nucleotide in the transcript (e.g., chr8: 4,399–4,400; the length of the region assignable should be more than 0). In the Sequence Retrieval Region Options, the "Add extra bases upstream (5′)" window and the "extra downstream" window specify suitable 5′- and 3′ boundaries of the requested sequence segments relative to a transcription start site (as it is the reverse strand, the values should be in the reverse order, e.g., 0 and –500).
11. Mark "Reverse complement (get "–" strand sequence)." Press "Get DNA" button.
12. The result will be the upstream sequence of the corresponding gene in the FASTA format.

3.2. Data for TFBS Recognition Method Training

3.2.1. Preparation of the Training Sets of Sequences That Are Known from Laboratory Experimentation to Interact with a Transcription Factor in Question

Creation of the training sample, that is, the aligned set of known binding sites for a transcription factor of interest, is one of the most complicated steps in the TFBS recognition workflow. It includes two steps: (a) retrieving the sequences of known binding sites and (b) the corresponding alignment. The creation of a reliable TFBS training sample requires reliable experimental data. A site could be used in the sample if binding of the transcription factor to the site has been demonstrated by one of the following methods: EMSA (electrophoretic mobility shift assay) with nuclear extract or specific antibodies, EMSA with purified or recombinant protein, or DNase I footprinting with purified or recombinant protein. This is important because indirect methods can lead to the inclusion of erroneous sequences in training sample sets (1). Also, consider the taxonomic origin of the site and transcription factor.

To retrieve known binding sites of transcription factors of interest, one can use several specialized information resources that compile this data, namely TRANSFAC (12), TRED (13), TRRD (14), ooTFD (15), and MPromDb (16). For example, TRANSFAC has links to RefSeq or EMBL (17) accession numbers of the sequences containing TFBS sequences. In addition, data on the degree to which the sites have been studied experimentally can be represented as either the quality of a site with an indication of the experiment type (TRED and TRANSFAC) or a digital code of the experimental technique used (TRRD). These allow the user to arrange the TFBS sequence sets according to a set of different criteria. One should avoid taking binding sites for transcription factors from species that are too distantly related from an evolutionary viewpoint into one training set.

The increasing efficiency of experimental techniques for TFBS detection has lead to the ever growing information on newly discovered TFBSs. This makes it promising to retrieve from scientific literature reliable TFBS sequences as well as ready-to-use TFBS training sets. In particular, development of new technologies for in vitro selection procedures (e.g., SELEX) has yielded ample data on the structures of binding sites for various transcription factors, both eukaryotic and prokaryotic. Several databases compile this information, namely TRANSFAC, JASPAR (18), and TRRD-ARTSITE. However, sequences selected artificially in vitro should be used with care, as these data in some cases poorly reflect the genuine structures of natural binding sites (19–21).

(a) To retrieve a binding site for a particular transcription factor from the *TRED* database:

1. Enter TRED at http://rulai.cshl.edu/TRED/.
2. Choose Retrieve transcription factor Motifs.
3. Select the type of search key: Factor name.
4. Enter search terms – the acronym of the transcription factor of interest.
5. Select Binding Quality: known (known is assigned in TRED as the binding quality level to a binding that has been proven by gel-shift competition, DNase I footprinting, etc.).
6. Press "SEARCH" button. As a result, you get a table list of experimentally confirmed TFBS sequences. Links in the "motif" row will lead a user to the site information page, where site sequence, its chromosome coordinates, and links to the sequence(s) of the "promoters with this site" are accessible. Also, the page contains links to information concerning the transcription factor, binding quality level (must

be 1, *experimentally verified directly*), species, and references (*see* **Notes 4** and **5**).

After collecting the proper set of TFBS sequences, the alignment is next. This process has not been formalized yet, and in some cases the best alignment can be made manually, with regard to various pieces of supplementary information, depending on the particular transcription factor and sequence set. The more accurate the alignment, the more accurate the detection of common contextual characteristics; consequently, it allows better recognition quality (less recognition errors). Nevertheless, application of tools available for the alignment of TFBS sequences can provide satisfactory results (22).

Example of aligned TFBS training sample of dioxin response element (DRE) in FASTA format (23):

```
> mCyp1a1 Site a
caagctcGCGTGagaagcg
> mCyp1a1 Site b
cctgtgtGCGTGccaagca
> mCyp1a1 Site d
cggagttGCGTGagaagag
> mCyp1a1 Site e
ccagctaGCGTGacagcac
> mCyp1a1 Site f
cgggtttGCGTGcgatgag
> mCyp1b1 XRE5
ccccttGCGTGcggagct
> rCyp1a1 XRE1
cggagttGCGTGagaagag
> rCyp1a1 XRE2
gatcctaGCGTGacagcac
> rAldh3
cactaatGCGTGccccatc
> rNqr1
tccccttGCGTGcaaaggc
> rSod1
gaggcctGCGTGcgcgcct
> rGstya
gcatgttGCGTGcatccct
> rUgt1a1
agaatgtGCGTGacaaggt
```

(b) Alignment of the TFBS sequences with the *info-gibbs* tool (24):

1. Enter RSAT server at http://rsat.ulb.ac.be/rsat/.
2. Choose "info-gibbs" in the "*Motif discovery*" menu at the left of the page.

3. Paste the TFBS sequences collected for the training set into the appropriate window and point the format used in the upper menu "format" (e.g., FASTA).
4. Uncheck "search both strands" if necessary.
5. Modify the options available to optimize the alignment quality.
6. As a result, find the numerous alignment result indicators together with the resulting aligned TFBS training sample and the frequency matrix derived from it.

In some cases, division into subsamples is a promising approach. A particular transcription factor can interact with its binding sites in a different fashion, thus making possible the situation when binding sites are present, for example, in the form of either direct or inverse repeats (25, 26) or conserved motifs with varying lengths of the spacer between them (27). In some cases, the methods for separation into subsamples are unclear; however, the need for such partition is evident.

3.2.2. Retrieving Frequency Matrix

A frequency matrix is a derivative of TFBS sequences, describing the frequencies of four nucleotides at each position of a TFBS training set. Tools based on PWM and consensus approaches can utilize frequency matrices (*see* **Note 6**). Frequency matrices are often used in a tab-separated text format, indicating the number of occurrences of each residue (each row per matching nucleotide) at each position (column = position) of the TFBS training set. Below is an example of a frequency matrix for DRE derived from the corresponding training sample:

A |	1	2	0	0	0	0	0	6
C |	1	1	0	13	0	0	0	7
G |	2	0	13	0	13	0	13	0
T |	9	10	0	0	0	13	0	0

Extraction of the *TRANSFAC* frequency matrix and consensus sequence from *ALLGEN PROMO* (28):

1. Enter *ALLGEN* at http://alggen.lsi.upc.es/ and choose *PROMO* from the list of main projects.
2. Click "ViewMatrices" at the left of the page.
3. Select the transcription factor of interest from the list of the matrices and click "Submit."
4. The result will be the frequency matrix together with its consensus sequence (*see* **Note 6**).

3.2.3. Retrieving Consensus Sequence

A consensus sequence (*see* **Note 3**) is a derivative from TFBS sequences or from a frequency matrix and shows which residues are most abundant in the alignment at each position.

It is usually presented as a word written in the generalized 15-letter IUPAC alphabet: {A, T, G, C, R = G/A, Y = T/C, M = A/C, K = T/G, W = A/T, S = G/C, B = T/C/G, V = A/G/C, H = A/T/C, D = A/T/G, N = A/T/G/C} (29).

3.3. Binding Site Recognition for Transcription Factors, Proposed by the Tool

3.3.1. Binding Site Recognition Using ***ALLGEN PROMO*** *(See* **Note 7***)*

1. Enter ALLGEN at http://alggen.lsi.upc.es/ and choose PROMO from the list of main projects.
2. Go through step 1: click "select species." Here the user can select the taxonomic level for the binding site and/or the transcription factor to be more specific in the search. Choose the appropriate taxonomic level for the search. In most cases, selection at the "site" level alone will be enough. Click the "Submit" button when done.
3. Click "Select factors": Here the user can select the transcription factors of interest from the list of factors (hold CTRL key to select multiple entries). Click "Submit" button when done.
4. Go through step 2: click the "SearchSites" link to analyze a single sequence or click "MultiSearchSites" to analyze a set of sequences. The MultiSearchSites user can choose to view results on the binding site recognitions that appear in a minimum number (determined by the user) of input sequences. Choose the appropriate option at the top of the page in that case.
5. Choose the maximum matrix dissimilarity rate. This parameter controls how similar a sequence must be to the matrix to be reported as a true binding site and appear in the results. Choosing a high dissimilarity rate will lead to the recognition of an excessive number of transcription factor-binding sites with a low reliability. Choosing a low dissimilarity rate will lead to a smaller number of the putative TFBSs being recognized, but with higher reliability. Default is 15% (85% similarity), but it can be modified by the user to specify the value most suitable for the task.
6. Input the regulatory sequence(s) to be analyzed in FASTA format into the only window or access the corresponding file at user's PC by the "Browse" command and press the "SUBMIT" button to run the program.
7. At the results page, one can find the following:
   - A link to this results page at the top of the page (7 days limit for storage of the result);

- Links to each of the transcription factors of interest. Clicking the link will lead to a page with a detailed view (positions, sequences, dissimilarity rates, and expectation values for each of the binding sites predicted for this transcription factor). Note that the expectation value (*E* value) gives a measure of the reliability of each recognition. The *E* value shows the probability of finding each of the matches by chance in a random sequence of 1,000 nucleotides and depends on the matrix used and the similarity level of the sequence to the matrix. Thus, a lower *E* value indicates better reliability of the recognition.
- The distribution of potential TFBSs of interest from sequence(s) submitted is visualized through a graphical representation: Potential TFBSs predicted are shown at the corresponding positions of the query sequence(s) in the table view.
- Distribution of the nucleotides among all the given chains.
- Distribution of the nucleotides for each one of the given chains.

3.3.2. Binding Site Recognition Using TFSiteScan (See **Note 8***)*

1. Enter *TFSiteScan* at http://www.ifti.org/cgi-bin/ifti/Tfsitescan.pl.
2. Input the regulatory sequence to be analyzed in one of the common sequence formats (IG, GenBank, EMBL, GCG, DNAStrider, or FASTA) at the only window (maximum sequence length allowed is 1,500 bp).
3. Mark the "IFTI Tfmatrix" menu item to make recognitions based on PWM from ooTFD.
4. Choose the appropriate clade in the menu at the right.
5. Press the "Submit" button.
6. The resulting window is divided into three parts. In the upper part, one can obtain a list of TFBSs recognized. Each line contains data on a potential site, including matrix similarity score values, positions, transcription factor name, and the accession number in ooTFD:
   a. The lower part contains an image map in association with the sequence analysis results, which is linked to individual Sites entries.

3.3.3. Binding Site Recognition Using SITECON

1. Enter SITECON (30) at http://wwwmgs.bionet.nsc.ru/mgs/programs/sitecon.
2. Select a particular transcription factor from the menu at the top of the page (*see* **Note 9**).
3. Press the "Recognition errors count" button. Press the "Recognition errors table" link in the window that opens

automatically. Here, type I errors show the fraction of potential sites missed during the recognition at a corresponding threshold. Type II errors allow for assessing the fraction of the sites recognized accidentally and, therefore, reflect the reliability that the site found is actually the site for binding of a given transcription factor. Choice of a low threshold will lead to the recognition of an excessive number of transcription factor-binding sites with a low reliability. The choice of a high threshold will lead to a smaller number of putative TFBSs being recognized, but with higher reliability. Choose the threshold with the desired level of recognition errors that is most suitable for the task.

4. Press "Return" at the main window to return to the SITECON starting page at http://wwwmgs.bionet.nsc.ru/mgs/programs/sitecon. A particular transcription factor should be selected in the menu at the top of the page.
5. Enter the chosen threshold value in "cut threshold." The cutoff threshold value can be corrected upon completion of the calculation by the recognition program; the value of the cutoff threshold is bounded below by the "minimal threshold" parameter. Enter the desired "minimal threshold" value.
6. Input the regulatory sequence(s) to be analyzed in the FASTA format into the lower window or access the corresponding file at user's PC by the "Browse" command.
7. Press "Recognition" to start the program.
8. Get the program output. Data on potential sites are preceded by the name of the sequence where they were found. Each line contains data on a potential site: position, level of conformational similarity, orientation relative to the beginning of sequence, and the sequence that was recognized as the site.

3.4. TFBS Recognition with User's Data for Training

3.4.1. TFBS Recognition with User's Consensus Using SCPD Analysis Tools

1. Enter the SCPD (31) homepage at http://rulai.cshl.edu/SCPD/.
2. Choose the link to "Search for user-defined consensus sequences" from the *Analysis tools* list.
3. Input the regulatory sequence(s) to be analyzed in the FASTA format into the upper window.
4. Input the consensus sequence into the lower window.
5. Press "Submit."
6. In the results page: Below the header of each of sequences analyzed, find a list of motifs matching the matrix found in this particular sequence in the following order: strand where

it was found (+/−), positions of the putative TFBS in the sequence analyzed, and putative TFBS sequence.

3.4.2. TFBS Recognition with User's Frequency Matrix Using SCPD Analysis Tools

1. Enter the SCPD homepage at http://rulai.cshl.edu/SCPD/.
2. Choose the link to "Search for user-defined matrix" from the *Analysis tools* list.
3. Input the regulatory sequence(s) to be analyzed in the FASTA format into the upper window.
4. Input the frequency matrix into the lower window (*see* **Note 6**). Enquire about the right format at the "example format" link on this page.
5. Specify a cutoff value for matrix similarity rate between 0 and 1. This parameter controls how similar a sequence must be to the matrix to be reported as a true binding site and to appear in the results. The choice of a low cutoff value will lead to the recognition of an excessive number of transcription factor-binding sites with a low reliability. The choice of a high cutoff value will lead to a smaller number of putative TFBSs being recognized but with higher reliability. The default value is 0.8 similarity, but it can be modified by the user. Choose the value most suitable for your task.
6. Press "Submit."
7. In the results page: Below the header of each of the sequences analyzed, find a list of motifs matching the matrix found in this particular sequence, in the following order: strand where it was found (+/−), positions of the putative TFBS in the sequence analyzed, putative TFBS sequence, and matrix similarity rate for this putative TFBS sequence.

3.4.3. TFBS Recognition with the UGENE Stand-alone Tool

1. Download the version of the program at http://ugene.unipro.ru/download.html for the appropriate OS. Install the package at your computer conventionally.
2. Start UGENE at your computer.
3. Open a file containing the regulatory sequence to be analyzed in FASTA format (menu File → Open).
4. Call the menu Actions → Analyse → search TFBS with matrices (*see* **Note 10**).
5. To start the analysis, call the menu Action→Analyse→Search TFBS with matrices. To search using the matrices from the JASPAR database, click the button "Search JASPAR database" (*see* **Note 11**). Choose the desired matrix for the appropriate taxonomic level.
6. Select the score threshold ("score" slider). This parameter controls how similar a sequence must be to the matrix to be

reported as a true binding site and to appear in the results. The choice of a low score threshold value will lead to the recognition of an excessive number of transcription factor-binding sites with low reliability. The choice of a high-score threshold value will lead to a smaller number of the putative TFBSs being recognized, but with higher reliability. The default value is 75% similarity, but it can be modified by the user. Choose the value most suitable for the task. Push "Search."

7. The recognition results will be shown in the lower window of this menu as a list of detected putative TFBSs, showing the position of a putative TFBS in the sequence analyzed, strand, and similarity score. To achieve better tuning of the score threshold for the task, the user can adjust the ("score" slider) and restart the recognition.
8. To view the results in the graphical representation in the browser, save the recognition results to the user's PC by pushing the button "Save as annotations." Here one can choose an optional annotation name, group of annotation, and project name for the convenience of result storage. Push the "Create" button.
9. The putative TFBS will be depicted in the graphical view in the browser.

3.5. TFBS Recognition by the Phylogenetic Footprinting Approach

3.5.1. Retrieving a Set of Upstream Sequences of Orthologous Genes in EnsEMBL Using RSAT

1. Enter *RSAT* at http://rsat.ulb.ac.be/rsat/.
2. Choose "Retrieve EnsEMBL sequence" in the "Sequence tools" menu at the left of the page.
3. In the "query organism" menu, choose the organism of interest.
4. Check "Multiple organisms," at the "Optional filters," for the "Homology type" choose "Orthologs."
5. Specify the ID from a gene of interest. These IDs can be *EnsEMBL* gene, transcript or protein IDs, or IDs from other databases (Uniprot, RefSeq, Flybase, SGD, etc.).
6. Under the "Type of sequence to retrieve" menu for the "Sequence type," choose "upstream/downstream."
7. Under the "Options for upstream or downstream sequence" menu for the "Sequence position," choose "upstream" and specify suitable 5′ and 3′ boundaries of the requested sequence segments relative to the transcription start site (e.g., from –500 to –1). Under "Relative to feature" choose "mRNA."
8. As a result, find the upstream sequences of orthologous genes for a number of species where orthologs for the gene chosen are known to date. The species name from where the sequence originates is indexed in the annotation after

the ">" symbol. A pair of upstream sequences of orthologous genes for a pair of species can be easily chosen from the whole set retrieved.

3.5.2. TFBS Recognition with CONREAL

1. Enter the CONREAL homepage (32) at http://conreal.niob.knaw.nl/.
2. Paste a pair of upstream sequences of orthologous genes (see **Section 3.5.1** for guidance) for a pair of species in FASTA format to the main window (max. 100 kb per sequence) or access the corresponding file at the PC of user by the "Browse" command.
3. Select search parameters: Specify the "threshold for PWMs," indicating a matrix similarity rate, between 70 and 90%. This parameter controls how the sequence must be similar to the matrix to be recognized by the program as a true binding site. Choice of a low threshold for PWMs will lead to the recognition of an excessive number of TFBSs with a low reliability. The choice of a high threshold for a PWM value will lead to a lesser number of the putative TFBSs being recognized, but with higher reliability. The default value is 80%, but it can be modified by the user. The user can also define "length of flanks to calculate homology" and "threshold for homology" to the preferred values.
4. Four possible aligners as well as both JASPAR and TRANSFAC vertebrate TFBS dataset are used as defaults; the user can change this optionally.
5. Press "Search."
6. At the results page, the user obtains the alignment of the sequences. The results are summarized in a graphical output, showing the positions of aligned hits and the distribution/concentration of conserved TFBSs along the sequences. The graphs are followed by sequence-alignment data and tables of conserved TFBSs linked to TransFac entries. The CONREAL Web interface also provides access to the LAGAN-based phylogenetic footprinting approach so that the two methods and their results can be easily compared.

4. Notes

1. The set of tools presented here were chosen for the sake of usability. Some existing tools, not mentioned here, may surpass them in performance.

2. In the traditional PWM-based methods, it is assumed that positions within a motif site are mutually independent. However, recent biological experiments have shown that nucleotides of transcription factor-binding sites exert interdependent effects on the binding affinities of transcription factors (33).
3. A consensus sequence is better used for rough initial annotation of the sequence analyzed (34). The PWM approach can provide far better recognition quality.
4. The sequence of "promoters with this site" can be used for retrieving TFBS flanking sequences of desired length if it is necessary for TFBS set construction.
5. Natural (not in vitro selected) TFBS flanking sequences usually also contain information that can also be used by recognition methods leading to an increase in accuracy (35). So making the training sample of the longer TFBS sequences (not only core sequences) and the sequential varying of the length to achieve lower recognition errors could allow a considerable increase in the accuracy of prediction. Of course, ready-made matrices and consensi do not allow this optimization.
6. The rows in the frequency matrix (A C G T) may differ from those used in other programs.
7. ALLGEN PROMO currently uses version 8.3 of TRANSFAC. This version contains about 400 matrices classified by taxa, mostly eukaryotic.
8. TFSiteScan is integrated with ooTFD. It can currently utilize 634 matrices, classified by taxa.
9. SITECON utilizes 220 high-quality training sets for mammalian TFBSs from TRRD. It can also utilize a user's TFBS training sample. Parameters "window size" (*see* **Note 5**) and "apply weight" can be modified in that case to achieve better recognition quality. Use the "Recognition errors count" option to compare them.
10. One can use SITECON integrated into UGENE. Call the menu Tools → SITECON→Build new SITECON model from alignment to use your own TFBS training set. Call the menu Action→Analyse→Search TFBS with SITECON to use it for putative site recognition with ready-made and user's TFBS training sets.
11. A user can construct a matrix of his/her own from a TFBS training set with UGENE and use it for putative site recognition. To calculate a new matrix, call the menu Tools → Weight matrix→Build weight matrix. Subsequently, it can be used through the menu Action→Analyse→Search

TFBS with matrices. More matrices for recognition are available via browse ("...") option in this menu. Analysis of multiple sequences is also available. Call the menu Tools → "Workflow designer."

References

1. Kolchanov, N. A., Merkulova, T. I., Ignatieva, E. V., et al. (2007) Combined experimental and computational approaches to study the regulatory elements in eukaryotic genes. *Brief Bioinform* 8, 266–274.
2. Elnitski, L., Jin, V. X., Farnham, P. J., et al. (2006) Locating mammalian transcription factor binding sites: a survey of computational and experimental techniques. *Genome Res* 16, 1455–1464.
3. Schneider, T. D., Stormo, G. D., Gold, L., et al. (1986) Information content of binding sites on nucleotide sequences. *J Mol Biol* 188, 415–431.
4. Day, W. H., McMorris, F. R. (1992) Threshold consensus methods for molecular sequences. *J Theor Biol* 159, 481–489.
5. MacIsaac, K. D., Fraenkel, E. (2006) Practical strategies for discovering regulatory DNA sequence motifs. *PLoS Comput Biol* 2, e36.
6. Schmid, C. D., Perier, R., Praz, V., et al. (2006) EPD in its twentieth year: towards complete promoter coverage of selected model organisms. *Nucleic Acids Res* 34, 82–85.
7. Karolchik, D., Hinrichs, A. S., Kent, W. J. (2009) The UCSC Genome Browser. *Curr Protoc Bioinform* 28, 1.4.1–1.4.26.
8. Yamashita, R., Wakaguri, H., Sugano, S., et al. (2010) DBTSS provides a tissue specific dynamic view of Transcription Start Sites. *Nucleic Acids Res* 38, 98–104.
9. Pruitt, K. D., Tatusova, T., Klimke, W., et al. (2009) NCBI Reference Sequences: current status, policy and new initiatives. *Nucleic Acids Res* 37, 32–36.
10. Flicek, P., Aken, B. L., Ballester, B., et al. (2010) Ensembl's 10th year *Nucleic Acids Res* 38, 557–562.
11. Thomas-Chollier, M., Sand, O., Turatsinze, J. V., et al (2008) RSAT: regulatory sequence analysis tools. *Nucleic Acids Res* 36, 119–127.
12. Matys, V., Kel-Margoulis, O. V., Fricke, E., et al. (2006) TRANSFAC and its module TRANSCompel: transcriptional gene regulation in eukaryotes. *Nucleic Acids Res* 34, 108–110.
13. Jiang, C., Xuan, Z., Zhao, F., et al. (2007) TRED: a transcriptional regulatory element database, new entries and other development. *Nucleic Acids Res* 35, 137–140.
14. Kolchanov, N. A., Ignatieva, E. V., Ananko, E. A., et al. (2002) Transcription Regulatory Regions Database (TRRD): its status in 2002. *Nucleic Acids Res* 30, 312–317.
15. Ghosh, D. (2000) Object-oriented transcription factors database (ooTFD). *Nucleic Acids Res* 28, 308–310.
16. Sun, H., Palaniswamy, S. K., Pohar, T. T., et al. (2006) MPromDb: an integrated resource for annotation and visualization of mammalian gene promoters and ChIP-chip experimental data. *Nucleic Acids Res* 34, 98–103.
17. McWilliam, H., Valentin, F., Goujon, M., et al. (2009) Web services at the European Bioinformatics Institute—2009. *Nucleic Acids Res* 37, 6–10.
18. Sandelin, A., Alkema, W., Engström, P., et al. (2004) JASPAR: an open-access database for eukaryotic transcription factor binding profiles. *Nucleic Acids Res* 32, 91–94.
19. Robison, K., McGuire, A. M., Church, G. M. (1998) A comprehensive library of DNA-binding site matrices for 55 proteins applied to the complete *Escherichia coli* K-12 genome. *J Mol Biol* 284, 241–254.
20. Whyatt, D. J., deBoer, E., Grosveld, F. (1993) The two zinc finger-like domains of GATA-1 have different DNA binding specificities. *EMBO J* 12, 4993–5005.
21. Shultzaberger, R. K., Schneider, T. D. (1999) Using sequence logos and information analysis of Lrp DNA binding sites to investigate discrepancies between natural selection and SELEX. *Nucleic Acids Res* 27, 882–887.
22. Fu, Y., Weng, Z. (2005) Improvement of TRANSFAC matrices using multiple local alignment of transcription factor binding site sequences. *Genome Inform* 16, 68–72.
23. Sun, Y. V., Boverhof, D. R., Burgoon, L. D., et al. (2004) Comparative analysis of dioxin response elements in human, mouse and rat genomic sequences. *Nucleic Acids Res* 32, 4512–4523.

24. Defrance, M., van Helden, J. (2009) Info-gibbs: a motif discovery algorithm that directly optimizes information content during sampling. *Bioinformatics* 25, 2715–2722.
25. Schoenmakers, E., Alen, P., Verrijdt, G., et al (1999) Differential DNA binding by the androgen and glucocorticoid receptors involves the second Zn-finger and a C-terminal extension of the DNA-binding domains. *Biochem J* 341, 515–521.
26. Kim, J. B., Spotts, G. D., Halvorsen, Y. D., et al. (1995) Dual DNA binding specificity of DD1/SREBP1 controlled by a single amino acid in the basic helix–loop–helix domain. *Mol Cell Biol* 15, 2582–2588.
27. Khorasanizadeh, S., Rastinejad, F. (2001) Nuclear-receptor interactions on DNA-response elements. *Trends Biochem Sci* 26, 384–390.
28. Messeguer, X., Escudero, R., Farré D, et al. (2002) PROMO: detection of known transcription regulatory elements using species-tailored searches. *Bioinformatics* 18, 333–334.
29. Cornish-Bowden, A. (1985) Nomenclature for incompletely specified bases in nucleic acid sequences: recommendations 1984. *Nucleic Acids Res* 13, 3021–3030.
30. Oshchepkov, D. Y., Vityaev, E. E., Grigorovich, D. A., et al. (2004) SITECON: a tool for detecting conservative conformational and physicochemical properties in transcription factor binding site alignments and for site recognition. *Nucleic Acids Res* 32, 208–212.
31. Zhu, J., Zhang, M. Q. (1999) SCPD: a promoter database of the yeast *Saccharomyces cerevisiae*. *Bioinformatics* 15, 607–611.
32. Berezikov, E., Guryev, V., Cuppen, E. (2007) Exploring conservation of transcription factor binding sites with CONREAL. *Methods Mol Biol* 395, 437–448.
33. Zhou, Q., Liu, J. S. (2004) Modeling within-motif dependence for transcription factor binding site predictions. *Bioinformatics* 20, 909–916.
34. Mikkelsen, T. (1993) Interpreting sequence motifs: a cautionary note. *Trends Genet* 9, 159.
35. Levitsky, V. G., Ignatieva, E. V., Ananko, E. A. et al. (2007) Effective transcription factor binding site prediction using a combination of optimization, a genetic algorithm and discriminant analysis to capture distant interactions. *BMC Bioinformatics* 8, 481.

Chapter 17

In Silico Prediction of Splice-Affecting Nucleotide Variants

Claude Houdayer

Abstract

It appears that all types of genomic nucleotide variations can be deleterious by affecting normal pre-mRNA splicing via disruption/creation of splice site consensus sequences. As it is neither pertinent nor realistic to perform functional testing for all of these variants, it is important to identify those that could lead to a splice defect in order to restrict experimental transcript analyses to the most appropriate cases. In silico tools designed to provide this type of prediction are available. In this chapter, we present in silico splice tools integrated in the Alamut (Interactive Biosoftware) application and detail their use in routine diagnostic applications. At this time, in silico predictions are useful for variants that decrease the strength of wild-type splice sites or create a cryptic splice site. Importantly, in silico predictions are not sufficient to classify variants as neutral or deleterious: they should be used as part of the decision-making process to detect potential candidates for splicing anomalies, prompting molecular geneticists to carry out transcript analyses in a limited and pertinent number of cases which could be managed in routine settings.

Key words: Unknown variants, splice, in silico prediction, diagnosis.

1. Introduction

The accuracy of intron excision and exon junction during pre-mRNA splicing is determined by recognition of well-known consensus sequences, i.e. the 5′ donor and 3′ acceptor splice sites and the branch site (**Fig. 17.1**). More discrete elements are also involved such as exonic splicing enhancers (ESEs) that enhance pre-mRNA splicing when present in exons (1–3).

Several lines of evidence suggest that all types of nucleotide variations are potentially deleterious by affecting normal pre-mRNA splicing via disruption of consensus sequences or creation of cryptic sequences. As a result, each nucleotide variation should be considered to be a potential candidate for splicing alterations;

B. Yu, M. Hinchcliffe (eds.), *In Silico Tools for Gene Discovery*, Methods in Molecular Biology 760,
DOI 10.1007/978-1-61779-176-5_17, © Springer Science+Business Media, LLC 2011

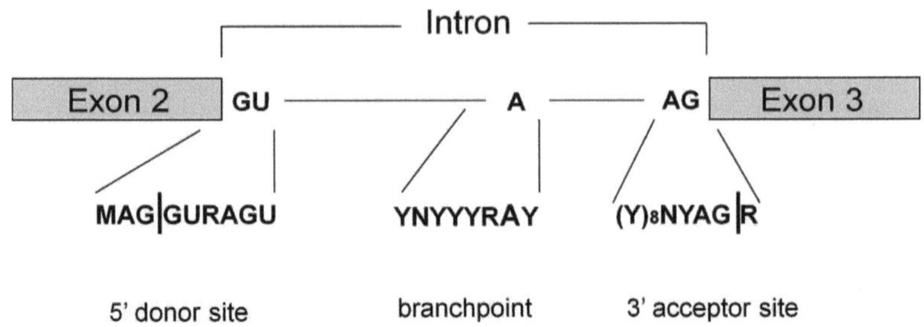

Fig. 17.1. Schematic representation of the splicing consensus sequences. Exons are *boxed* and the intron is drawn as a *line* (not scaled). M stands for A or C, R for G or A, Y for T or C and N for any base.

not only intronic but also nonsense, missense and translationally silent variants may impact splicing (3–5). Therefore, one of the key issues raised in molecular diagnosis is the correct interpretation of the biological consequences of so-called variants of unknown significance (UV), for example, their putative impact on splicing. Unfortunately, testing all nucleotide variants at the RNA level is a tremendous task that cannot be performed in routine diagnostic settings. The use of algorithms allowing correct and reliable predictions of the impact of nucleotide variations on splicing would therefore be of utmost importance (*see* **Notes 1** and **2**).

Some web-based tools designed to provide this type of prediction are available, such as Splice Site Prediction by Neural Network (NNSplice) (6), Splice Site Finder (SSF), MaxEntScan (MES) (7), ESE Finder (8), Relative Enhancer and Silencer Classification by Unanimous Enrichment (RESCUE-ESE) (9) and more tools described in **Note 3**. NNSplice, SSF and MES use current knowledge on base composition of the splice site sequences (10) but run distinct algorithms that generate a score matrix for each splice site (donor, acceptor for SSF, NNSplice and MES, plus branch site for SSF). The algorithms used in SSF are based on Refs. (10, 11). The availability of statistics for a large number of splice sites makes it possible to rate each location in a gene for its potential as a splice site. Hence SSF was developed to predict potential exons in a sequence, using a scoring and a ranking scheme based on nucleotide weight tables. NNSplice uses a computer-learning method based on neural networks that identifies sequence patterns once it is trained with a set of real splicing signals. The larger the set of real splicing signals used, the better the predictions obtained (6). The MES framework is based on the maximum entropy principle and uses large datasets of human splice sites and takes into account adjacent and non-adjacent dependencies. These splice site models assign a log–odd ratio (MaxENT score) to a 9-bp (5′ splice site) or a 23-bp (3′ splice site) sequence. The higher the score, the higher the probability that the sequence is a true splice site (12). RESCUE-ESE identifies candidate ESEs as hexanucleotides significantly enriched in human exons and/or located with a significant frequency in the vicinity of weak 3′ and 5′ splice sites. ESE Finder uses functional Systematic Evolution of Ligands by EXponential enrichment (SELEX) and position-weight matrices to score ESEs specific for a subset of Ser/Arg-rich proteins, a family of splicing factors.

These in silico prediction tools are available as either stand-alone programs or part of commercial (Alamut, Interactive Biosoftware) or free web-based application [Human Splicing Finder (13).

Of note, SSF is no longer supported but Alamut uses algorithms based on Alex Dong Li's Splice Site Finder (hereinafter designed as SSF-like). A major advantage of MES running under Alamut (hereinafter designed as MES-Alamut) is that the user no longer needs to indicate a dedicated analysis window with intron/exon junctions. Alamut scores the entire sequence, automatically moving the window with a 1 bp shift. As a result, all positions can be analysed with the MES-Alamut implementation, as opposed to the stand-alone program. This has to be underlined as it circumvents the limitation of the stand-alone program which cannot always be used as a first-line tool (14). Branch point prediction is available in Alamut and uses matrixes developed by Zhang (15). Alamut also integrates GeneSplicer (16). However, in our hands, it does not give reliable splicing predictions and therefore is neither presented nor discussed.

For routine molecular diagnostic applications, in silico predictions are, at this time, useful for variants that decrease the strength of wild-type sites or create a cryptic splice site. Importantly, in silico predictions are not sufficient to classify variants as neutral or deleterious: they should be used as part of the decision-making process, to detect potential candidates for splicing anomalies, prompting molecular geneticists to carry out experimental transcript analyses in a limited and pertinent number of cases which could be managed in routine settings (*see* **Note 4**). We believe these tools should improve in the coming years as new algorithms should be designed, based on the increasing number of transcript studies available. In this chapter, we present a step-by-step protocol for Alamut as well as some general rules for other tools (**Section 3.1**). Guidelines for interpretation are provided in **Section 3.2**. Recommendations made in this chapter mostly rely on previous literature and a set of 337 *BRCA1* and *BRCA2* variants from the French splice consortium Génétique et Cancer, providing in-depth transcript analyses with their corresponding in silico modelling (submitted elsewhere for publication).

2. Materials

Alamut software is available from Interactive Biosoftware (http://www.interactive-biosoftware.com/, Rouen, France). Alamut is a software application that runs on Windows XP/Vista/7, Mac OS X and Linux. It requires Internet access for connection with the Interactive Biosoftware's servers, from which regularly updated sequence and annotation data are provided. Installing the software does not require administrator privileges. If installed behind an institution's firewall, web proxy information must be provided (generally available through the IT Department).

3. Methods

3.1. Application of Alamut Software

1. Open the Alamut software.
2. Connect to the Alamut server.
3. Select the gene, then the transcript of interest (if different transcripts are available). We recommend choosing a favourite transcript by ticking the appropriate box in order to avoid potential confusion.
4. Right click on the base(s) of interest to enter the variant(s) to be tested (*see* **Note 5**).
5. Click the 'Splicing' button from the variant annotation window (**Fig. 17.2**) for splicing predictions.
6. The splicing window displays the reference (wild-type) and mutated sequences (in the range displayed in the main window when the Splicing button was clicked) and the predicted 5′ and 3′ splice sites are reported above and below each sequence, respectively (**Fig. 17.3**). Exons are drawn as grey boxes. Hits from Splice Site Finder-like, MaxEntScan, NNSPLICE and GeneSplicer are displayed as dark vertical bars for 5′ (donor) sites and as grey vertical bars for 3′ (acceptor) sites. The height of each bar is proportional to the maximum possible score computed by the corresponding algorithm. Known constitutive signals are displayed as small dark (5′) or grey (3′) triangles, close to the sequence letters. When moving the mouse over each vertical bar or triangle, a tooltip appears with the corresponding score. You can display score numbers for each hit bar by just clicking the bar itself.

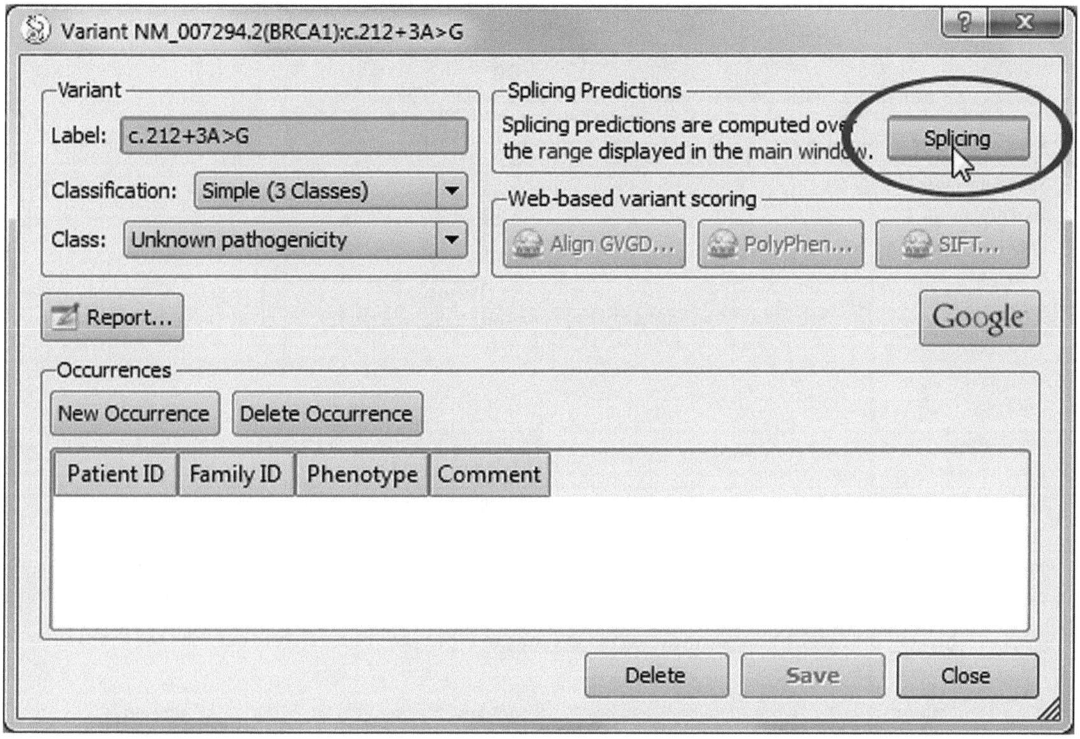

Fig. 17.2. Alamut analysis window. Splicing predictions are available by clicking the Splicing button (*upper right*). Nomenclature of the variant under study (according to Human Genome Variation Society guidelines) appears in the *upper left* part of the screen. Other Alamut features are available in this screen but are beyond the scope of this chapter (e.g. summary report for the variant, web-based scoring using SIFT, Align-GVD and PolyPhen).

7. Branch points appear as white vertical bars. However, great care has to be taken regarding interpretation as the prediction reveals a huge number of putative signals (*see* **Section 3.2**).
8. To reveal differences between wild-type and mutated scores, click on the 'Highlight Differences' button. Unchanged scores get dimmed, while score numbers are displayed beside those that differ (**Fig. 17.4**). This is a useful and fast way to analyse variants because a vast number of pseudo-splicing signals surround real splicing signals, clearly demonstrating that consensus sequences per se are not sufficient for exon definition. This exemplifies the need to work by comparison between mutant and wild-type sequences.
9. To display ESE predictions, click the 'ESE Predictions' button. ESE hits from ESE Finder are now displayed above each sequence and appear as rectangles of different colours depending on the ESEs. RESCUE-ESE hexamers are drawn under them and appear as a square with a solid line (**Fig. 17.5**).

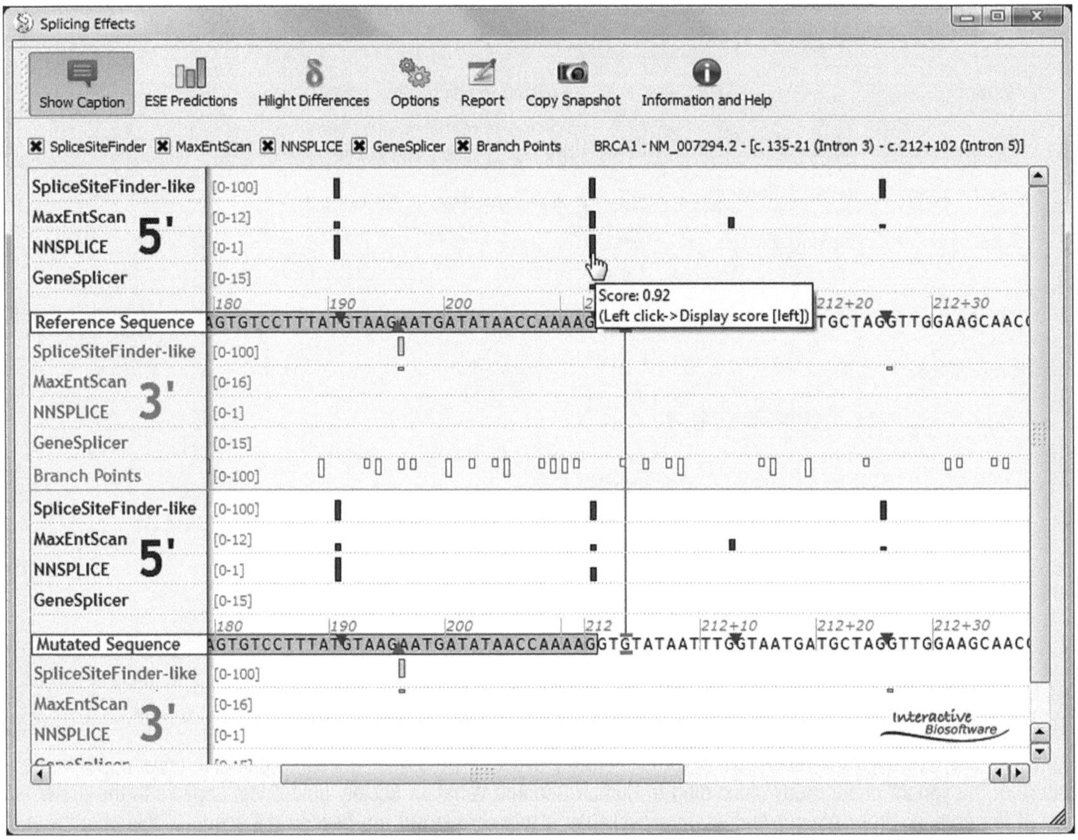

Fig. 17.3. Alamut splicing window. Options are available at the top of the screen, including ESE prediction, options for advanced users and report in HTML format. By default, all matrices are used for calculation and shown as *ticked boxes*. The gene under study and the analysis range are indicated in the *upper right part* of the screen. Tools integrated in Alamut are indicated in the *left part* for 5′ and 3′ splice sites. The variant nucleotide is indicated by a *vertical line* (see text for details).

10. For advanced users, an 'Option' button is available. It allows personal definition of the thresholds (*see* **Note 6**).
11. To generate a tabular report of splicing predictions, click the 'Report' button. The report, generated in HTML format, can be opened and edited by most word processors.

3.2. Prediction Data Analysis

In our hands, MES-Alamut and SSF-like provide the best predictions in that a decisional threshold can be defined. Therefore, this analysis section will be based on these tools.

3.2.1. Preliminary Step

Before testing the impact of the variant, the first step is to check that surrounding wild-type splice sites are correctly identified with an expected high score. As an example, in the case of exons with 'GC' donor sites, these algorithms do not work properly and consequently the impact of variants cannot be analysed (*see* **Note 7**). Anyway, the user should be aware that there is no strict correlation

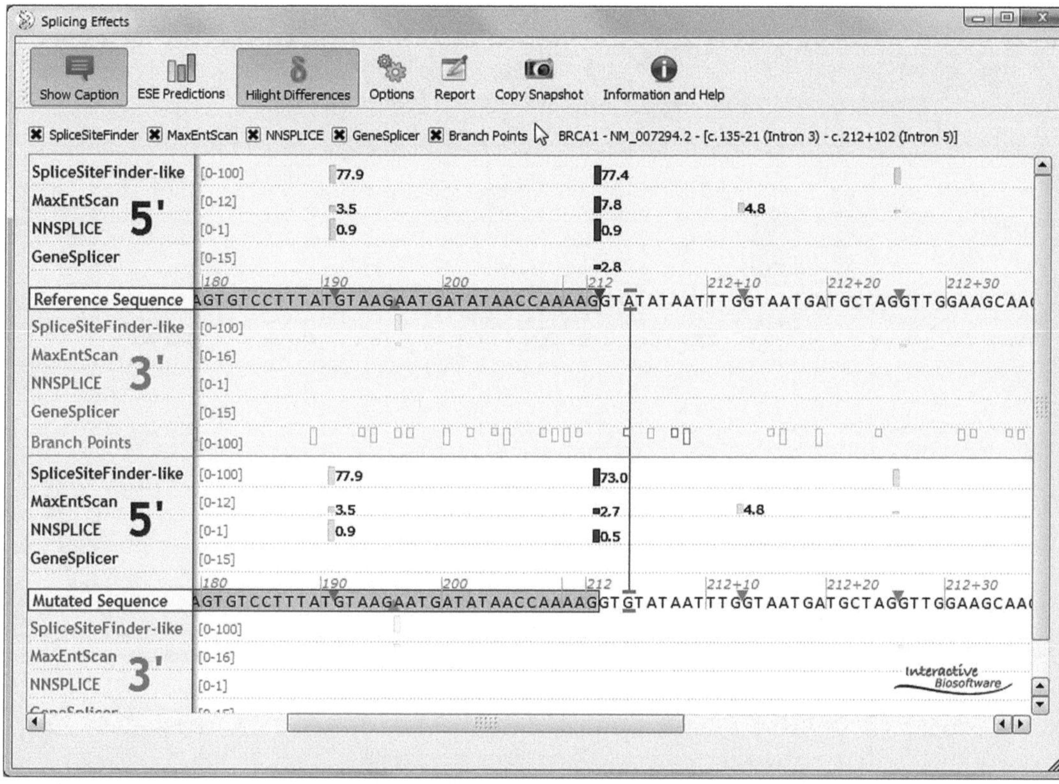

Fig. 17.4. Alamut splicing window with differences highlighted. This screenshot shows the scores of the predicted splice sites. A significant decrease is observed between the wild-type and mutant 5′ splice sites with all tools. Putative cryptic sites are located upstream and downstream from the wild-type site (see text for details).

between the tools (some may provide a high score, others a lower one), with these discrepancies reflecting the differences in the algorithms used.

3.2.2. Interpretation

In order to facilitate in silico interpretations, it is recommended to look at the score variations rather than the scores themselves and to set a limit of significance for score variations (*see* **Notes 4** and **8**). The reason is that many factors other than splice sites are also involved in the splicing process. These thresholds depend on the tools used and may even depend on the local sequence context. Anyway, some general rules emerge (*see* **Note 9**):

1. *Variations occurring at the AG/GT consensus canonical site* can be considered as impacting splicing; predictions are good but this is not surprising as this deleterious impact has been widely recognized for a long time and this knowledge was probably taken into account when designing the algorithms running in these tools. It does not provide any supplementary information to the user.
2. *Variations occurring at loosely defined consensus positions* are also reliable. Using MES-Alamut, we recommend that the

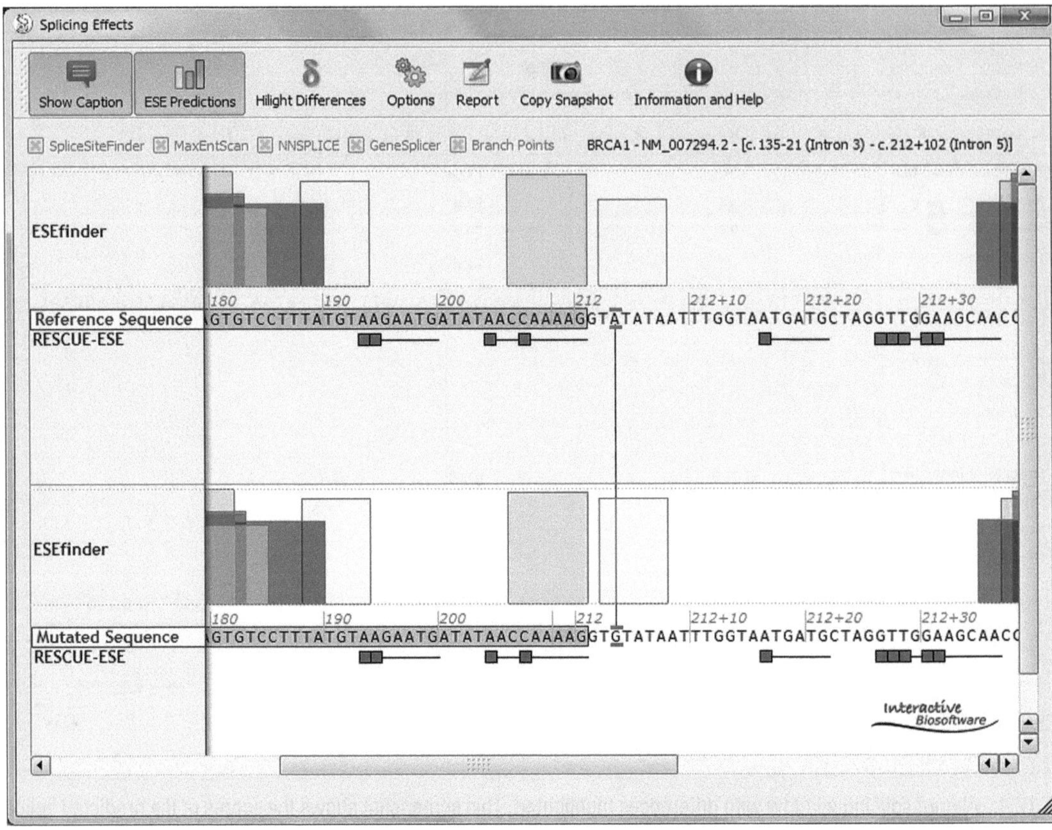

Fig. 17.5. Alamut splicing window with ESE predictions. ESE hits from ESE Finder and RESCUE-ESE appear as rectangles of different colours and as a square with a solid line, respectively. As detailed in the text, a large number of distinct ESEs are predicted.

mutant score should be at least 15% lower than the wild-type score in order to consider the prediction as positive and deleterious. Using SSF-like, this threshold should be 5%. Using our dataset, these thresholds provide 96% sensitivity and 74% specificity with MES-Alamut and 91% sensitivity and 87% specificity with SSF-like.

3. *Variations located outside the consensus positions* are less reliable with specificity issues mainly. Creation of a cryptic splice site should be interpreted in a context-dependant manner. If it is close to a wild-type splice site, competition should be evaluated (*see* **Notes 8** and **10**). If it is a deep intronic cryptic site, the user has to look for other nearby consensus sites needed for intronic exonization (5). As a result, deep intronic mutations are rarer because a combination of 5′ and 3′ splice sites, branch point and discrete elements concurring to exon definition (such as ESEs) is needed for exonization and this favourable context is rarely found in introns. On the other hand, an exonic cryptic site will use existing, wild-type

consensus sites. Using MES-Alamut, we would consider a cryptic site as a putative competitor if it reaches at least 80% of the score of the wild-type one.

4. *Branch point* prediction reveals a huge number of putative signals. As a result, specificity is too poor to be used in diagnostic procedures; similarly this applies to ESE predictions (see below).
5. *ESE.* It is generally inappropriate to perform RNA studies on the basis of ESE prediction alone due to a major lack of specificity (*see* **Note 11**). In reality, the objective is not to detect ESE loss for a given variant but to determine whether or not this ESE is used by the splicing machinery of the exon under study. Unfortunately this cannot be predicted at the present time. In other words, we cannot predict whether or not a modified ESE pattern is deleterious. Therefore, at the present time, it appears unrealistic to use ESE tools for diagnosis unless functional mapping of exonic splicing regulatory elements have been done for the gene of interest.

4. Notes

1. In silico tools are not used to classify variants but to detect candidates for splicing anomalies. However, impacting splicing does not necessarily mean pathogenic. In the extreme case of AG/GT disruptions (obviously impacting splicing), we recommend looking for putative cryptic splice sites located in the vicinity of the disrupted, wild-type one. The reason is that if a strong cryptic 5′ site is located, let us say 12 bp from the disrupted wild-type GT, this cryptic may be used by the splicing machinery, thereby resulting in deletion (or insertion, depending on the cases) of four amino acids, rather than the skipping of an entire exon. As a result, biological interpretation could not be the same. Therefore, in this specific (and rare) situation, where a neighbouring in-frame cryptic site could rescue splicing to a certain extent, AG/GT disruption should be investigated at an RNA level to check splicing outcome.
2. Quantitation is an important point to consider in splicing assays. Hence, variations leading to isoform imbalance or a low level of an abnormal transcript are not necessarily deleterious. But the point is that very few quantitative splicing data are available yet (17, 18) and as a result alteration levels cannot be predicted by in silico tools. More generally, in silico tools cannot yet be used to define splicing

outcome (e.g. exon skipping versus use of a cryptic splice site) because it results from a complex interplay between consensus sequences and other factors from the splicing machinery. This is illustrated in **Fig. 17.4**. The *BRCA1* c.212+3A>G mutation actually leads to the use of the 22-bp upstream cryptic site (scored 3.5) rather than the intronic 13-bp downstream cryptic site (scored 4.8).

3. A number of other in silico tools are available. Among them, Automated Splice Site Analyses (14, 19) and Human Splicing Finder (13) have been tested. Prediction is done by copying and pasting wild-type and variant sequences in dedicated windows or by entering variant nomenclature with the corresponding reference sequence. They are not as user-friendly as Alamut and output from Human Splicing Finder is sometimes complex to interpret. The reason is that it provides the user with a very complete analysis integrating a number of available matrices (e.g. MES, ESE Finder but also algorithms aiming at detecting silencer elements) as well as new, proprietary ones.
4. To use in silico predictions for diagnostic purposes, a decision threshold must be selected. At this point in time, there is no threshold allowing 100% sensitivity while keeping proper specificity. In other words, too many false positives need to be tested to reach maximum sensitivity. In this chapter, thresholds are proposed, based on present knowledge. However, these thresholds may vary depending on the user who has to define the optimum specificity/sensitivity combination meeting his/her objectives (balance between the time and cost required by RNA analysis and the risk of missing a deleterious mutation).
5. Alamut splicing predictions are computed over the range displayed in the main window. This range should be large enough to allow reliable calculation by the tools (e.g. MES needs 23 bp for 3′ splice site score calculation) but a minimum range of 100 bp upstream and downstream from the variant should be analysed to give a useful view of the sequence context. The user may enlarge this range if needed and then get back to the main window.
6. Alamut's default settings are appropriate for diagnostic purposes. On the other hand, setting thresholds to zero could be useful for research projects. It also allows detection of poorly defined consensus splice sites. Surprisingly, setting zero as a threshold for NNSplice will lead to aberrant predictions: we therefore recommend using 0.1 as the minimum.
7. The better the definition of the consensus site (i.e. the higher the score), the better the reliability of predictions.

In other words, if the wild-type consensus site is not scored or poorly defined, the tool should not be used (e.g. see above the 'GC' donor sites). As an example, a wild-type site scored 3 with MES or 60 with SSF-like is poorly defined and predictions will therefore not be reliable (mainly specificity problems). To define these 5′ and 3′ reliability thresholds for a given gene, we would suggest defining the mean score and standard deviation (SD) for all 5′ and 3′ splice sites of this gene and set the reliability threshold at mean–2SD.

8. Using MES-Alamut, a cryptic site is considered as a putative competitor if it reaches at least 80% of the score of the wild-type one. Of note, no such threshold could be found using SSF-like and as a result no recommendation could be made. As explained above, this threshold will not avoid false positives, mainly in introns, but should be a good compromise between sensitivity and specificity.

9. Rather than using each tool separately, the user may choose to combine them to tentatively increase overall performance. In all cases, we recommend first-line analysis with MES-Alamut using a 15% threshold. Then candidate variants could be selected using SSF-like with a 5% threshold. This way, and in our hands, specificity reaches 83% while keeping the 96% sensitivity (**Fig. 17.6**).

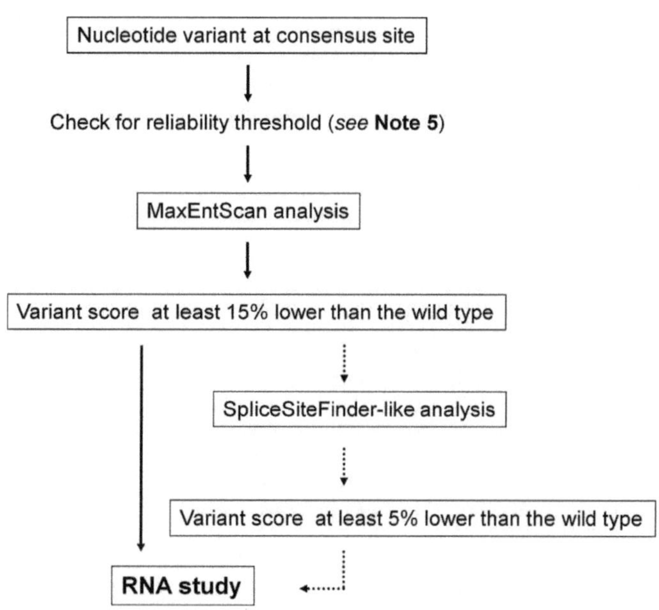

Fig. 17.6. Tentative MES-Alamut in silico analysis pipeline (*solid line*) and in combination with SSF-like (*dotted line*).

10. Creation of a putative competitive cryptic site should be interpreted in the context of the surrounding splicing signals. As an example, creation of an intronic 3′ cryptic site close to the 5′ wild-type one is not relevant.
11. The role of ESE in splicing defects has been clearly demonstrated. However, ESE predictions cannot be used in routine diagnostic practice for reason of specificity. Alternatively, they could be used in research settings to explain a splicing defect already found. This might be the case for the above-mentioned *BRCA1* mutation (**Fig. 17.4**). The use of a weaker cryptic site might be explained by the co-occurrence of ESEs that might provide better exon definition (**Fig. 17.5**).

Acknowledgements

The author wishes to thank the Groupe Génétique et Cancer, Virginie Moncoutier, Laurent Castéra and André Blavier for helpful support.

References

1. Hastings, M. L., and Krainer, A. R. (2001) Pre-mRNA splicing in the new millennium. *Curr Opin Cell Biol* 13, 302–309.
2. Cooper, T. A., and Mattox, W. (1997) The regulation of splice-site selection, and its role in human disease. *Am J Hum Genet* 61, 259–266.
3. Cartegni, L., Chew, S. L., and Krainer, A. R. (2002) Listening to silence and understanding nonsense: exonic mutations that affect splicing. *Nat Rev Genet* 3, 285–298.
4. Zatkova, A., Messiaen, L., Vandenbroucke, I., et al. (2004) Disruption of exonic splicing enhancer elements is the principal cause of exon skipping associated with seven nonsense or missense alleles of NF1. *Hum Mutat* 24, 491–501.
5. Dehainault, C., Michaux, D., Pages-Berhouet, S., et al. (2007) A deep intronic mutation in the RB1 gene leads to intronic sequence exonisation. *Eur J Hum Genet* 15, 473–477.
6. Reese, M. G., Eeckman, F. H., Kulp, D., and Haussler, D. (1997) Improved splice site detection in Genie. *J Comput Biol* 4, 311–323.
7. Yeo, G., and Burge, C. B. (2004) Maximum entropy modeling of short sequence motifs with applications to RNA splicing signals. *J Comput Biol* 11, 377–394.
8. Cartegni, L., Wang, J., Zhu, Z., et al. (2003) ESEfinder: A web resource to identify exonic splicing enhancers. *Nucleic Acids Res* 31, 3568–3571.
9. Fairbrother, W. G., Yeh, R. F., Sharp, P. A., and Burge, C. B. (2002) Predictive identification of exonic splicing enhancers in human genes. *Science* 297, 1007–1013.
10. Shapiro, M. B., and Senapathy, P. (1987) RNA splice junctions of different classes of eukaryotes: sequence statistics and functional implications in gene expression. *Nucleic Acids Res* 15, 7155–7174.
11. Senapathy, P., Shapiro, M. B., and Harris, N. L. (1990) Splice junctions, branch point sites, and exons: sequence statistics, identification, and applications to genome project. *Methods Enzymol* 183, 252–278.
12. Eng, L., Coutinho, G., Nahas, S., et al. (2004) Nonclassical splicing mutations in the coding and noncoding regions of the ATM Gene: maximum entropy estimates of

splice junction strengths. *Hum Mutat* 23, 67–76.

13. Desmet, F. O., Hamroun, D., Lalande, M., et al. (2009) Human Splicing Finder: an online bioinformatics tool to predict splicing signals. *Nucleic Acids Res* 37, e67.
14. Houdayer, C., Dehainault, C., Mattler, C., et al. (2008) Evaluation of in silico splice tools for decision-making in molecular diagnosis. *Hum Mutat* 29, 975–982.
15. Zhang, M. Q. (1998) Statistical features of human exons and their flanking regions. *Hum Mol Genet* 7, 919–932.
16. Pertea, M., Lin, X., and Salzberg, S. L. (2001) GeneSplicer: a new computational method for splice site prediction. *Nucleic Acids Res* 29, 1185–1190.
17. Walker, L. C., Whiley, P. J., Couch, F. J., et al. Detection of splicing aberrations caused by BRCA1 and BRCA2 sequence variants encoding missense substitutions: implications for prediction of pathogenicity. *Hum Mutat* 31, E1484–1505.
18. Rouleau, E., Lefol, C., Moncoutier, V., et al. A missense variant within BRCA1 exon 23 causing exon skipping. *Cancer Genet Cytogenet* 202, 144–146.
19. Nalla, V. K., and Rogan, P. K. (2005) Automated splicing mutation analysis by information theory. *Hum Mutat* 25, 334–342.

Chapter 18

In Silico Tools for qPCR Assay Design and Data Analysis

Stephen Bustin, Anders Bergkvist, and Tania Nolan

Abstract

qPCR instruments are supplied with basic software packages that enable the measurement of fluorescent changes, calculations of quantification cycle (C_q) values, the generation of standard curves and subsequent relative target nucleic acid quantity determination. However, detailed assessments of the technical parameters underlying C_q values and their translation into biological meaningful results require validation of these basic calculations through further analyses such as qPCR efficiency correction, normalization to multiple reference genes, averaging and statistical tests. Some instruments incorporate some of these features, while others offer additional tools to complement the basic running software, in many cases providing those that are described below. In this chapter, there is a detailed description of some of these programs and recommended strategies for the design of robust qPCR assays. Some of the packages available for validation of the resulting C_q data and detailed statistical analysis are described.

Key words: Assay design, real-time PCR, RT-qPCR, PCR efficiency, normalization.

1. Introduction

The broad division of real-time quantitative PCR (qPCR) assays into those that are used within life science research and those used for diagnostic purposes entails two fundamentally different approaches to qPCR assay design (*see* **Note 1**). Research projects tend to be relatively low throughput, but with a requirement for great flexibility with respect to experimental and assay designs. Furthermore, individual researchers have highly variable requirements and coupled with their independence and creativity, this means that they use a wide variety of design and analysis tools, as well as optimization and validation protocols for qPCR assay design. In general, therefore, assays are designed using either

B. Yu, M. Hinchcliffe (eds.), *In Silico Tools for Gene Discovery*, Methods in Molecular Biology 760,
DOI 10.1007/978-1-61779-176-5_18, © Springer Science+Business Media, LLC 2011

no computer assistance or relatively low-powered assay design software, with data analysis software remaining optional and most statistical analysis being performed using tools available in spreadsheets such as Microsoft Excel or Apple's Numbers. Those involved in clinical diagnostics, on the other hand, are increasingly making use of the growing public availability of pathogen genome sequences to implement qPCR assays that rely on sequence-based pathogen identification. Assays must be unique to the pathogen with respect to all other non-target genomes; hence the design of pathogen diagnostic assays is a high throughput activity that involves the computationally expensive comparison of multiple target genomes with all known non-target sequences. Furthermore, accurate, reliable and robust data analysis is essential, resulting in data analysis software with clear process tracking function being an absolute necessity.

This diversity of practice, coupled with the flexibility of qPCR itself, means that numerous in silico tools have been developed to guide the design of qPCR assays and analyse any resulting quantitative data. Many tools are freely available online, while others are bundled with qPCR instruments or are available from various software houses. The most comprehensive information for accessing and evaluating these programs is available at http://www.gene-quantification.de/main-bioinf.shtml, along with additional links to detailed reviews and other publications dealing with qPCR data analysis. With so many different tools available, it is impossible to overview them all and do them justice. Hence this chapter describes an example of assay design to demonstrate the steps involved at every stage of the process, utilizing the tools we are familiar with and consider to be the best available. This does not mean, of course, that other tools are not equally capable of performing the task.

The MIQE guidelines (1, 2) provide clear guidance on the steps that are important for assay design, and we shall follow these guidelines to design this example assay. The selected target is the human vitamin D receptor (VDR) mRNA. VDR mediates the effects of 1,25-dihydroxyvitamin D3 [1,25-(OH)2D3] and is specified by the *VDR* gene; transcription is directed by distinct promoters that can generate unique transcripts with major N-terminal differences (3).

2. Materials

A computer, access to the Internet and ideally assay design software such as Beacon Designer and data analysis software such as GenEx or qbasePLUS are required for qPCR design and data analysis. However, as described, there are free online alternatives to these programs. It is also useful to have access to a spreadsheet program such as Microsoft Excel or Apple's Numbers.

3. Methods

3.1. qPCR Target Information

A search of any sequence repository for a specific nucleic acid target often reveals a number of variants, making it challenging to deduce which particular pathogen, DNA or RNA has been targeted. Providing an accession number is the most basic, yet frequently omitted piece of information. Common starting points for qPCR target searches are the National Center for Biotechnology Information (NCBI) nucleotide search site (http://www.ncbi.nlm.nih.gov/sites/nuccore) and gene search (http://www.ncbi.nlm.nih.gov/gene) websites, where a search for "human VDR" provides a link to VDR (*Homo sapiens*): vitamin D (1,25-dihydroxyvitamin D3) receptor, with the unique GeneID 7421 and official symbol VDR, both of which are essential MIQE requirements. Following this link opens up a page providing detailed, summarized information on this gene, including a link to Ensembl's genome browser (*see* below). A section labelled "Genomic regions, transcripts, and products" provides a link to the reference sequence with the all-important accession numbers, which confirms that there is more than one transcript. Variant 1 lacks an alternate exon in the 5′-UTR when compared with variant 2; both variants specify the same protein. Following the links to GenBank reveals two reference mRNA sequences, NM_0000376.2 (variant 1) and NM_001017535.1 (variant 2). The requirements of the experiment are crucial considerations at this stage. In some cases, there is a requirement to detect all sequences, regardless of splicing, and so the conserved region is selected as the target. Alternatively, as in this case, the requirement is to distinguish between sequences and so individual assays are designed to target each of the variants. In this case we will design two assays, one targeting each of the two variants.

Both mRNA sequences are imported into the CLC Sequence Viewer (http://www.clcbio.com), a free software package developed for Windows, Mac and Linux platforms that allows basic nucleic acid and protein analysis. An alternative would be to use ClustalW, one of the free tools provided by the European Bioinformatics Institute (EBI) (http://www.ebi.ac.uk/Tools/clustalw2/index.html). The sequences are aligned to reveal the differences at the 5′-end of the mRNA, with the rest of the sequences being identical (**Fig. 18.1**). An analysis of the alignment shows that the first 76 nucleotides from the 5′-end are

```
                                      20                                      40                                      60
NM_000376.2     ctgcttgtca aaaggcggca gcggagccgt gtgcgccggg agcgcggaac agcttgtcca  60
NM_001017535.1  ctgcttgtca aaaggcggca gcggagccgt gtgcgccggg agcgcggaac agcttgtcca  60
                                      80                                     100                                     120
NM_000376.2     cccgccggcc ggacca---- ---------- ---------- ---------- ----------  76
NM_001017535.1  cccgccggcc ggaccagggc tcctgaacct agcccagctg gacggagaaa tggactctag 120
                                     140                                     160                                     180
NM_000376.2     ---------- ---------- ---------- ---------- ---------- ----------  76
NM_001017535.1  cctcctctga tagcctcatg ccaggccccg tgcacattgc tttgcttgcc tccctcaatc 180
                                     200                                     220                                     240
NM_000376.2     ---------- --------ga agcctttggg tctgaagtgt ctgtgagacc tcacagaaga 118
NM_001017535.1  ctcatagctt ctctttggga agcctttggg tctgaagtgt ctgtgagacc tcacagaaga 240
                                     260                                     280                                     300
NM_000376.2     gcacccctgg gctccactta cctgccccct gctccttcag ggatggaggc aatggcggcc 178
NM_001017535.1  gcacccctgg gctccactta cctgccccct gctccttcag ggatggaggc aatggcggcc 300
                                     320                                     340                                     360
NM_000376.2     agcacttccc tgcctgaccc tggagacttt gaccggaacg tgccccggat ctgtggggtg 238
NM_001017535.1  agcacttccc tgcctgaccc tggagacttt gaccggaacg tgccccggat ctgtggggtg 360
```

Fig. 18.1. Alignment of the 5′-ends of the two reference sequences specifying the VDR. Two blocks of identical sequences surround the 122-bp sequence (*highlighted*) unique to variant 2. A GC-rich sequence (nucleotides 70–72) precedes the splice junction at position 75.

identical, with variant 2 having a 122-bp insert. This is the critical region of differentiation that provides useful anchors for the variant-specific assay design. An upstream primer centred on nucleotide 76 should allow the generation of variant 1-specific amplicons, whereas an upstream primer located within the variant 2-specific sequence should result in a variant 2-specific amplicons. In either case, the primers will be intron spanning, minimizing any problems associated with genomic DNA (gDNA) contamination.

Ensembl (http://www.ensembl.org/index.html) and the UCSC Genome Bioinformatics Site (http://genome.ucsc.edu/) provide alternative means of acquiring and handling sequence information. Which toolkit to use is down to personal preference, but in our experience, the relative simplicity of NCBI's sites makes them the tools of choice for simple sequence acquisition and browsing of information that is critical for high-quality qPCR assay designs.

3.2. Primer/Probe Design

In theory it should be easy to utilize tens of thousands of published qPCR assays to obtain suitable primer and probe sequences. The Quantitative PCR Primer Database (QPPD) (http://web.ncifcrf.gov/rtp/gel/primerdb/) provides an assembly of assay details from published articles, and in compliance with the MIQE guidelines, it provides information on primer location, amplicon size, assay type, positions of single-nucleotide polymorphisms (SNPs) as well as literature references. However, these assays have not been independently optimized or validated and so may not generate reliable quantitative data. RTPrimerDB (http://medgen.ugent.be/rtprimerdb/) contains more than 8,000 qPCR assays for over 5,500 genes. When an assay is submitted, there is a requirement for appropriate validation and optimization data, with the option for further users to leave feedback (4–6). The use of such properly validated assays has numerous advantages, obviating the requirement for time-consuming primer design and empirical optimization and critically introducing more uniformity and standardization among different laboratories. RTPrimerDB is particularly flexible and can be queried using the official gene name or symbol, Entrez or Ensembl Gene identifier, SNP identifier or oligonucleotide sequence. Queries can be restricted to a particular application, e.g. mRNA quantification, gDNA copy number quantification, SNP detection, organism or detection chemistry.

However, these databases cannot accommodate every gene or variant; new variants may have been identified, or suitable assays may never have been designed for the organism of interest. Consequently, there are a large number of conditions where a proficiency in good assay design is indispensable. Happily, there are numerous options available if an assay needs to be designed from scratch; less propitiously, the many choices available can be confusing. Several software tools provide comprehensive facilities for designing primers and probes for standard and bisulphite modification qPCR assays, as well as multiplex designs that permit the design of multiple primers simultaneously. Many allow detailed control over numerous features, including assay location, primer and amplicon sizes, probe modifications, annealing temperatures, ionic conditions, GC content and dimer formation. Some can design assays if the sequences of only one primer or probe are provided. We have found two programs to be consistently useful: (i) Premier Biosoft Beacon Designer, which can be used to design single template as well as multiplex assays and supports all common chemistries such as SYBR Green I, standard hydrolysis as well as locked nucleic acid (LNA)-modified probes, hybridization probes, Molecular Beacons and Scorpions. Beacon Designer can predict CpG islands, or CpG regions can be delineated manually, thus permitting the design of MethyLight hydrolysis probes and methyl-sensitive PCR primers, together with suitable control primers and probes for unmethylated and untreated DNA sequences. Beacon Designer is particularly useful for designing high-resolution melting analysis assays, as it uses proprietary algorithms for designing the best primers and the shortest possible amplicons (*see* **Note 2**). (ii) Premier Biosoft AlleleID supports hydrolysis minor grove binding (MGB) probe design and can design assays across exon junctions. Its particular power applies to the design of qPCR-based diagnostic assays for pathogen detection. For cross-species assays, AlleleID identifies the conserved regions to design a universal probe. When it is not possible to identify a significant conserved region for a set of sequences, AlleleID helps design a “mismatch tolerant” probe. Also included is a "minimal set" option that helps design a minimum number of probe sets that uniquely identify a sequence reducing the overall assay cost. This functionality is also useful to help study gene expression when genomic sequences of the organism under study are not available.

The power of both Beacon Designer and AlleleID lies in the customization both programs permit the user. Details are outside the scope of this chapter, but both contain the facility to check primer specificity by avoiding significant cross-homologies identified by automatically interpreting BLAST search results, maximize annealing efficiency by avoiding template structures identified by in silico folding prediction of the template (using mfold, *see* below), can design up to five multiplex hydrolysis probe assays by checking for cross-homologies with all probes and primers to prevent competition, allow the evaluation of predesigned primers and probes and can design wild-type and mutant probes for SNP identification. Previously designed assays can be evaluated and AlleleID can be used to align multiple sequences and select target regions for pathogen detection assay design.

If there is no need for the additional specificity inherent in a probe-based assay, the use of double-stranded DNA-binding dyes such as SYBR Green is recommended. This has several advantages: (i) costs should be lower as there is no need to order a probe; (ii) there are fewer constraints on the location of the primers and consequently (iii) assay design is easier and may result in a more efficient and sensitive assay. An SYBR Green assay for the VDR would be designed so that amplification of the two variants results in different amplicon lengths which could be easily distinguished through the analysis of the resulting melt curves. Quantification relative to variant-specific dilution curves would then permit accurate quantification of the two variants relative to each other. However, SYBR Green is not an option for diagnostic assays, hence there will be numerous occasions when probe-based assays represent the only recourse and this can mean having to design suboptimal assays that are likely to require extensive empirical optimization without any guarantee of success. Nevertheless, while suboptimal assays may not be accurately quantitative, they will always be qualitative, which often is sufficient in a clinical context.

The difficulty with designing a primer set specific for a probe-based assay detecting VDR variant 1 is that the sequence around the unique splice site is very GC rich (**Fig. 18.1**). Since the forward primer must span the splice junction, the Beacon Designer program feature permitting the use of a predesigned primer is used, allowing Beacon Designer to specify a downstream primer and a probe. The only additional stipulation is a limit on amplicon size of 70–100 bp. The program output is shown in **Fig. 18.2**. The program suggests five alternative probes, and a sequence

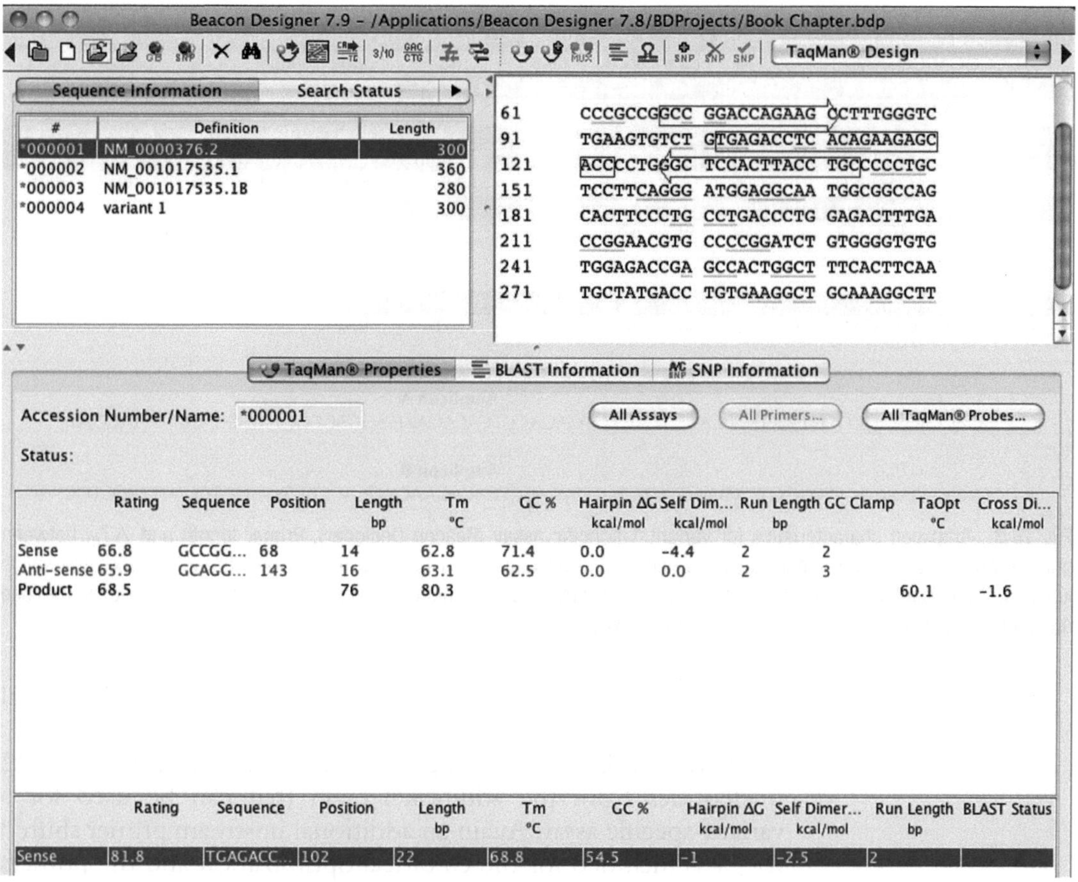

Fig. 18.2. Beacon Designer output following a design for an assay that is variant 1 specific and used a predetermined upstream primer spanning the splice junction.

analysis reveals one possible sense primer dimer (unavoidable), no antisense primer dimer, no primer hairpins, two weak cross-dimers, no runs of greater than two and no repeats (**Fig. 18.3**). Primers and probe are categorized as good and best, respectively. In principle, therefore, this should be an acceptable assay for the specific detection of variant 1. Testing an additional upstream primer, obtained by shifting the binding site by +1 nucleotide, gives the sense primer a slightly higher rating, resulting in a better primer pair rating. Care must be taken with the interpretation of the ratings. These are a measure of how well the assay fits to the criteria defined by the user, hence if a huge tolerance of conditions is permitted, the assay will be rated higher than if a narrower tolerance is permitted. For empirical testing, it is best to test more than one primer set per amplicon, hence both sense primers will be tested against the reverse primer. Primers, probe and their characteristics are shown in **Fig. 18.3**. Alternatively, it would have been possible to designate the reverse primer as the variant-specific primer, with the forward primer in the common

Variant 1 Sense Primer A	Length	Tm	GC%	Rating	Position	Pair Quality	Pair Rating	Product Length	Product Tm	Product TaOpt
GCCGGACCAGAAGC	14	62.8	71.4	66.8	68	Good	68.5	76	80.3	60.1
Anti-sense Primer A	**Length**	**Tm**	**GC%**	**Rating**	**Position**					
GCAGGTAAGTGGAGCC	16	63.1	62.5	65.9	143					

Sense Primer B	Length	Tm	GC%	Rating	Position	Pair Quality	Pair Rating	Product Length	Product Tm	Product TaOpt
CCGGACCAGAAGCC	14	61.9	71.4	73.5	69	Best	71.4	75	80	59
Anti-sense Primer B	**Length**	**Tm**	**GC%**	**Rating**	**Position**					
GCAGGTAAGTGGAGC	15	59.7	62.5	78.8	143					

Probe Sequence	Length	Tm	GC%	Rating	Position	Quality
TGAGACCTCACAGAAGAGCACC	22	68.8	54.5	81.8	102	Best

Amplicon A

GCCGGACCAGAAGCCTTTGGGTCTGAAGTGTCTGTGAGACCTCACAGAAGAGCACCCCTGGGCTCCACTTACCTGC

Amplicon B

CCGGACCAGAAGCCTTTGGGTCTGAAGTGTCTGTGAGACCTCACAGAAGAGCACCCCTGGGCTCCACTTACCTGC

Fig. 18.3. Amplicon characteristics for variant 1-specific assay (Beacon Designer). Primer length and ΔT_m between primers and probe are not ideal, but governed by the absolute need to place the forward primers across the splice junction. If the resulting assay is not optimal, it is important to note this during the analysis step and, for example, use the data in a qualitative rather than a quantitative way.

5′-region. Designing a splice junction-specific probe with general primers is another possibility.

Variant 2 is a more straightforward design, as there are 122 nucleotides from the additional exon that can be used for a variant-specific assay. Again an additional upstream primer shifted to +1 is included for the empirical optimization and the primers and probe are shown in **Fig. 18.4**.

Variant 2 Sense Primer A	Length	Tm	GC%	Rating	Position	Pair Quality	Pair Rating	Product Length	Product Tm	Product TaOpt
CACATTGCTTTGCTTGCC	18	62.2	50	73.2	153	Best	80	75	76.1	56.8
Anti-sense Primer A	**Length**	**Tm**	**GC%**	**Rating**	**Position**					
CTCACAGACACTTCAGACC	18	61.2	52.6	84.9	227					

Sense Primer B	Length	Tm	GC%	Rating	Position	Pair Quality	Pair Rating	Product Length	Product Tm	Product TaOpt
ACATTGCTTTGCTTGCCT	18	62.4	44.4	72.5	154	Best	78.7	90	77.4	58
Anti-sense Primer B	**Length**	**Tm**	**GC%**	**Rating**	**Position**					
TGCTCTTCTGTGAGGTCTC	19	62.6	52.6	83.8	243					

Probe Sequence	Length	Tm	GC%	Rating	Position	Quality
TTCTCTTTGGGAAGCCTTT	19	70.2	42.1	62.8	189	Good

Amplicon A

CACATTGCTTTGCTTGCCTCCCTCAATCCTCATAGCTTCTCTTTGGGAAGCCTTTGGGTCTGAAGTGTCTGTGAG

Amplicon B

ACATTGCTTTGCTTGCCTCCCTCAATCCTCATAGCTTCTCTTTGGGAAGCCTTTGGGTCTGAAGTGTCTGTGAGACCTCACAGAAGAGCA

Fig. 18.4. Amplicon characteristics for variant 2-specific assay. The two primer sets described here are just two of many possible combinations. Alternatively it would have been possible to design exon-spanning primers or have the antisense primer in the common upstream sequence. There are no hard and fast rules and importantly, what gets the highest ratings in silico must be tested empirically as primer sequences that look very unpromising on paper can perform well and conversely, those that should result in optimal assays may not perform adequately.

Since it may be desirable to detect both transcripts simultaneously and determine the relative quantities of each, it would be useful to design a multiplex assay. The problem here is that the constraint of having to place the forward primer for variant 1 places severe limitations on assay design. Hence one option is to design a set of primers that detect both variants, with the second set being variant 2 specific. This provides no direct information with respect to variant 1 but allows some inference from a comparison of variant 2 and total mRNA copy numbers. This kind of assay is easily designed in BD, as shown in **Figs. 18.5** and **18.6**.

AlleleID generates a slightly different assay for variant 1, with the same probe but a different reverse primer (**Fig. 18.7**). In order to maximize the chances of obtaining an optimal assay, this sequence should also be tested empirically.

For anyone who would like the assurance of a well-designed assay but prefers not to tackle these programs, there are freely available design service options. Sigma Genosys offers a free consultancy-based option; scientists submit their sequence and

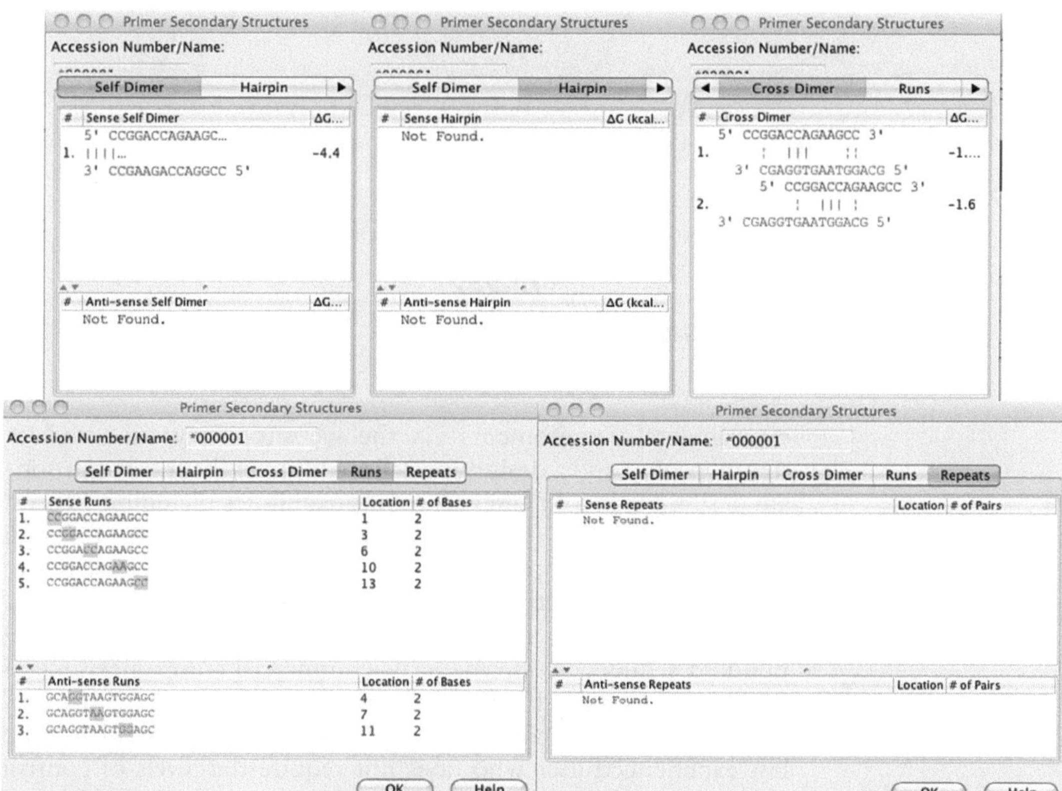

Fig. 18.5. Beacon Designer analysis of primer secondary structure. The program checks for self-dimers, hairpins, cross-dimers, single-nucleotide runs and repeats. These data, together with the ratings, help to base primer choice on more rational criteria.

NM_0000376.2 Sense Primer	Length	Tm	GC%	Rating	Pair Quality	Pair Rating	Product Length	Product Tm	Product TaOpt
GACCCTGGAGACTTTGAC	18	63.2	55.6	65.6	Good	69	89	81.3	60.8
Anti-sense Primer	**Length**	**Tm**	**GC%**	**Rating**					
CAGGTCATAGCATTGAAGTG	20	62.6	45	72.5					
Probe Sequence	**Length**	**Tm**	**GC%**	**Rating**	**Quality**				
TCCACACACCCCACAGATCC	20	69	60	64.9	Good				

NM_001017535.1 Sense Primer	Length	Tm	GC%	Rating	Pair Quality	Pair Rating	Product Length	Product Tm	Product TaOpt
TCCCTCAATCCTCATAGC	18	61.7	50	74.2	Good	69.8	72	76	56.8
Anti-sense Primer	**Length**	**Tm**	**GC%**	**Rating**					
GCTCTTCTGTGAGGTCTC	18	62.9	55.6	68.9					
Probe Sequence	**Length**	**Tm**	**GC%**	**Rating**	**Quality**				
TTCAGACCCAAAGGCTTCCCA	21	69.1	52.4	77.1	Best				

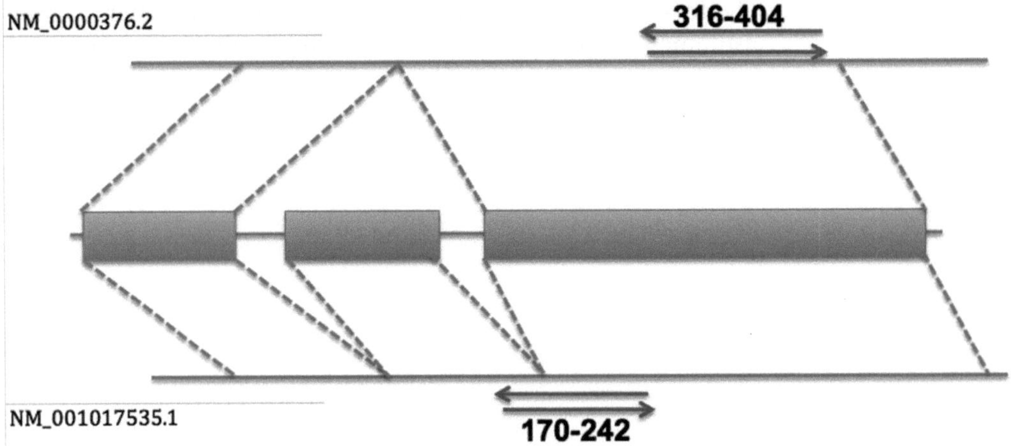

Fig. 18.6. Multiplex assay for general VDR/variant 2-specific assay.

experimental requirements via the website (www.sial.com/designmyprobe) and a design specialist will apply the most appropriate design protocol from a suite of possibilities including Beacon Designer, AlleleID (as described above) and Roche FRET design software. All of the options described for these packages are therefore available from this service. A dedicated bioinformatics scientist team can also manage huge alignment projects of several hundred sequences. Alternatively, commercial companies such as Roche and Biosearch offer real-time design tools (e.g. http://www.biosearchtech.com/realtimedesign) that are useful for the less experienced user who does not require the levels of control offered by the above two heavyweight programs. The Biosearch option can be used to design assays for both standard quantification and SNP genotyping and can be used to design up to 10 different assays simultaneously. It offers default and moderate

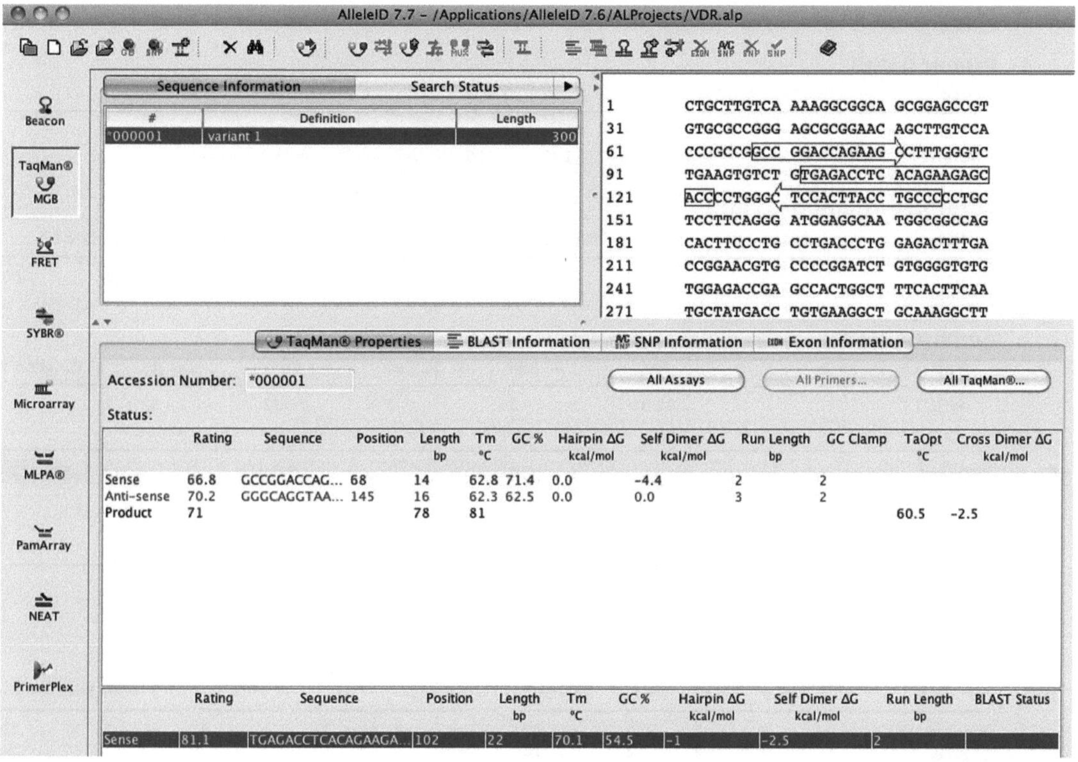

Fig. 18.7. Amplicon characteristics for variant 1-specific assay (AlleleID). This program suggests a different downstream primer, confirming that there are a large number of possible primer sites on a target, depending on user-defined settings, making it essential that assays are published with primer and probe sequences.

user-modifiable modes (amplicon length, GC content, mononucleotide run length and dimers) and links directly to NCBI to retrieve sequences according to accession number and to confirm priming specificity. For our current assay, the need to place the forward primer for variant 1 at a very specific site precludes its use for the design of a variant 1-specific assay, but it can be used to design a variant 2-specific assay. Using the custom mode, the program offers a wide range of primer options, from which we initially choose three (**Fig. 18.8**).

3.3. In Silico Validation

Primer specificity and target accessibility are two important parameters that must be reviewed prior to commencing empirical assay optimization and validation. When using Beacon Designer or AlleleID, these functions can be performed within the process. Primer specificity is most easily and rapidly checked using Primer-BLAST (http://www.ncbi.nlm.nih.gov/tools/primer-blast/) (*see* **Chapter 6** for more discussion on the application of Primer-BLAST). The program can analyse an amplicon, or one or both primer sequences. However, if a single primer is entered, the template sequence is also required. For the

0032	62	164	81.03

Primer Detail

Oligo	Tm	GC%	Length	5' Pos	3' Pos	5'-Sequence-3'
Forward	66.5	61	18	164	181	GCTTGCCTCCCTCAATCC
Reverse	65.4	48	21	225	205	CACAGACACTTCAGACCCAAA

Identified Mis-Alignments

Self Align	Dimer	3'Align	Hairpin	Total ΔG°	Pair Align	Dimer	3' Align	Bi-ΔG°
Forward	3	2	3	-11.07	Forward/Reverse	3	3	.00
Reverse	2	2	2	-11.04				

Amplicon Detail

Amplicon	Rank	AT Run	GC Run	GC%	Length	Variation
Allele 1	82.31	3	3	52	62	

GCTTGCCTCC CTCAATCCTC ATAGCTTCTC TTTGGGAAGC CTTTGGGTCT GAAGTGTCTG TG

0039	64	164	80.97

Primer Detail

Oligo	Tm	GC%	Length	5' Pos	3' Pos	5'-Sequence-3'
Forward	66.5	61	18	164	181	GCTTGCCTCCCTCAATCC
Reverse	67.5	48	23	227	205	CTCACAGACACTTCAGACCCAAA

Identified Mis-Alignments

Self Align	Dimer	3'Align	Hairpin	Total ΔG°	Pair Align	Dimer	3' Align	Bi-ΔG°
Forward	3	2	3	-11.07	Forward/Reverse	3	3	.00
Reverse	2	2	2	-11.10				

Amplicon Detail

Amplicon	Rank	AT Run	GC Run	GC%	Length	Variation
Allele 1	84.11	3	3	52	64	

GCTTGCCTCC CTCAATCCTC ATAGCTTCTC TTTGGGAAGC CTTTGGGTCT GAAGTGTCTG TGAG

0332	63	163	80.85

Primer Detail

Oligo	Tm	GC%	Length	5' Pos	3' Pos	5'-Sequence-3'
Forward	67.4	55	20	163	182	TGCTTGCCTCCCTCAATCCT
Reverse	65.4	48	21	225	205	CACAGACACTTCAGACCCAAA

Identified Mis-Alignments

Self Align	Dimer	3'Align	Hairpin	Total ΔG°	Pair Align	Dimer	3' Align	Bi-ΔG°
Forward	3	2	3	-11.10	Forward/Reverse	3	3	.00
Reverse	2	2	2	-11.04				

Amplicon Detail

Amplicon	Rank	AT Run	GC Run	GC%	Length	Variation
Allele 1	83.75	3	3	51	63	

TGCTTGCCTC CCTCAATCCT CATAGCTTCT CTTTGGGAAG CCTTTGGGTC TGAAGTGTCT GTG

Fig. 18.8. Primers and probes for variant 2 suggested by the Biosearch online program. These differ from those obtained using Beacon Designer and AlleleID but are similar to each other. Since primers are cheap, it is best to have these assays synthesized without the probe, determine which one works best and only then order the probe. This has the added advantage of not jeopardizing the probe with primer contamination.

highest level of sequence specificity, the source organism and the smallest database that is likely to contain the target sequence are selected; for broadest coverage, it is best to choose the nr database and not to specify an organism. The results show potential additional targets, with sequence information to allow the researcher to decide whether the chosen primer pairs are acceptable. For VDR variant 1, primer choice is very limited due to the need to target a GC-rich splice junction. The Primer-BLAST results (**Fig. 18.9**) reflect the potential for mis-amplification.

Target accessibility is the second important parameter that must be checked in silico as it is important that primers anneal to areas of minimal secondary structure. This can be quite difficult to achieve when reverse priming from RNA, as RNA is characterized by extensive secondary structure. DNA templates, on the other hand, are less structured, making it easier to identify primer/target combinations that are located in open structures. The most useful analysis tools for determination of optimal and suboptimal secondary structures of RNA or DNA molecules are found on the mfold web server (http://mfold.bioinfo.rpi.edu/) (7). There are mfold tools ("m" simply refers to "multiple"), allowing the folding of DNA (http://mfold.bioinfo.rpi.edu/cgi-bin/dna-form1.cgi) and RNA (*see* **Chapter 19** for RNA folding prediction). RNA folding can be carried out at a fixed temperature of 37°C (version 3.2, http://mfold.bioinfo.rpi.edu/cgi-bin/rna-form1.cgi) or at variable temperature, using the

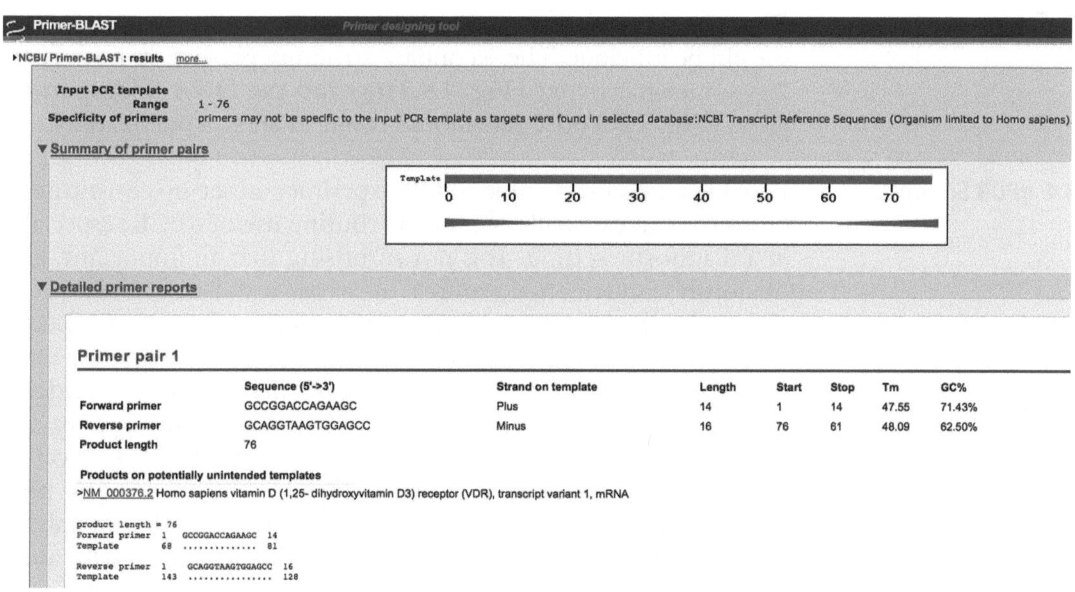

Fig. 18.9. Primer-BLAST output warning of potential non-specificity of primers. The designer needs to analyse the output in detail to decide whether his designs are sufficiently specific.

version that we recommend (version 2.3, http://mfold.bioinfo.rpi.edu/cgi-bin/rna-form1-2.3.cgi). User-definable parameters are significantly more flexible for DNA folding analysis, with an option to fine-tune folding temperature as well as ionic conditions (Na^+ and Mg^{2+}). RNA folding is carried out at 1 M Na^+, with no Mg^{2+}. Folding predictions are based on energy rules specific for DNA (8–14) or RNA (15–18) as well as unpublished parameters. Since any predicted optimal secondary structure for an RNA or a DNA molecule depends on the model of folding and the specific folding energies used to calculate that structure, different optimal folding may be calculated if the folding energies are changed. Because of uncertainties in the folding model and the folding energies, the "correct" folding may not be the "optimal" folding determined by the program. It is important to view several potential optimal and suboptimal structures within a few percent of the minimum energy and use the variation among these structures to determine which regions of the secondary structure can be predicted reliably (7).

Both amplicons chosen for the VDR variants are analysed using the RNA and DNA folding prediction programs. The problem with the assay is that the splice junction dictates the choice of target sequence resulting in determination of a relatively poor secondary structure prediction for the mRNA (**Fig. 18.10a**), which precludes a re-design. Instead, it may be possible to use a higher temperature for the reverse transcription (RT) protocol to optimize the efficiency and reliability of the RT step. The prediction for the folding of the DNA structure looks reasonable (**Fig. 18.10c**) and so it is acceptable to predict that the PCR should be efficient. The secondary structure prediction for variant 2 is somewhat better (**Fig. 18.10b**) and the DNA folding looks good (**Fig. 18.10d**), and should result in an acceptable assay.

3.4. qPCR Set-up

Reliable and reproducible qPCR experimental set-up constitutes a serious technical challenge for the routine use of qPCR, especially in a diagnostic setting. It is not surprising that an important, and obviously fundamental, source of errors associated with qPCR experiments arises from mistakes made during the set-up process. Furthermore, pre-analysis considerations such as testing for template quality, PCR inhibition and optimizing the assay considerations are important contributors to a successful assay but are not generally implemented, and certainly not automated. Prexcel-Q (P-Q) is an interesting tool that addresses these issues by providing a template to allow the user to carry out these analyses systematically and comprehensively. Prexcel-Q is not a data analysis program, it is an extensive qPCR validation, set-up and protocol printout program for each step of the qPCR experimental set-up process. It comprises 35 inter-linked Excel files and can be obtained by contacting Dr. Dario Valenzuela at Iowa State

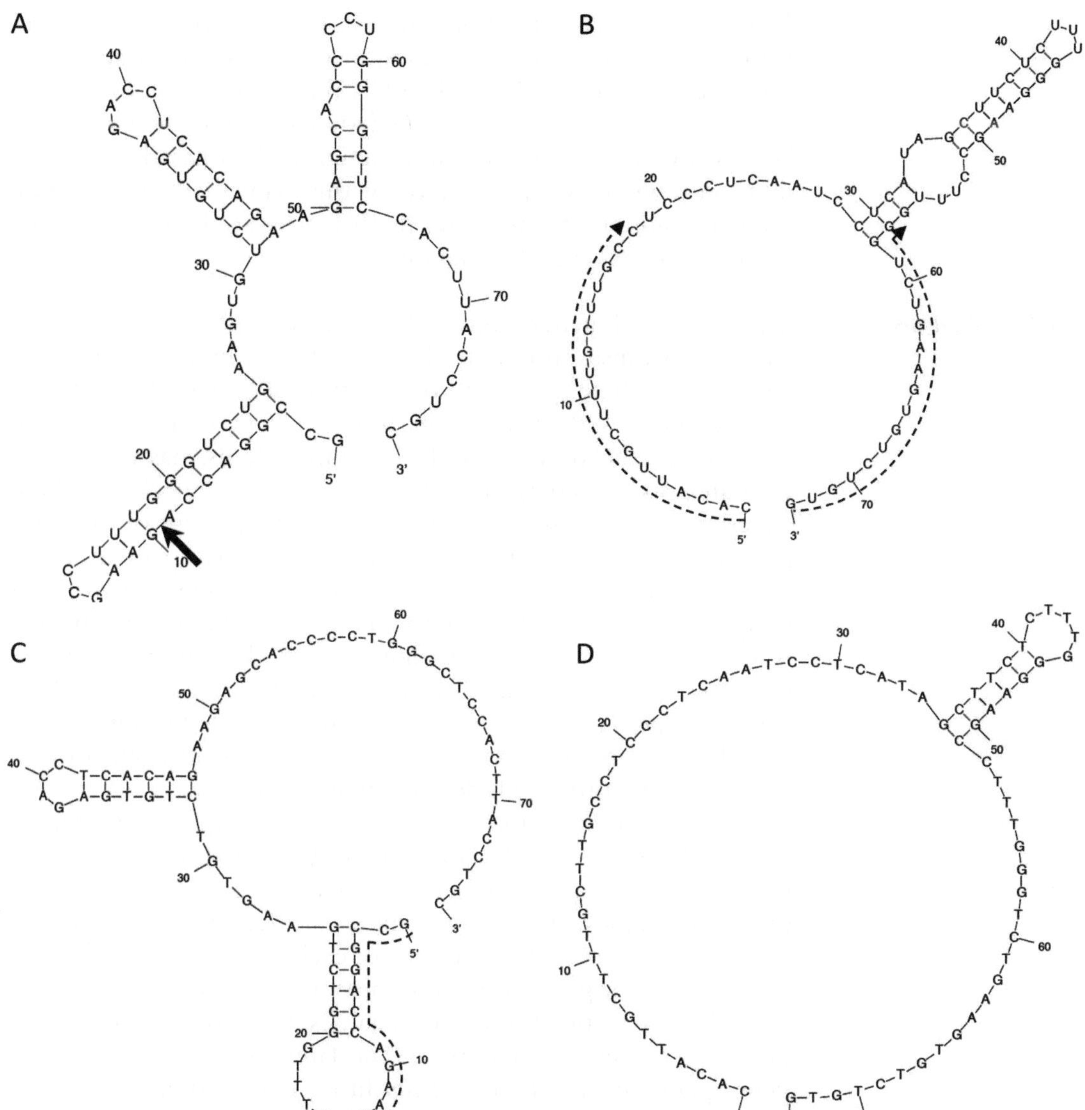

Fig. 18.10. mfold RNA/DNA folding of VDR variants. (**a**) The folding structure of mRNA variant 1 is severely handicapped by the need to place one of the primers over the splice junction (indicated by an *arrow*). The Beacon Designer software warns of this limitation and designs this assay only after manual override of basic primer design guidelines. However, the downstream primer-binding site is reasonably accessible and should be accessible to the primer for reverse transcription. (**b**) Both upstream and downstream primer-binding sites in mRNA variant 2, indicated by *dashed lines* with an *arrow*, are accessible, and it would have been easy to design slightly longer amplicons to reduce the secondary structure at the 3′-end of the amplicons even further. (**c**) The upstream primer-binding site in DNA amplicon 1, indicated by the *dashed line* with an *arrow*, lies within a hairpin, although there is a large loop that will help destabilize the secondary structure at high temperatures. The optimal annealing temperature for this assay has been kept high at 60°C, and it may be possible to empirically determine assay conditions that overcome the secondary structure problem. (**d**) There is no secondary structure at either end of DNA amplicon 2, with a very minor potential hairpin in the middle. This assay would be predicted to be efficient.

University Research Foundation (ISURF) at dariov@iastate.edu. P-Q automatically calculates amounts of all reagents required for nuclease treatments, RT and qPCR reactions, provides an estimate of total sample material needed, assists directly with calculations involving standard curve designs, identifies the dynamic dilution range of sample material within which qPCR inhibition is absent and target amplification efficiencies are highest and even estimates the total cost of the assay.

3.5. Data Analysis

The successful generation of high-quality qPCR experimental runs and acquisition of C_q values is followed by the critical data analysis step. The increasing penetration of 384-well and higher throughput qPCR instruments, together with PCR array methods such as the Biotrove and Fluidigm systems, has resulted in data analysis becoming one of the biggest bottlenecks in qPCR experiments. Data analysis is an essential component of the complete assay and this step needs to be handled with care and precision. Many biologists are statistically challenged and may not be able to analyse and interpret the quantitative data from their qPCR assays appropriately. In this context, dedicated data analysis software provides valuable guidance, although it is no substitute for expert consultations with knowledgeable biostatisticians. A wide range of analysis packages can be accessed from http://www.gene-quantification.de/download.html.

One of the first tools was REST (relative expression software tool) (19), which was developed to address the problem of comparing target gene expression levels relative to reference genes in different samples. Importantly, these calculations also accommodated differences in the efficiency of each of the PCR assays. The use of ratios for gene expression measurements makes it complex to perform traditional statistical analysis, as ratio distributions do not have a standard deviation. The latest REST (http://www.gene-quantification.de/rest-2009.html) is a stand-alone software package and has been extended with advanced algorithms using randomization and bootstrapping techniques to take into account issues of multiple reference gene normalization and quantification of the uncertainty inherent in any measurement of expression ratios. The program also allows measurement of not only the statistical significance of deviations but also their likely magnitude, even in the presence of outliers. A visually attractive graphing ability provides a visual representation of variation for each gene, highlighting potential issues such as distribution skew.

In terms of power and sophistication, two commercial software tools stand out: GenEx and qbase PLUS.

GenEx (http://www.multid.se/) (*see* **Note 3**) is a powerful tool for processing and analysing qPCR data. It offers a vast range of tools, ranging from basic data editing and management to advanced, cutting-edge data analysis including selection and validation of reference genes, classification of samples, gene grouping, monitoring of time-dependent processes and basic and sophisticated statistical and graphic capacity. Statistical features include parametric and non-parametric tests, clustering methods, principal component analysis and artificial neural networks. Most qPCR experimental processes have a nested design with technical replicates at each step, where each step introduces more variance to the data. The noise contribution from each step can be analysed and used to optimize the experimental design for future experiments. One interesting feature is the experimental design optimization module, which calculates how to minimize the total variation for the experimental design with consideration of the experimental budget. GenEx can be used for the analysis of both relative quantification ($\Delta\Delta C_q$) and "absolute" quantification, i.e. relative to a dilution curve, with powerful presentation tools generating visually attractive illustrations. For accurate and robust normalization of qPCR data, GenEx has the advantage of incorporating both NormFinder (20) and geNorm (21) in the software. geNorm (http://medgen.ugent.be/~jvdesomp/genorm/) is used to select an optimal set of reference genes from a larger set of candidate genes. It is critical that the tested candidate genes are not co-regulated. The geNorm process performs a reiterative calculation of the *M* value, which describes the variation of a potential reference gene compared with all other candidate genes. The gene with highest *M* value is eliminated until there are only two reference genes left. Usually the last two or three remaining genes are recommended as the optimum candidate reference genes. NormFinder (http://www.mdl.dk/publicationsnormfinder.htm) is also used to find the optimum reference genes but, in contrast to geNorm, takes information of expression in groupings of samples into account. The result is an optimum pair of reference genes that might have compensating expression so that one gene is slightly overexpressed in one group but the other gene is correspondingly underexpressed in the same group.

qbasePLUS (http://www.biogazelle.com/products/qbaseplus) is a relatively new software tool developed by members of the group that invented the geNorm algorithms (21, 22). It is the only non-web-based software tool that can run natively on Mac, Linux and Windows operating systems. The basic concept of qbasePLUS is similar to that of GenEx in that the emphasis is on validation of all technical parameters using appropriate statistical and quality control metrics. It contains four levels of quality control analysis: PCR replicate variation, assessment of positive and negative control samples, determination of reference gene expression stability and evaluation of deviating normalization factors.

Technical replicates (repeated measurements of the same sample in the same run) are useful as they allow for quality control of the technical reproducibility of the qPCR data, provide better accuracy and allow the generation of results when individual qPCR reactions fail. Low reproducibility of the qPCR reaction is often the first indication of an unstable assay that requires optimization. qbasePLUS and GenEx automatically deal with technical replicates or repeated measurements. Outliers can be excluded so that they do not contribute to a significant bias and large errors. However, it is important to note that biological variability is often much larger than RT technical variability which is also much larger than PCR technical variability.

The second type of quality control allows an evaluation of the positive and negative sample controls. An amplification signal in the NTC sample indicates a potential contamination issue or formation of primer dimers; hence both packages flag suspicious no-template control (NTC) samples based on a user-defined or default thresholds.

Reference gene or normalization factor stability is the third type of quality control. The user is able to choose a minimal acceptable normalization factor stability by defining a threshold value for two indicators of expression stability of the used reference genes: the geNorm expression stability value of the reference gene (*M*) (21) and the coefficient of variation of the normalized reference gene relative quantities (CV) (22). qbasePLUS has extended and improved the functionality of geNorm by allowing ranking of candidate reference genes up to the single most stable gene, by combining the calculation of relative quantities and geNorm analysis and by allowing the processing of experiments with missing data in a way that has the lowest impact on the overall analysis through intelligent retention of as many data points as possible.

Inspection of normalization factors is a very useful feature and constitutes a fourth type of quality control. qbasePLUS displays the geometric mean of selected reference genes (the normalization factor) for each sample. These factors should be similar for all samples if approximately equal amounts of equal quality input material were used. High variability of the normalization factors indicates large differences in starting material quantity or quality, or a problem with one of the reference genes, which may be either not stably expressed or not adequately measured.

There are alternative, usually web-based tools available: QPCR (https://esus.genome.tugraz.at/rtpcr/) allows storage, management and analysis of qPCR data (23). It comprises a parser to import data from qPCR instruments and includes a variety of analysis methods to calculate cycle threshold and amplification efficiency values. The analysis pipeline includes technical and biological replicate handling, incorporation of sample- or gene-specific efficiency, normalization using single or multiple reference genes, inter-run calibration and fold change calculation. Moreover, the application supports an assessment of error propagation throughout all analysis steps and allows the conduction of statistical tests on biological replicates (*see* **Note 4**). Results can be visualized in customizable charts and exported for further investigation. Calculation of amplification efficiencies for RT-PCR experiments (CAmpER) (http://camper.cebitec.uni-bielefeld.de) is a limited, not very user-friendly web-based tool for the basic analysis of qPCR assay runs on Roche's LightCycler, the Biorad Opticon and the Qiagen Rotor-Gene.

Currently, transparent data interchange between instrument software and third-party data analysis packages, colleagues and collaborators, and between authors, peer reviewers, journals and readers is difficult. One solution to this problem is the development of the Real-time PCR Data Markup Language (RDML), a structured and universal data standard for exchanging qPCR data (24). The aim is to enable transparent exchange of annotated qPCR data by providing sufficient information for a third party to be able to understand the experimental set-up, re-analyse the data and interpret the results. A useful tool for converting instrument-specific data to the RDML format for convenient data interchange is found on the RDML website (http://medgen.ugent.be/rdml/chooseTool.php).

As qPCR moves from the realm of a cutting-edge technology to becoming a routine technique, there is the danger of losing the attention to experimental detail that is required to ensure that the C_q values generated accurately reflect the original biology under examination. When handling large numbers of samples, these details become even more difficult to manage. When sample sets are divided between several plates, or processed independently, additional factors such as variability between these individual runs must also be accommodated. While this can be carried out using some instrument packages, such as the Stratagene (Agilent) MxPro suite, it is only a small matter of scale before management of these data sets requires sophisticated data management and processing. The publication of the MIQE guidelines is testament to the drive towards improving the quality, uniformity and transparency of qPCR experiments. There is a clear requirement for open access to qPCR data in a system analogous to those developed for microarray users. This would promote a heightened awareness of the requirement for diligent experimental procedure and also make it possible for scientists to re-analyse combined data sets. These are also essential factors to consider when selecting software to use for assistance in designing experiments and analysing data. Software packages should be considered as scientific tools and applied intelligently, using processes that are absolutely transparent to the user.

4. Notes

1. Arguably the most common biostatistical trap for many users is failing to distinguish between exploratory and confirmatory biostatistical studies. For a study to arrive at a statistically significant conclusion, its hypothesis needs to be defined *before* data collection and analysis; this is a confirmatory study. In an exploratory study, data are collected and analysed for various patterns and trends. The exploratory study *may* produce hypotheses, but due to conscious or subconscious manipulation of the data, multiple testing issues will be raised and statistical significance will risk being unreliable at best. A correct approach for a complete statistical analysis involves first an exploratory study to generate one or a few hypotheses that are subsequently validated or discarded in a confirmatory study based on a freshly collected data set. An exploratory study may be of value on its own, but authors should stress that the results produced by such a study have not been verified statistically and only constitute hypotheses pending statistical confirmation.
2. Beacon Designer is our preferred assay design program, and there are a few considerations we would like to share: Designs of primer or probe oligonucleotide sequences often involve trade-off issues between potentially conflicting parameters such as melting temperature, self-hybridization and cross-hybridization risks, and GC content. The Beacon Designer program does a very good job at finding optimal balances between these parameters for a list of different detection chemistries. However, in many applications, primer or probe sequences are restricted to specific locations on the target sequence. The primer or probe location is a parameter that no predesigned algorithm can take into account; it is something that depends on the specific target of the assay. One example is a desire to have a primer or a probe covering an exon–exon junction to avoid amplification of genomic DNA. Another example is a desire to have a primer or a probe in a conserved region of a sequence alignment to allow detection of all species in a group of species. Conversely, it may be desired to have a primer or a probe in a unique region of a sequence alignment to allow detection of only one species in the group of species. The "Alternate Assays" setting in Beacon Designer is a useful feature as it allows the user to specify the number of assay designs that Beacon Designer will generate. The default setting is 5 (for normal assays) or 2 (for LNA assays) and the maximum setting is 50. By using the maximum 50, the list

of additional design alternatives often allows users to find designs at desired locations.

It is worth noting that Beacon Designer has a limit of sequence length range of 1200 bp for calculations of target secondary structure features that may inhibit PCR efficiency. For longer target sequences, the first 1200 bp are used by default for the calculation. However, the location and the length of the calculated interval can be adjusted. By shortening the interval and locating it around a desired location, the algorithm is driven to produce assay designs near the desired location.

One feature available in Beacon Designer is an algorithm to identify assay designs for SNP classification. This feature drives the assay design algorithm to the location of the SNP. Although this is the intended purpose of the feature in Beacon Designer, users can also use this feature to drive the assay design algorithm to any location on the target sequence by introducing fake SNPs at desired locations.

To some extent, several of the unique features available in AlleleID can also be accomplished in Beacon Designer. Sequence alignment performed in a sequence alignment program such as CLC viewer or ClustalW can be used to identify conserved or unique target sequence regions. Using the "limit assay design location" function in Beacon designer, it is possible to find suitable designs at desired locations such that they do target a multitude of species or a unique subset of the sequence alignment.

Under circumstances that an assay design fails to produce any results, this may not necessarily be cause to abandon the attempt to create an assay design for this particular target. Beacon Designer reports which parameter limit was crossed and relaxation of the limiting parameter may enable a new calculation to come up with results. The introduced trade-off may very well be reasonable, given the specifics of the target and the assay. However, this procedure requires detailed understanding of each parameter's consequence on assay performance and a careful balance between opposing desires. The report from Beacon Designer on failing parameters may thus be a useful item to look out for.

3. One of the advantages with the GenEx software is that two reference gene validation algorithms have been made easily available through the common user interface of GenEx. Using several reference gene validation algorithms enables the methods to be cross-validated against each other for more confident identification of preferred reference genes.

   A nice feature of GenEx is that the NormFinder algorithm has been supplemented with an analysis of accumulated standard deviations. The analysis thus not only provides a ranking of preferred reference genes but also estimates the optimal number of reference genes for the assay. Multivariate data are inherently difficult to visualize due to the high dimensionality of the data. GenEx has capabilities to produce all of 1D, 2D and 3D graphs. Grouping subsets of the data and assigning specific colours and symbols to them may add additional visual cues to facilitate visual understanding of the data. A specific tip is to use variation in colour to distinguish categories of one data set dimension (for example, time after induction) and variation in plot symbol to distinguish categories of another data set dimension (for example, dose).

Replicates can be used to reduce confounding variability from technical handling steps in the assay. Taking advantage of a pilot study, GenEx has tools to determine optimal distribution of replicates in a nested experimental design under conditions of economics and limits to total number of samples. Another important use of replicates is to evaluate statistical significance. The larger the number of biological replicates, the smaller the treatment effect verified at a given statistical significance. Based on estimates of standard deviations within each sample group, which may have been obtained from a pilot study, GenEx has a feature to calculate the necessary number of biological replicates for validation of a given observed treatment effect and level of statistical significance. This is useful to ensure that enough samples are collected to validate the studied hypothesis.

Optimal statistical tests often depend on the underlying sample distribution. Choices include the parametric *t* test and non-parametric tests. GenEx provides automatic tests of the underlying sample distribution and provides recommendations of the most suitable statistical test depending on sample distribution features. It should be kept in mind, though, that the tests of the underlying sample distribution become unreliable for small sample sizes and the recommendations provided by GenEx should only be considered tentative pending deeper analysis by a trained biostatistician. The easy access of several different types of statistical tests within GenEx is particularly useful during exploratory studies. Careful consideration of underlying sample distributions and choice of suitable statistical test is critical only for confirmatory statistical studies.

Visualization of expression profiles and hierarchical clustering are recommended first steps in exploratory studies of multivariate data sets. The modular design of GenEx's user interface allows for easy transitions between different analysis methods on the same data set. The data set can thus, for example, be tentatively analysed with hierarchical clustering to identify related groups, these groups assigned specific colours and the groups analysed in one of the more advanced multivariate data analyses methods available in GenEx. An interesting trick is to transpose the data in order to toggle analysis between the perspective of genes and the perspective of the sample groups.

4. Biological replicates are often the most expensive among the steps in a nested design, but they are necessary for development and confirmation of statistical tests. More biological replicates are needed if high statistical significance is desired; the assay has a high confounding variability and/or the studied effects are small. Technical replicates are valuable to reduce confounding variability due to the technical handling. However, the optimal distribution of replicates will depend on the sensitivities of each of the technical handling steps to the introduction of confounding variabilities and the amplitude of the studied effect in the assay. It is therefore recommended that a *pilot study* be performed and used as an exploratory study. The pilot study is then used to
   - evaluate the amplitude of confounding variabilities within each technical handling step so that the optimal distribution of replicates can be determined;
   - estimate the amplitude of the studied effect in the assay so that the number of biological replicates necessary for the desired degree of statistical significance is attainable;
   - optimize assay experimental conditions and
   - validate reference genes for data normalization.

Acknowledgements

S.A.B. would like to thank the charity B&CR (Charity Number 1119105) for support.

References

1. Bustin, S. A., Benes, V., Garson, J. A., et al. (2009) The MIQE guidelines: minimum information for publication of quantitative real-time PCR experiments. *Clin Chem* 55, 611–622.
2. Bustin, S. A. (2010) Why the need for qPCR publication guidelines? – The case for MIQE. *Methods* 50, 217–226.
3. Crofts, L. A., Hancock, M. S., Morrison, N. A., and Eisman, J. A. (1998) Multiple promoters direct the tissue-specific expression of novel N-terminal variant human vitamin D receptor gene transcripts, *Proc Natl Acad Sci USA* 95, 10529–10534.
4. Lefever, S., Vandesompele, J., Speleman, F., and Pattyn, F. (2009) RTPrimerDB: the

portal for real-time PCR primers and probes. *Nucleic Acids Res* 37, D942–D945.
5. Pattyn, F., Robbrecht, P., De Paepe, A., et al. (2006) RTPrimerDB: the real-time PCR primer and probe database, major update 2006. *Nucleic Acids Res* 34, D684–D688.
6. Pattyn, F., Speleman, F., De Paepe, A., and Vandesompele, J. (2003) RTPrimerDB: the real-time PCR primer and probe database. *Nucleic Acids Res* 31, 122–123.
7. Zuker, M. (2003) Mfold web server for nucleic acid folding and hybridization prediction. *Nucleic Acids Res* 31, 3406–3415.
8. SantaLucia, J., Jr. (1998) A unified view of polymer, dumbbell, and oligonucleotide DNA nearest-neighbor thermodynamics. *Proc Natl Acad Sci USA* 95, 1460–1465.
9. Bommarito, S., Peyret, N., and SantaLucia, J., Jr. (2000) Thermodynamic parameters for DNA sequences with dangling ends. *Nucl Acids Res* 28, 1929–1934.
10. Peyret, N., Seneviratne, P. A., Allawi, H. T., and SantaLucia, J., Jr. (1999) Nearest-neighbor thermodynamics and NMR of DNA sequences with internal A.A, C.C, G.G, and T.T mismatches. *Biochemistry* 38, 3468–3477.
11. Allawi, H. T., and SantaLucia, J., Jr. (1998) Nearest-neighbor thermodynamics of internal A.C mismatches in DNA: sequence dependence and pH effects. *Biochemistry* 37, 9435–9444.
12. Allawi, H. T., and SantaLucia, J., Jr. (1998) Thermodynamics of internal C.T mismatches in DNA. *Nucleic Acids Res* 26, 2694–2701.
13. Allawi, H. T., and SantaLucia, J., Jr. (1998) Nearest neighbor thermodynamic parameters for internal G.A mismatches in DNA. *Biochemistry* 37, 2170–2179.
14. Allawi, H. T., and SantaLucia, J., Jr. (1997) Thermodynamics and NMR of internal G.T mismatches in DNA. *Biochemistry* 36, 10581–10594.
15. Mathews, D. H., Sabina, J., Zuker, M., and Turner, D. H. (1999) Expanded sequence dependence of thermodynamic parameters improves prediction of RNA secondary structure. *J Mol Biol* 288, 911–940.
16. He, L., Kierzek, R., SantaLucia, J., Jr., et al. (1991) Nearest-neighbor parameters for G.U mismatches: [formula; see text] is destabilizing in the contexts [formula; see text] and [formula; see text] but stabilizing in [formula; see text]. *Biochemistry* 30, 11124–11132.
17. SantaLucia, J., Jr., Kierzek, R., and Turner, D. H. (1991) Stabilities of consecutive A.C, C.C, G.G, U.C, and U.U mismatches in RNA internal loops: Evidence for stable hydrogen-bonded U.U and C.C.+ pairs. *Biochemistry* 30, 8242–8251.
18. SantaLucia, J., Jr., Kierzek, R., and Turner, D. H. (1990) Effects of GA mismatches on the structure and thermodynamics of RNA internal loops. *Biochemistry* 29, 8813–8819.
19. Pfaffl, M. W., Horgan, G. W., and Dempfle, L. (2002) Relative expression software tool (REST) for group-wise comparison and statistical analysis of relative expression results in real-time PCR. *Nucleic Acids Res* 30, e36.
20. Andersen, C. L., Jensen, J. L., and Orntoft, T. F. (2004) Normalization of real-time quantitative reverse transcription-PCR data: a model-based variance estimation approach to identify genes suited for normalization, applied to bladder and colon cancer data sets. *Cancer Res* 64, 5245–5250.
21. Vandesompele, J., De Preter, K., Pattyn, F., et al. (2002) Accurate normalization of real-time quantitative RT-PCR data by geometric averaging of multiple internal control genes. *Genome Biol* 3, 0034.0031–0034.0011.
22. Hellemans, J., Mortier, G., De Paepe, A., et al. (2007) qBase relative quantification framework and software for management and automated analysis of real-time quantitative PCR data. *Genome Biol* 8, R19.
23. Pabinger, S., Thallinger, G. G., Snajder, R., et al. (2009) QPCR: Application for real-time PCR data management and analysis. *BMC Bioinformatics* 10, 268.
24. Lefever, S., Hellemans, J., Pattyn, F., et al. (2009) RDML: structured language and reporting guidelines for real-time quantitative PCR data. *Nucleic Acids Res* 37, 2066–2069.

Chapter 19

RNA Structure Prediction

Stephan H. Bernhart

Abstract

The prediction of RNA structure can be a first important step for the functional characterization of novel ncRNAs. Especially for the very meaningful secondary structure, there is a multitude of computational prediction tools. They differ not only in algorithmic details and the underlying models but also in what exactly they are trying to predict. This chapter gives an overview of different programs that aim to predict RNA secondary structure. We will introduce the ViennaRNA software package and web server as a solution that implements most of the varieties of RNA secondary structure prediction that have been published over the years. We focus on algorithms going beyond the mere prediction of a static structure.

Key words: RNA secondary structure, RNA structure prediction, consensus structures, local structures.

1. Introduction

Form follows function is a basic principle in most parts of biology, from zoology to molecular biology. For functional characterization of novel ncRNA genes, knowing the structure of an RNA molecule is therefore a good starting point. There are several levels of structure description for RNA. The sequence itself is called the primary structure, while the Watson–Crick (GC and AU) and wobble (GU) base pairs realized by the sequence constitute the secondary structure. Other contacts between bases, knots, and the spatial arrangement of the helices are part of the tertiary structure.

For the in silico prediction of RNA structure, we make use of the fact that RNA folding is a hierarchical process. The secondary structures, Watson–Crick and wobble base pairs, form first, and the spatial arrangement is a subsequent step. Furthermore, the

B. Yu, M. Hinchcliffe (eds.), *In Silico Tools for Gene Discovery*, Methods in Molecular Biology 760,
DOI 10.1007/978-1-61779-176-5_19, © Springer Science+Business Media, LLC 2011

main part of the folding energy of an RNA molecule is realized by the stacking of the base pairs to form the secondary structure. As a consequence, the comparison of secondary structures is usually sufficient to evaluate the differences between RNA structures.

Because secondary structure is such a powerful descriptor for the overall RNA structure, it is fortunate that it is easier to predict than, for example, is the protein secondary structure. The stacking of the π-electron systems of the bases that lead to the stabilization of the RNA secondary structures is understood quite well. If pseudo-knots are forbidden (they are defined to be tertiary structure motifs), the secondary structure of an RNA molecule can be predicted in reasonable time, even for large RNA molecules like ribosome subunits. However, the quality of the prediction deteriorates with the length of the RNA molecule.

In this contribution, we will describe how a secondary structure is predicted given a specific RNA sequence, what can be done to analyze the confidence of parts of the various predicted structures, what possibilities there are to improve the quality of predictions, and how to get some additional information about the RNA structures of interest.

1.1. Visualization of RNA Molecules

The visualization of an RNA secondary structure inspires research much more than a list of base pairs does. For many people, pictures make it easier for new thoughts to occur. In addition, publications become more comprehensive through the use of good graphics.

There are several approaches to RNA secondary structure visualization (*see* **Fig. 19.1** for examples). There is the classical graphical drawing (top left of **Fig. 19.1**), which is usually most comprehensive but not easily read by computer programs, for example, if you want to use the structure prediction of one program as an input for another one. For larger sequences, the mountain plot (top right of **Fig. 19.1**), also a graphical representation, is easier to analyze. The arrangement of tops and valleys of a mountain plot, as it is linear, is independent of the size of the molecules. In **Fig. 19.1**, you can see the typical three peaks on a plateau shape that always identify a clover leaf. For exchange between computer programs, there are two commonly used formats. The bpseq/ct format is a list of the bases with the number of bases paired to them, while the dot-bracket format is a one-line representation that uses dots for unpaired nucleotides, ")" for bases paired upstream, and "(" for bases paired downstream (see bottom of **Fig. 19.1**). Using the standard mathematical rules for brackets, this format is unambiguous.

1.2. Prediction of a Single Secondary Structure

The most basic task for RNA structure prediction is predicting a single secondary structure, the structure with the minimum free energy (mfe). There are two approaches: one, henceforth

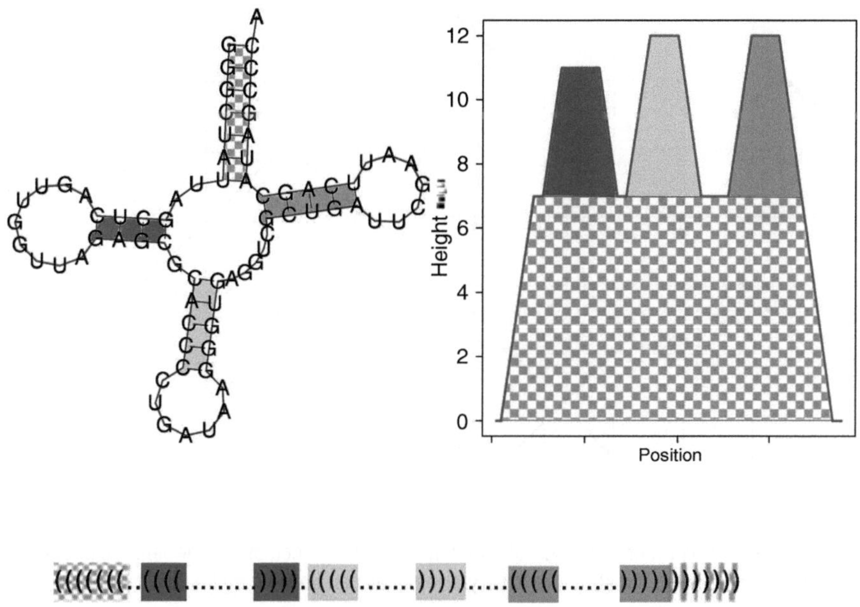

Fig. 19.1. Visualization of RNA secondary structure. Three types of structural representation are shown: *top left*, graphical drawing; *top right*, mountain plot; *bottom*, dot-bracket string. Identical stems are represented by the same *shades of gray*.

called the thermodynamic approach, uses the Zuker–Stiegler (1) algorithm and a mixture of experimentally derived and modeled energy parameters. The other approach uses stochastic context-free grammars (SCFGs) or generalizations thereof, where the probabilities of structural features are computed out of their frequency in known RNA structures (2).

1.3. An Ensemble of Structures Instead of a Single Structure

The minimum free energy structure is much too static to always give a good description of the structures active in nature. The energy gained by the stacking of base pairs is in the same range as the thermal energy at room temperature. This means that RNA molecules can and will take many different structures in time, constantly refolding. Every possible structure has a probability of occurring that is proportional to its Boltzmann factor. Accordingly, the minimum free energy structure is the most probable of all structures. However, there may exist many significantly different structures that together are much more probable. As a result, it is recommended to consider this ensemble of structures instead of focusing on a static picture as is the case with the mfe structure.

A way to obtain this information is the so-called partition function. In the secondary structure context, the partition function of an RNA molecule is the sum of the Boltzmann weights for all possible secondary structures of the molecule. It can be computed with relative ease with both the thermodynamic (3) and the SCFG approaches to folding.

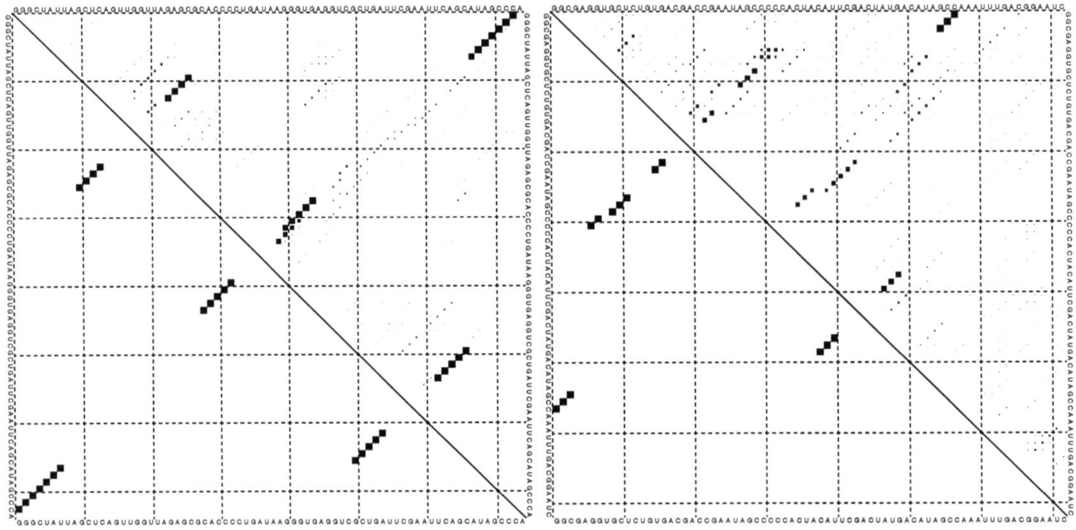

Fig. 19.2. Dot plots. The *dot plot* representation of two different RNA molecules. To the *left*, a clover leaf shape with a well-defined structure. To the *right*, the structure is very diverse, as can be seen by the great number of smallish dots.

A practical way to represent a partition function is via the probabilities of the single base pairs in the dot plot (**Fig. 19.2**). In this matrix, the sequence is written from left to right and from top to bottom. A dot in a cell represents a base pair. At the bottom left triangle, the minimum free energy structure is represented. At the top right triangle, the size of the dots is proportional to the probability of a base pair. Helices are represented as rows of dots perpendicular to the main diagonal.

If the top right triangle contains only a small number of big dots, the structure is well defined. If, on the other hand, there are many smallish dots spread over the whole area, the ensemble is very diverse. Furthermore, the dot plot shows what structures or at least structural features are part of the ensemble with what probability. Properly interpreted, the dot plot can hence give a comprehensive account over the structural ensemble, containing literally millions of different structures.

As the proper interpretation of a dot plot needs practice, there are several ways to generate a single structure to represent the ensemble of structures computed via the partition function. CONTRAfold (4) and others use a maximum likelihood approach. A generalized centroid structure for the CONTRAfold or the Zuker–Stiegler model is used by Centroidfold (5).

These approaches lead to a slight increase in the quality of the prediction for a single structure. However, remember that the partition function can be used to get much more information than a single structure. This way of thinking about RNA structure is highly recommended, as it may inspire better ideas for molecular mechanisms than the simplistic “one molecule one structure” dogma.

1.3.1. Suboptimal Structures

Using stochastic backtracking, the probability of any (combination of) structural feature(s) can be computed. There is a stochastic backtracking option for the RNAsubopt program of the ViennaRNA package. For many sophisticated applications around stochastic backtracking, one can use Sfold (6).

In principle, stochastic backtracking generates a number of suboptimal structures. The probability of these structures is their respective probability in the structural ensemble. There are two other approaches to generate a set of suboptimal structures. One, introduced by Zuker and part of the mfold package and web server, is to look at every possible base pair within the sequence and generate the optimal structure that contains this base pair. As many of these structures will be redundant, this gives you a small but diverse sample of structures. The Wuchty algorithm (7), as used in the ViennaRNA package, generates a set of all structures within a certain energy distance to the minimum free energy (**Fig. 19.3**). This set may better represent the structural ensemble, but as the number of structures grows exponentially with sequence length, the list may become very long. For example, in an energy band of 3 kcal/mol, there are several hundred structures for 100 nt and several thousand for 200 nt.

1.4. Additional Programs

While RNA secondary structure prediction using the tools introduced above works reasonably well, there are some limitations. In comparison to known structures, about 75% of the base pairs are correctly predicted by the single sequence structure prediction tools. This mean number is lower for large RNA molecules (about 50 and 55% for SSU and LSU ribosome subunits, respectively) and higher for smaller molecules (e.g. 80% for tRNA) (8). Some small comments going beyond secondary structure are at the back of this chapter (*see* **Notes 4** and **5**).

1.4.1. Pseudo-knots

About 20% of the known biologically relevant RNA structures contain pseudo-knots, where the percentage of knotted base pairs varies between 43% for RydC and 0.2% for LSU ribosomal subunit. Therefore, trying to predict a structure containing pseudo-knots can be worthwhile. One of the programs that can cope with the most prevalent pseudo-knot types is pknotsRG.

However, including pseudo-knots does not necessarily improve the quality of the prediction. Most of the programs that predict pseudo-knots have a bias toward pseudo-knotted structures.

1.4.2. Predicting Local Structures

There are several reasons for looking at local secondary structure elements instead of the global secondary structure of a given sequence. Due to some general properties and assumptions shared by all the prediction programs, they predict long-range

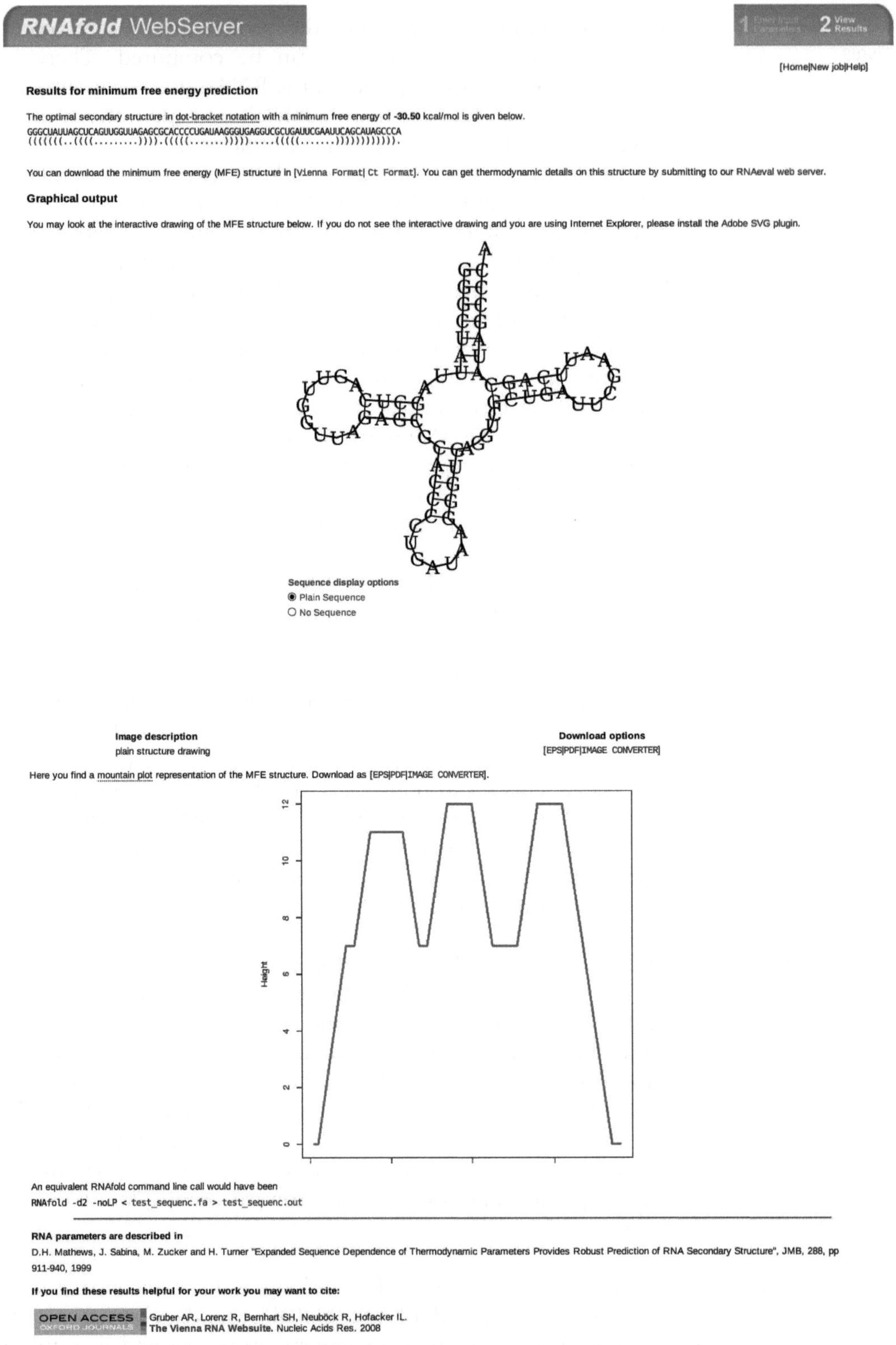

Fig. 19.3. Example output page of the ViennaRNA web server.

base pairs more often than they exist in known RNA structures. Accordingly, the prediction of, for example, the SSU ribosomal RNA structure can be improved by simply making long-range (over 200 nt) base pairs impossible.

On the other hand, a cell is packed with molecules that interact with RNA molecules. As an example, mRNAs are bound to ribosomes and smaller complexes, but most RNA molecules are known to be bound to proteins, other RNA molecules, or small ligands. As these bound molecules are likely to prevent the formation of long-range base pairs, it is advisable to predict locally stable secondary structures for longer RNA sequences.

As for global structure prediction, there are programs for minimum free energy structure prediction and variants for partition function computation. The RNALfold algorithm of the ViennaRNA package will predict local minimum free energy structures, while RNAplfold will predict local partition functions using a sliding window approach.

As these programs are designed to cope with very long RNA sequences (up to bacterial genome or chromosome size) and the exchange of huge amounts of data is inconveniently expensive, there is no web server available for the ViennaRNA version at the moment. Local folding however is part of the download version of the ViennaRNA package and can be chosen as an option at the mfold web server.

RNAplfold predicts not only base pair probabilities but also accessibilities of RNA molecules. The accessibility is the probability of a stretch of an RNA molecule to be single stranded and thus accessible for binding to other RNA molecules (or other ligands). For example, siRNAs are more effective if they target highly accessible parts of RNA molecules (9). Accordingly, accessibility can give additional information to sequence motifs found in an RNA molecule. These sequence motifs usually require a certain pairing state (either single strandedness or double strandedness) for their biological function. The accessibility can therefore be used to confirm suspected sequence motifs.

1.4.3. Consensus Structure Prediction

If one has a set of evolutionary-related RNA sequences which are expected to share a common structure or at least common structural features, one can use evolutionary information to greatly improve the quality of the structures predicted. Generally, if a structure is functionally important, there will be evolutionary pressure to conserve it. This pressure can be observed via a distinct pattern of mutations: consistent mutations, which retain the possibility to form a base pair (GU to AU base pair, for example), and compensatory mutations, where both bases are mutated to keep the pairing possible after one base has mutated (e.g. GC to CG and AU to GC).

There are three ways to look for common secondary structures for a set of RNA molecules. (1) Align the sequences first, then predict the structures, (2) predict structures and then align these structures afterward, or (3) align and fold simultaneously (*see* **Note 3**).

Looking for signals for structural conservation is used as an approach for in silico discovery of non-coding RNA genes. As an example, RNAz, available on the ViennaRNA server, uses machine learning approaches to find structures that are much more conserved than would be expected by chance.

1.4.4. Integrating Existing Knowledge or Assumptions About the Structure of RNA Molecules

In some cases, there already is a certain idea about at least a part of a structure of a sequence of interest. There might, for example, be information about single or double strandedness established by chemical probing. Scientists may make educated guesses, finding, for example, a combination of an H and an ACA box and therefore expect the sequence in question to be an H/ACA snoRNA. In this case, one wants the bases of these two boxes to be unpaired. Several programs, e.g., mfold, allow the introduction of structural constraints to reflect such knowledge or assumptions.

2. Materials

For the most part, we will describe the use of the ViennaRNA software package, as we are most familiar with it. There are many other tools of roughly the same quality that are run in a very similar fashion. An overview page that links to some of them can be found at http://en.wikipedia.org/wiki/List_of_RNA_structure_prediction_software

The following web server provides an easy-to-use interface for the ViennaRNA package: http://rna.tbi.univie.ac.at/

In this chapter, we focus on an audience that has no expertise in in silico prediction of RNA secondary structure. We will therefore mostly describe how to use this web server to encourage gaining of experience with RNA structures. An additional reason for this decision is that the graphical representation of the results is better for the web server. For serial experiments, it is preferable to use locally installed programs. There are several tutorials around that introduce the command line versions of the ViennaRNA package and most other tools recommended here. The command line commands that generate the respective results can be seen at the result page of the web server. To install the local version of the ViennaRNA package, download the latest tar.gz file at http://www.tbi.univie.ac.at/~ivo/RNA/

Untar it writing

```
$ tar -xzf ViennaRNA-X.Y.Z.tar.gz
```

After changing to the ViennaRNA directory created by untaring the archive, type

```
$ ./configure
$ make
$ sudo make install
```

to compile and install the package. Note that you will need root permissions for the global installation.

The ViennaRNA binaries should now be installed in /usr/local/bin/

Pre-compiled binaries for Windows can also be downloaded from http://www.tbi.univie.ac.at/~ivo/RNA/ (*see* **Note 1**).

3. Methods

3.1. Single Secondary Structure Prediction

There are several online tools that can be used for predicting secondary structures, for example, the web server of the SCFG-based CONTRAfold: http://contra.stanford.edu/contrafold/server.html

Mfold, a thermodynamics-based structure prediction web server, can be found at http://mfold.bioinfo.rpi.edu/cgi-bin/rna-form1.cgi. The input pages of most web applications resemble BLAST. There is a field to paste your sequence into and there are different options that can be selected or changed below. At the ViennaRNA RNAfold server (10) (http://rna.tbi.univie.ac.at/cgi-bin/RNAfold.cgi), you can see the input page containing the sequence field and several buttons for the options. If the question marks are clicked, a short explanation for the respective option is given.

First, to get a sample sequence, click onto the "this sample sequence." The input field should now read as follows:

```
>test_sequence
GGGCUAUUAGCUCAGUUGGUUAGAGCGCACCCCU
GAUAAGGGUGAGGUCGCUGAUUCGAAUUCAGCAU
AGCCCA
```

To get the minimum free energy structure only, mark the "minimum free energy (MFE) only" button, then click "proceed" at the bottom of the page. After a visit to a page showing you some statistics and how many people are before you in the queue, you will be redirected to the results page.

The mfe of the test sequence is –30.5 kcal/mol, and you will see a structural representation in dot-bracket format below the sequence, as well as a graphical and a mountain plot representation. The images can be downloaded in different formats.

The structure shown is a classical tRNA clover leaf, as the sequence indeed is a tRNA from *Chlorella ellipsoidea*. At the bottom of the page, the equivalent RNAfold command line call can be seen:

RNAfold -d2 -noLP < test_sequence.fa > test_sequence.out

If you are interested in what parts of the molecule contribute how much to the overall energy, you can follow the submit to "our RNAeval web server" link. After clicking proceed, you get a table showing the individual contributions of the secondary structure modules.

If you go back to the start page (http://rna.tbi.univie.ac.at/cgi-bin/RNAfold.cgi) and click the "show advanced options" link, a number of additional parameters that can be changed appear. The default parameters used are applicable for the most frequent problems of structure prediction. Mostly, changing them will not have a positive impact on the results.

Allowing non-canonical base pairs, i.e., base pairs that are not directly adjacent to other base pairs, or disallowing GU base pairs at the end of stacks will usually only slightly change the results. In the example, you will see that allowing non-canonical base pairs will result in a shift changing two of the arms of the clover leaf. The quality of the mfe structure prediction may be slightly increased if the parameter for dealing with so-called dangling bases (bases that are directly adjacent to a stack but do not belong to this stack) is set to coaxial stacking possible. This means that an energy bonus for the stacking of helices that are in close vicinity – as in the tRNA molecule – will be used. However, this is not supported for the partition function version of RNAfold (see below) and is not recommended. Disregarding the dangling end stabilization, on the other hand, will destroy the clover leaf fold of the test sequence.

If you want to fold DNA, you should choose the appropriate energy parameters. Using the Andronescu RNA parameters (11), which are extracted from known structures much as it is done for SCFG-based approaches, will sometimes increase the quality of the predictions.

3.2. Characteristics of the Ensemble

Go back to the start page of the ViennaRNA RNAfold server and select the "minimum free energy (MFE) and partition function" button. Then click proceed at the bottom of the page.

At the result page, we get a lot of additional information about the secondary structure of the RNA molecule.

In addition to the dot-bracket string of the structure of minimal free energy, the centroid structure is shown. The centroid structure is the structure with minimal base pair distance to all other structures of the ensemble of structure. It is simply the structure containing all base pairs with a probability higher than 0.5. While for the test sequence, the centroid structure is identical to the mfe structure, for very diverse ensembles, the centroid structure can also be a very unstable structure. Furthermore, the Gibbs free energy of the ensemble, the frequency of the mfe structure in the ensemble, and the ensemble diversity (the average base pair distance between the structures of the ensemble) can be seen.

In the graphical view, we can color the picture by either base pair probability (which is the default state) or positional entropy by selecting the respective button. The example structure is, for the most part, extremely well defined. The red markings of the base pairs mean that 90% of all structures realize this particular base pair, while the green base pairs are present in only about 50% of all structures. For unpaired bases, the probability of being unpaired is used for the coloring. Similar information is shown by the positional entropy coloring, where a higher positional entropy means that a base has many different reasonably probable base pairings.

For the mountain plot, the distance between the blue (mfe) and the green (partition function) line is a good indicator of how well the minimum free energy structure represents the characteristics of the whole ensemble of structures. A bigger distance between the lines indicates a poorer description.

Following one of the three links will get you the dot plot representation of the structural ensemble. You can see that there is not much structural flexibility for this RNA molecule, as there are only a small number of tiny dots that represent alternative structures. The only main alternative structure can be seen almost at the center of the dot plot. Here, the inner part of the helix is shifted, leading to a tetraloop instead of a hexaloop hairpin, and one C nucleotide bulges out (*see* **Note 2**). The existence of an alternative structure can be deduced by the green or the blue coloring of the helix in the base pair or positional entropy coloring scheme. The different graphical representations can be downloaded in several formats.

3.3. Consensus Structure Prediction

For RNAalifold, an alignment of the structures in question in Clustal format is needed (**Fig. 19.4**). This alignment is best created by an alignment program that takes RNA structure into account, e.g., MAFFT (12), but other programs such as Clustal (13) work almost as well. The alignment can be pasted in the entry field at http://rna.tbi.univie.ac.at/cgi-bin/RNAalifold.cgi.

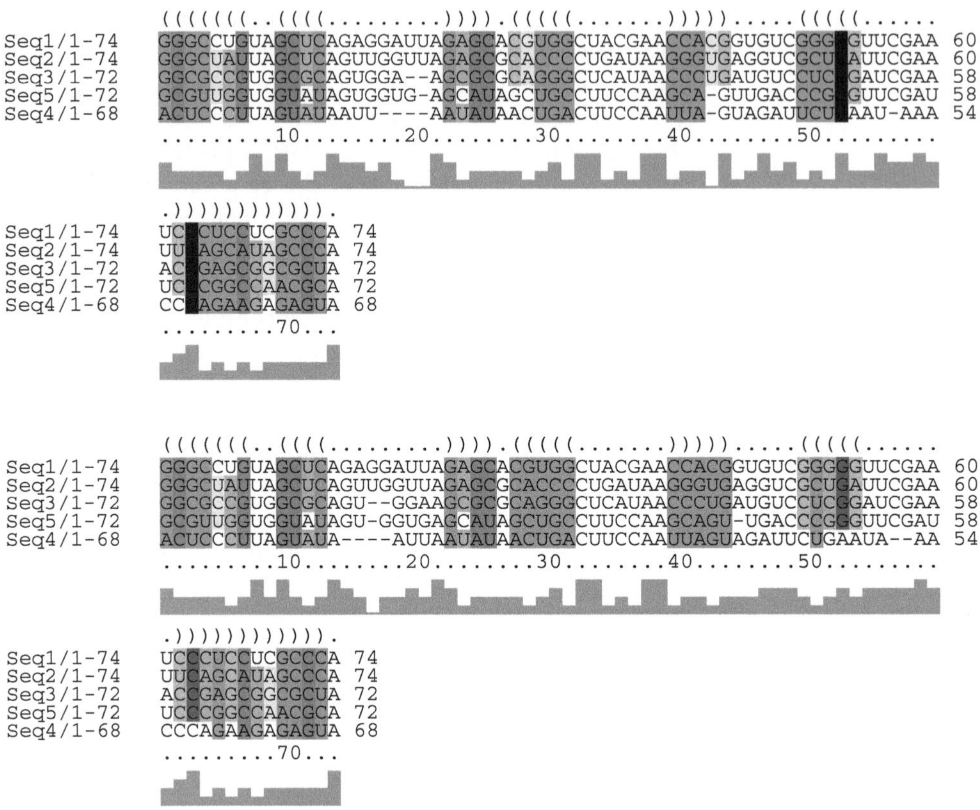

Fig. 19.4. Comparison of two structure-annotated alignments created by RNAalifold. *Top*, Clustal alignment; *bottom*, LocARNA alignment. The third stem looks better in the LocARNA and the fourth in the Clustal alignment.

For now, we will use the sample alignment and not change the default parameters. After clicking "proceed" at the bottom of the page, we get the result page that is similar to the one for RNAfold. However, it shows a graphical representation with an evolutionary conservation color scheme. The colors correspond to the number of different base pairs (of the six possible) that have been encountered at the corresponding positions of the alignments. Pale colors indicate that there are sequences where the respective base pair cannot be formed.

The impact of the additional information about evolutionary conservation can best be seen if the base pair probability or positional entropy color schemes are used. The only major uncertainty that remains is around the possible AU base pair at the bottom (middle) loop. In the dot plot, which is colored using the evolutionary conservation color scheme, it can be seen that there are no compensatory mutations at either of the two possible base pairs (the two directly adjacent small red dots closest to the diagonal in the approximate center represent the two possible AU base pairs). As the color scheme for evolutionary conservation is used in the mountain plot also, it can be easily seen which plateau or step of the mountain plot corresponds to which base pair.

The RNAalifold web server also provides a structure-annotated alignment, where the compatibility of single sequences to the consensus structure can be easily seen by the lack of coloring if a base pair cannot be formed (**Fig. 19.4**).

Back at the start page, some unique parameters can be used. The RNAalifold versions that can be chosen mostly differ in the energy evaluation for the evolutionary conservation. The RIBOSUM scoring scheme uses a score based on observed frequencies for ribosomal RNA alignments, while the other variant uses a rather ad hoc scoring scheme. The old RNAalifold version is available for backward compatibility; however, its use is not recommended. For alignments of many (more than 15) sequences, the RIBOSUM scoring is to be preferred, as it also gives a slight bonus to totally conserved base pairs.

The simultaneous folding and aligning approach is realized, e.g., by LocARNA (http://rna.tbi.univie.ac.at/cgi-bin/LocARNA.cgi). As these approaches are computationally much more expensive than the subsequent aligning and folding of the RNAalifold kind, the length of the sequences that can be used is limited. We will use the example sequences (which are the same as the ones in the RNAalifold example); after clicking "proceed" at the bottom of the page, we get to the results page. The result consists of a Clustal type sequence alignment with the predicted secondary structure in dot-bracket format. The result can be downloaded or it can be submitted to the RNAalifold web server by clicking the respective link. After clicking proceed at the RNAalifold web page, we can compare the result with the one we earlier obtained using the Clustal alignment.

The ambivalence of the results can be easily spotted by comparing the two structure-annotated alignments. While the middle stem is aligned better by LocARNA than in the Clustal alignment, the 3′ stem of sequence 4 (bottom sequence) does not look as good.

3.4. Local Folding

Getting local substructures of long RNA molecules is done via the command line at the local version of the ViennaRNA package. For minimum free energy folding, if you want to restrict base pairs to a length of X, type

$ RNALfold -L X

You will get to an input prompt where you can paste your sequence:

```
Input string (upper or lower case); @ to quit
....,....1....,....2....,....3....,....4....,....5....,
....6....,....7....,....8
```

If you hit return, you get a list of local secondary structure elements that can be formed by the molecule.

The format of this list is as follows: structure in dot-bracket notation, minimum free energy, and starting point on the sequence:

```
.((((((((....)))))))). (-10.60) 973
.(((((((((((....))))))).)))). (-12.00) 970
.((((((.....)))))) ( -5.20) 957
.(((......)).). ( -0.90) 941
(((....))). ( -4.30) 937
.(((((((....))))))). ( -4.90) 932
.((((.....)))). ( -5.50) 926
```

As an alternative, you can also use the standard input redirector and a file name for all ViennaRNA programs:

$ RNALfold -L X < sequence.file

If you just want one structure with base pairs of restricted length, you can use the mfold web server.

To compute the partition function and pair probabilities in a sliding window approach, RNAplfold is called as follows:

$ RNAplfold -L X -W Y < sequence.file

Here, the Y stands for the window size (as opposed to the maximum size of a base pair X). As RNAplfold computes the mean over all windows a base pair can possibly appear in, it is advisable to use a window size bigger than the maximum size of a base pair to avoid taking the mean of a single value.

The output of RNAplfold is a cut out of a dot plot along its diagonal, turned 45°, usually called plfold_dp.ps. If you want to compute accessibilities, use the -u option:

$ RNAplfold -L X -W Y -u < sequence.file

This will give you an additional file called plfold_lunp, which contains a matrix of the probabilities to be unpaired (for stretches up to a length of 31 consecutive unpaired bases). The columns correspond to the length of the unpaired region, while the rows correspond to the last unpaired base. That is, in row 2 you will find the entry for an unpaired region for bases 1 and 2 in the second column and the probability for base 2 to be unpaired in the first column.

3.5. Suboptimal Structures

RNAsubopt is the ViennaRNA program that can generate suboptimal structures. It can be used to generate all structures within a certain energy band (-e energy option) and all Zuker-type suboptimal structures (-z option), and perform stochastic backtracking for x structures (-p x option):

$ RNAsubopt -e 2 -s < sequence.file

The -s option sorts the output according to its energy. The output is a list of suboptimal structures and, except for stochastic backtracking, their respective energies:

AUGCUAGCAUGCUAGGGAUGCGUAGCUAGUGCGGAU GGUG -1240 200

```
..((((((((((.......)))).))))))..........  -12.40
.(((((((((((.......)))).))))))).........  -12.00
..((((((((((.......)))).))))))((.....)).  -11.30
```

The first line contains the sequence, the minimum free energy, and the width of the energy band in units of 0.01 kcal/mol.

3.6. Constraint Folding

In most programs of the ViennaRNA package, bases can be constrained to be paired ("|"), unpaired ("x"), paired up- or downstream ("<,>"), or base pairs that have to be realized by the sequence can be specified ("(,)"). The dot "." is used to signalize unconstrained bases. The best structure that fulfills the constraints is then computed (*see* **Note 4**).

For the ViennaRNA web server, there is a link "show constraint folding" that will show you a second input field where a constraint string can be given. This constraint string always has to be as long as the respective sequence.

4. Notes

1. The ViennaRNA package (but not the web server) uses a reduced FASTA format, where every new line is considered to be a new sequence. A standard FASTA file can be converted by removing new lines and white spaces from the sequences.

   Recommended programs for RNA structure prediction that have to be locally installed are UNAfold (14) and RNAstructure (15):
   http://dinamelt.bioinfo.rpi.edu/download.php
   http://rna.urmc.rochester.edu/RNAstructure.html
   Centroidfold and CONTRAfold can be found at
   http://www.ncrna.org/centroidfold/ and
   http://contra.stanford.edu/contrafold/
2. For longer (100 nt +) sequences, mfe frequencies are usually very small, as the number of structures rises exponentially with sequence length. The postscript file format for dot plots can be easily parsed to get the values of the probabilities. Within the file, there is a list of number triples followed by a ubox command:

956 993 0.2215 ubox
957 992 0.1085 ubox
958 974 0.9302 ubox
959 973 0.9935 ubox

The list consists of the bases that pair and the *square root* of the base pairing probability.

3. The WAR web server (16) unifies many programs to predict consensus structure. It can be found at http://genome.ku.dk/resources/war/
4. Note that constraints can be violated if they are energetically unfavorable or impossible. As an example, specifying a base pair constraint will lead to a structure where the specified base pair can be added without violating the base pairing rules for secondary structures, but it will contain the base pair only if it is energetically favorable.
5. There are several tools for the de novo prediction of three-dimensional RNA structures. As this problem is much harder than the prediction of secondary structure, most of today's programs are restricted to short RNA molecules (≤50 nt). A very interesting tool for three-dimensional prediction is Assemble (http://www.bioinformatics.org/assemble/index.html). It provides the possibility of using known tertiary structure motifs such as kink turns to combine with predicted helices. Furthermore, the torsion angles of all bases can be varied so that a tertiary structure can be created. There is a very good online tutorial (http://www.bioinformatics.org/assemble/screencasts.html). However, this way of semi-automated generation of a tertiary structure requires expert knowledge in the field.
6. Biological cells usually operate far from the thermodynamic equilibrium. As a consequence, biopolymers may never reach their mfe structure during their life time. Folding kinetics can be used to identify long-living meta-stable structures with biological function (17). Further interesting questions concern the structure of the folding landscape in terms of local minima and the energy barriers between them. These questions can be investigated using the ViennaRNA barrier server: http://rna.tbi.univie.ac.at/cgi-bin/barriers.cgi

References

1. Zuker, M., Stiegler, P. (1981) Optimal computer folding of large RNA sequences using thermodynamics and auxiliary information. *Nucleic Acids Res* 9, 133–148.
2. Eddy, S., Durbin, R. (1994) RNA sequence analysis using covariance models. *Nucleic Acids Res* 22, 2079–2088.
3. McCaskill, J. (1990) The equilibrium partition function and base pair binding

probabilities for RNA secondary structure. *Biopolymers* 29, 1105–1119.

4. Do, C., Woods, D., Batzoglou, S. (2006) Contrafold: RNA secondary structure prediction without physics-based models. *Bioinformatics* 22, 90–98.
5. Sato, K., Hamada, M., Asai, K., Mituyama, T. (2009) Centroidfold: a web server for RNA secondary structure prediction. *Nucleic Acids Res* 37(Web Server issue), 277–2780.
6. Chan, C., Lawrence, C., Ding, Y. (2005) Structure clustering features on the sfold web server. *Bioinformatics* 21, 3926–3928.
7. Wuchty, S., Fontana, W., Hofacker, I., Schuster, P. (1999) Complete suboptimal folding of RNA and the stability of secondary structures. *Biopolymers* 49, 145–165.
8. Mathews, D., Sabina, J., Zuker, M., Turner, D. (1999) Expanded sequence dependence of thermodynamic parameters improves prediction of RNA secondary structure. *J Mol Biol* 288, 911–940.
9. Tafer, H., Ameres, S., Obernosterer, G., et al. (2008) The impact of target site accessibility on the design of effective siRNAs. *Nat Biotechnol* 26, 578–583.
10. Gruber, A., Lorenz, R., Bernhart, S., et al. (2008) The Vienna RNA websuite. *Nucleic Acids Res* 36(Web Server issue), 70–74.
11. Andronescu, M., Condon, A., Hoos, H., et al. (2007) Efficient parameter estimation for RNA secondary structure prediction. *Bioinformatics* 23, 19–28.
12. Katoh, K., Kuma, K., Toh, H., Miyata, T. (2005) Mafft version 5: improvement in accuracy of multiple sequence alignment. *Nucleic Acids Res* 33, 511–518.
13. Larkin, M., Blackshields, G., Brown, N., et al. (2007) Clustal w and clustal x version 2.0. *Bioinformatics* 23, 2947–2948.
14. Markham, N., Zuker, M. (2008) Unafold: software for nucleic acid folding and hybridization. *Methods Mol Biol* 453, 3–31.
15. Mathews, D., Disney, M., Childs, J., et al. (2004) Incorporating chemical modification constraints into a dynamic programming algorithm for prediction of RNA secondary structure. *Proc Natl Acad Sci USA* 101, 7287–7292.
16. Torarinsson, E., Lindgreen, S. (2008) War: web server for aligning structural RNAs. *Nucleic Acids Res* 36(Web Server issue), 79–84.
17. Flamm, C., Hofacker, I.L. (2008) Beyond energy minimization: approaches to the kinetic folding of RNA. *Monatsh. f. Chemie* 139, 447–457.

Chapter 20

In Silico Prediction of Post-translational Modifications

Chunmei Liu and Hui Li

Abstract

Methods for predicting protein post-translational modifications have been developed extensively. In this chapter, we review major post-translational modification prediction strategies, with a particular focus on statistical and machine learning approaches. We present the workflow of the methods and summarize the advantages and disadvantages of the methods.

Key words: Mass spectrum, machine learning, post-translational modifications.

1. Introduction

Post-translational modification (PTM) is the chemical modification of a protein after its translation. Various amino acids can be incorporated in the process of protein biosynthesis. PTMs are covalent bond processing events that change the functions of a protein by either proteolytic cleavage, adding a modifying group to one or more amino acids, changing the chemical nature of an amino acid, or by making structural changes. The main PTMs include acetylation, acylation, and alkylation, as well as numerous others. PTMs of a queried protein affect its activity state, localization, turnover, and interactions with other proteins. These modifications allow the resulting protein to be involved in various molecular functions for cellular processes such as ligand binding, cell communication, cellular defense and immune regulation, enzymatic activation or inactivation, protein degradation, and blood coagulation. Losses or modifications of a normal protein modification site have been shown experimentally to be associated with many disease processes (1, 2). The role of PTMs

B. Yu, M. Hinchcliffe (eds.), *In Silico Tools for Gene Discovery*, Methods in Molecular Biology 760,
DOI 10.1007/978-1-61779-176-5_20, © Springer Science+Business Media, LLC 2011

in cell life activity is very important. For example, in the case of PTMs that are involved in signaling transduction, kinase cascades are turned on and off by the reversible addition and removal of phosphate groups (3, 4).

Accurate prediction of PTM sites can promote annotation of genome and proteome sequence data in order to meet the current demand of fast growing datasets and help understand the functions of proteins. Although there are a number of advanced biological technologies which have been applied to the proteomic research area, the identification of potential PTM sites and the characterization of complex protein structures still present enormous difficulties and continue to be challenging tasks (5).

Currently, mass spectrometry with modern ion separation technologies and computing algorithms represent the most powerful techniques for PTM site identification. In particular, with the development of proteomic technologies, PTM sites and protein sequence databases have increased dramatically, and algorithms for interpreting experimental data into referenced PTM sites have become more attractive. However, experimentally evident PTM sites, of which increasing numbers have been validated by proteomics, should be used to closely integrate computational prediction algorithms into proteomic PTM experiments. Public resources and tools for PTM prediction are listed in **Table 20.1**.

The types of methods that can enable in silico predictions of PTM sites can be summarized as follows:

1. *Sequence-based methods.* The identified PTM site information comes from the mass spectrum (MS) data via the amalgamation of protein sequence information.

2. *Sequence alignment-based approaches.* Those approaches predict PTMs by comparing the similarities between PTM sequences derived from MS. Each type of PTM site requires a different MS to meet the requirement. Different types of MS influence the quality of the data differently. Carrying out MS on certain PTMs can influence the quality of the amino acids and cause an offset in the MS or can make the peptide bond break. All of these influences will result in a change in the MS. Therefore, developing tools and algorithms that correctly identify PTM sites from the MS is a challenging task.

3. *Automatic discovery-based methods.* Those methods utilize the fact that each amino acid occupies a site that has a potential to be modified and focus on automatic PTM detection. Such approaches mainly focus on the alignment of a spectrum with a sequence to identify potential PTM sites. Another method that is similar to automatic PTM identification is the spectrum profile–profile-based method.

Table 20.1
Publicly available PTM web resources, databases, and prediction tools

Resource (Ref.)	Methods	URL	Comments
ChloroP (45)	Artificial neural network	http://www.cbs.dtu.dk/services/ChloroP/	Prediction of chloroplast transit peptides
ELM (46)	Consensus patterns	http://elm.eu.org/	Predicts eukaryotic linear motifs (ELMs) based on consensus patterns. Applies context-based rules and logical filters
PROSITE (47)	Consensus patterns	http://www.expasy.org/prosite/	Curated database of consensus patterns for many types of PTMs, including phosphorylation sites. Motif Scan feature allows for scanning of query sequence
HPRD (48)	Database	http://www.hprd.org	Human Protein Reference Database (HPRD). Highly curated database of disease-related proteins and their PTMs
RESID (49)	Database	http://www.ebi.ac.uk/RESID/	A comprehensive collection of annotations and structures for protein modifications including amino-terminal, carboxyl-terminal, and peptide chain cross-link post-translational modifications
Scansite (50)	Weight matrix	http://scansite.mit.edu	Based on peptide library studies. Predicts kinase- specific motifs and other types of motifs involved in signal transduction, e.g., SH2 domain binding
PREDIKIN (51)	Expert system	http://predikin.biosci.uq.edu.au/kinase/	The program produces a prediction of substrates for S/T protein kinases based on the primary sequence of a protein kinase catalytic domain
NetPhos (52)	Artificial neural network	http://www.cbs.dtu.dk/services/NetPhos/	Predicts general phosphorylation status based on sets of experimentally validated S, T and Y phosphorylation sites
NetPhosK (53)	Artificial neural network	http://www.cbs.dtu.dk/services/NetPhosK/	Predicts kinase-specific phosphorylation sites based on sets of experimentally validated S, T, and Y phosphorylation sites
PhosphoBase (54)	Database	http://phospho.elm.eu.org/	Curated database of validated phosphorylation sites
Phospho.ELM (54)	Database	http://phospho.elm.eu.org/	Curated database of in vivo validated phosphorylation sites

Table 20.1 (Continued)

Resource (Ref.)	Methods	URL	Comments
bigPI (55)	Statistic machine learning	http://mendel.imp.ac.at/gpi/gpi_server.html	Predicts GPI modification sites using a composite prediction function including a weight matrix and physical model. Provides a genome annotation and target selection tool
GlycoMod (56)	Lookup table	http://ca.expasy.org/tools/glycomod/	Predicts the possible oligosaccharide structures that occur on proteins from their experimentally determined masses
NetOGlyc (57)	Neural network	http://www.cbs.dtu.dk/services/NetOGlyc/	Predicts mucin-type CalNac O-glycosylation sites in mammalian proteins
DictyOGlyc (58)	Neural network	http://www.cbs.dtu.dk/services/DictyOGlyc/	The DictyOGlyc server produces neural network predictions for GlcNAc O-glycosylation sites in *Dictyostelium discoideum* proteins PMID:10521537
YinOYang (59)	Neural network	http://www.cbs.dtu.dk/services/YinOYang/	Predicts O-beta-GlcNAc attachment sites in eukaryotic protein sequences
TermiNator (60)	Prediction model	http://www.isv.cnrs-gif.fr/terminator3/index.html	predicts N-terminal methionine excision, N-terminal acetylation, N-terminal myristoylation, and S-palmitoylation of either prokaryotic or eukaryotic proteins originating from organellar or nuclear genomes
ProP (61)	Neural network	http://www.cbs.dtu.dk/services/ProP/	Predicts arginine and lysine propeptide cleavage sites in eukaryotic protein sequences using an ensemble of neural networks
NetPicoRNA (62)	Neural network	http://www.cbs.dtu.dk/services/NetPicoRNA/	Predictions of cleavage sites of picornaviral proteases
Myristoylator (63)	Neural network	http://www.expasy.org/tools/myristoylator/	Predicts N-terminal myristoylation of proteins by neural networks
GPS (64)	clustering	http://gps.biocuckoo.org/	Prediction of kinase-specific phosphorylation sites for 408 human protein kinases in hierarchy

Using peptide sequence information, an experimental MS can be matched to a theoretical MS from a protein database to screen for PTM sites. Based on established rules and the related criteria for forming a tag match, all possible PTM sites can be inferred from the database based on differences between the experimental MS and the theoretical MS.

As a result of the recent exponential growth in computational PTM site identification algorithms, computational prediction tools that utilize the resulting PTM databases have played important roles in proteomic research.

2. Materials

Computationally predicting PTMs using MS data is one of the most important methods. Because the performance of such prediction methods depends on the quality of experimental results, the prediction accuracy is greatly limited by noise and missing mass values in the dataset. Development of effective noise reduction methods and estimation of missing values are, therefore, keys for correctly identifying PTM sites. Many approaches have been proposed for PTM site recognition. Some methods, such as identifying physicochemical properties and searching motif patterns, have been developed and applied to the prediction of PTM sites. Among these methods, most of the successful algorithms are based on machine learning techniques, for example, NetPhosYeast (6), YinOYang (7), PredPhospho (8), AutoMotif (9, 10), KinasePhos 2.0 (11), PPSP (12), and SiteSeek (13). Many earlier approaches for identifying PTMs are based on amino acid information from the MS. These approaches have prominent differences in their computational complexities comparing the MS with all possible combinations of PTMs for each peptide from the database.

Currently, more than 30 PTM prediction servers for various processes, including phosphorylation, glycosylation, acetylation, sumoylation, palmitoylation, and sulfation, have been developed and are publicly available through the Internet. For example, dbPTM (14) integrates experimentally verified PTMs from several databases and annotates the predicted PTMs in Swiss-Prot proteins. dbPTM uses a knowledge base-based method that is comprised of the modified sites, the solvent accessibility of the substrate, the secondary and tertiary protein structures, as well as protein domains and protein variations. Literally related PTMs, protein conservations, and substrate site specificity can also be analyzed. dbPTM provides various computational tools to predict more than 10 types of PTMs, including phosphorylation, glycosylation, acetylation, methylation, sulfation, and sumoylation. PROSITE (15) consists of documentation entries describing protein domains, families and functional sites as well as associated patterns and profiles. Other databases such as NetAcet (16),

NetNGlyc (17), NetOGlyc (18), and NetPhos (19) can be used to predict phosphorylation sites. SulfoSite (20) is a tool for predicting substrates of *N*-acetyltransferase A, methylation sites, *N*-glycosylation sites in human proteins, mucin-type O-glycosylation, phosphorylation sites in eukaryotic proteins sites, and sulfation sites. PTM databases and prediction tools are listed in **Table 20.1**. Some of the data have been derived from ExPASy (21). Limitations of current PTM database developments are summarized in **Note 1**.

3. Methods

3.1. Mass Spectrum Alignment Algorithm-Based Methods

Spectrum alignment algorithms are one of the most common methods for PTM site prediction. These methods focus on protein sequence alignment that has been derived from a protein database by aligning a queried sequence with other known sequences to locate a site which has been modified. The queried sequence obtained from the experimental MS is compared with the corresponding theoretical MS. The difference between the experimental MS and the theoretical MS is used to predict PTM sites.

The common workflow of this method consist of (1) computing the similarity of the two sequences; (2) sorting their difference values which are based on the similarity scores between the two sequences; (3) comparing the query sequence with the protein database and extracting near-identical matches; and (4) running the obtained predictor on potential site features to output the prediction results. Many research directions, including similarity measures, scoring functions, and sequence alignment algorithms and database matching, are used in predicting the PTM sites. Novel scoring algorithms are constantly being developed to improve the identification ratio of PTM sites. To evaluate the validity of the predicted PTM sites, the queried protein is compared with homologous sites in closely related species. However, evolutionary information of this type does not always improve the performance of the methods of PTM prediction (22). Another alignment method aligns spectral and database sequences using dynamic programming (23). Experimental results show that the dynamic programming algorithm performs well for PTM identification. The general workflow of sequence alignment is shown in **Fig. 20.1**.

As shown in **Fig. 20.1**, the main task of spectrum alignment is the comparison of an experimental MS with a theoretical MS derived from the protein database. Through the whole alignment process of modifications, one of the most important steps

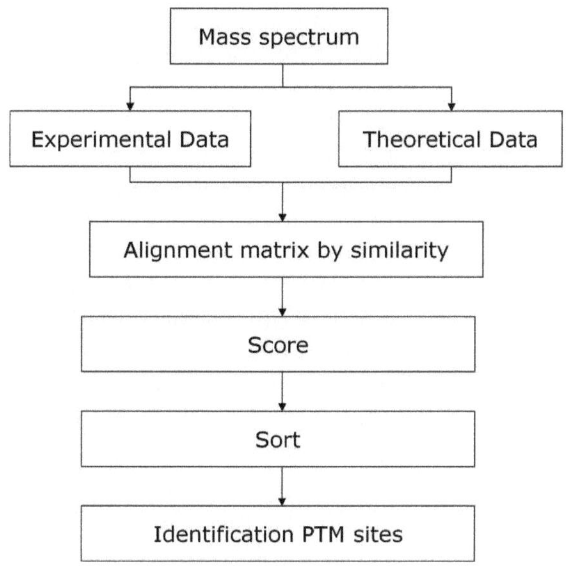

Fig. 20.1. Flowchart of the alignment algorithm.

is narrowing down the local regions where modifications may exist. Researchers use multiple sequence tags to effectively localize modified regions within a spectrum. Jung et al. (24) propose a PTM site identification method. Combining sequence patterns and evolutionary information as well as a noise-reducing algorithm improves the performance of the prediction. They further proposed a new scoring method to measure the similarity of the peptides. The work combines the similarity of the BLOSUM62 (25) matrix with the profile–profile alignment that contains the evolutionary information.

Na et al. (26) use a peptide sequence tag-based alignment and a single variable modification method to predict PTMs. Before the prediction, they optimize the alignment between the MS and the sequence with an unrestrictive search. A short sequence tag (2–4 amino acid stretch) from the MS was used to screen peptides in a protein database.

In recent studies involving computational proteomics, a major problem is distinguishing correct peptide identifications from false positives. Seungjin et al. (26) provided a good example of trying to resolve such issues. When modifications are included, the false-positive problem can be significantly exacerbated. The inclusion of many types of modifications can result in a large number of false positives due to the combinatorial increase in the number of possible matches (27).

3.2. Machine Learning-Based Method

Machine learning techniques have been broadly used in bioinformatics research fields including gene expression analysis, protein site prediction, and protein interaction network analysis. Machine learning and statistical approaches are very common tools and algorithms for PTM site prediction. Probabilistic frameworks and new kernel methods are also used. PPSP (12) is based on Bayesian decision theory to predict protein kinase (PK)-specific phosphorylation sites, and SiteSeek uses an adaptive kernel method with hydrophobic information (13). Machine learning is one of the most widely used methods in PTM prediction. Unsupervised machine learning is used for clustering and supervised machine learning is used for classification, especially for predictive model construction. Representative machine learning methods include artificial neural networks (ANNs), KinasePhos 1.0 (27), Bayesian neural networks (28), and SVM (support vector machine) (29). These PTM prediction approaches are viewed as a binary classification of protein fragments consisting of a candidate peptide. In this case, the known PTMs are positive samples and the others are negative samples. Feature selection is always used before extracting feature vectors.

3.2.1. The Prediction of PTM Sites Using SVM

The general steps of supervised machine learning in PTM prediction are (1) feature selection and (2) building a prediction model. Feature selection is feasible for dimension deduction. The prediction model is obtained by training with an SVM classifier. Thus, most of the related PTM prediction work using machine learning focuses on the two aspects to improve the performance of the prediction model. Ingrell et al. (6) present a publicly available model NetPhosYeast, which is based on a neural network method for the prediction of protein phosphorylation sites in yeast. They provide a public server that is available at http://www.cbs.dtu.dk/services/NetPhosYeast/. Blom et al. (30) propose NetPhosK (http://www.cbs.dtu.dk/services/NetPhosK/) which is also based on ANN together with sequence phosphorylation site prediction. Blom et al. use a Bayesian neural network model to mine the information contained in the MS data. Support vector machine-based methods are widely used in PTM prediction. For example, using a support vector machine, PredPhospho (8) predicts phosphorylation sites and kinase(s) that act at each site. AutoMotif (31) has been proposed by Plewczynski et al. It uses an SVM algorithm to train protein sets to predict a modification site. Lu et al. (32) use an SVM binary classifier to assess the correctness of phosphopeptide/spectrum matches. KinasePhos 2.0 (33) incorporates an SVM with the protein sequence profile to identify phosphorylation sites.

Normally a raw dataset is divided into a training set (to be used for model building) and a test set (to estimate the generalization power of the model) by randomly dividing the data. Various classification methods can be reliably benchmarked to gain insight into their capability to handle proteomic site prediction data.

SVMs are built on solid statistical learning theory. An SVM has minimal structural risk since the classification of the SVM depends on the support vectors. These features of SVMs make those methods work well on small samples that have a high dimensionality deduction and non-linear classification problem. Therefore, SVM is now a popular tool used for PTM site prediction. The workflow of the SVM is shown in **Fig. 20.2**.

The data used in the PTM prediction is the peptide sequence. The whole sequence is cut into fragments in which the target sites are centered among other constant amino acids in the sequence. A sliding window technique is used to select the feature vector using amino acid sequences of various lengths. **Figure 20.3** shows an example sequence of the O-GlcNAc protein. The red sites indicate serine and threonine residues in *N*-acetylglucosamine (GlcNAc).

For example, if we set the half window size of 20 (the sequence is truncated to fix segment sizes whose length depends on the sliding window size), the segment length of the feature vector is 41 amino acids. As shown in **Fig. 20.4**, the segment sequence in the middle with a red color is the abbreviation of serine and threonine amino acids which are OGlcNAcylated sites.

The feature vectors to input into the machine learning model are the predicted sites for T and S. The real PTM sites validated by experiments are positive sites. The other sites are negative. The

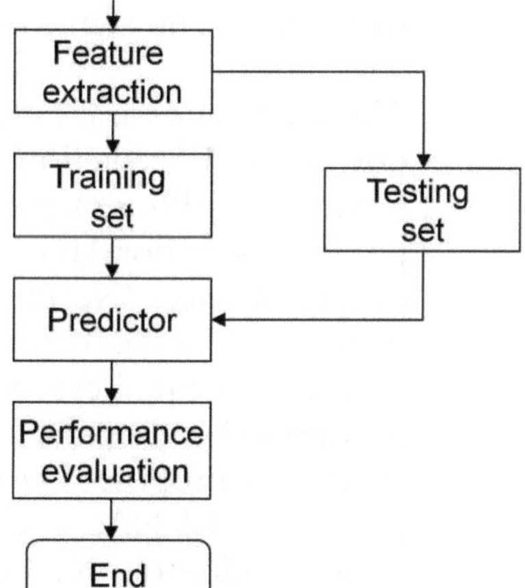

Fig. 20.2. Flowchart of a machine learning algorithm.

MPLNVSFTNR NYDLDYDSVQ PYFYCDEEEN FYQQQQQSEL
QPPAPSEDIW KKFELLPTPPLSPSRRSGLC SPSYVAVTPFSL
RGDNDGGG GSFSTADQLEMVTELLGGDM VNQSFICDPDDE
TFIKNIII QDCMWSGFSAAAKLVSEKLA SYQAARKDSG SPNP
ARGHSV CSTSSLYLQDLSAAASECID PSVVFPYPLN DSSSPK
SCAS QDSSAFSPSS DSLLSSTESS PQGSPEPLVLHEETPPTT
SS DSEEEQEDEE EIDVVSVEKR QAPGKRSESG SPSAGGHS
KP PHSPLVLKRC

Fig. 20.3. A sequence of an O-GlcNAc protein; the amino acids with *underlines* indicate they are GlcNAcylation site.

Half window size=20 Half window size=20

???????????????MPLNVSFTNR NYDLDYDSVQ PYFYCD
????????????? MPLNVSFTNRNYDLDYDSVQ PYFYCDEE
??MPLNVSFTNR NYDLDYDSVQPYFYCDEEENFYQQQQQS

Fig. 20.4. Feature vector for segment sequence.

dataset always has more negative sites than positive ones, which forms an imbalanced dataset. Different proportions of the positive and negative sites are mixed together to form the training and testing datasets. Next, feature selection is performed.

To illustrate the whole process of a machine learning approach, an example of the classic SVM method used by Webb-Robertson et al. (29) is given below. The dataset they used is from AMT studies for three diverse bacterial species (*Shewanella oneidensis*, *Salmonella typhimurium*, and *Yersinia pestis*). They use 35 features which capture the amino acid characteristics. Before SVM classification, these features are transformed based on the normalization factors used in the training phase. The feature selection they used is the Fisher criterion score (FCS) (34) which is a function that defines the distance between two distributions based on their means and standard deviations.

3.3. Artificial Neural Network-Based Method

The artificial neural network (ANN) is one of the earlier methods of PTM prediction. NetPhos 2.0 (http://www.cbs.dtu.dk/services/NetPhos/), proposed by Blom et al., utilizes an ANN to predict phosphorylation sites. NetPhosK 1.0 (http://www.cbs.dtu.dk/services/NetPhosK/) presented by Blom et al. (19) also uses an ANN-based program designed by training an ANN to find the potential cytoplasmic domains for their specificity to be phosphorylated by different kinases at Ser/Thr/Tyr. Plewczynski et al. (9) propose Yin-O-yang which uses an ANN model to predict O-GlcNAc and phosphate modifications sites of proteins. In addition, NetOGlyc 2.0 and 3.1 (35, 36) (http://www.cbs.dtu.dk/services/NetOGlyc/) predict O-glycosylation sites in mucin-type proteins; DictyOGlyc 1.1 (37) (http://www.cbs.dtu.dk/services/DictyOGlyc/) predicts O-a-GlcNAc sites in eukaryotic proteins. NetNGlyc 1.0 (http://www.cbs.dtu.dk/services/NetNGlyc/) predicts N-glycosylation sites. Each of these uses an ANN as the prediction model.

Before the MS data is transformed to a sequence, identifying the portion of the MS that refers to a certain peptide is the key step for identifying the PTM sites. Multiple sequence alignment is a simple and easy way to position the PTM sites. Positive and negative sites are divided into known and unknown modification sites. The known modification sites of Ser or Thr residues must be defined as positive sites, while the remaining sites are defined as false-positive sites. The sequence of the peptide is transformed into different feature vectors. This process is the encoding process. The binary encoding (38) method considers each amino acid as a binary vector with the 20 amino acids corresponding to 20 different binary strings. Each amino acid is denoted by 19 zeros and ones which correspond to the position of this amino acid in the sequence. For example, amino acids A, B, C are represented as binary strings: $A = \{1000000000\ 0000000000\}$, $B = \{0100000000\ 0000000000\}$, and $C = \{0010000000\ 00000\ 00000\}$. The binary format of the ABC sequence is the connection of the three binary strings and is presented as $ABC = \{1000000000\ 0000000000\ 0100000000\ 0000000000\ 0010000\ 000\ 000000000\}$. The sequence information is then transformed into binary information. Then the binary sequence string is inputted into the ANN to construct the predictor. Julenius and colleagues (39) extend the binary encoding method and explore various sequence encoding methods on a dataset consisting of 421 positive and 2,063 negative instances from 85 proteins. Another encoding method (40) counts the frequency of amino acids occurring at a certain position in the sequence. The size of the input vector depends on the window size of the truncated arbitrary sequence length. The predicted site is the center of the string. The center of each window is Ser or Thr. There are still other encoding methods including CKSAAP (41) which involves binary encoding with an SVM (42). These methods are capable of predicting PTM sites. After the data for the PTM is ready, the data will be divided into two parts: one is the training set and the other is the testing set. Ishtiaq et al. use ANN to predict O-GlcNAc and phosphorylation proteins. The dataset is extracted from the L-selectin sequence using the Entrez database No. A34015 and Swiss-Prot entry, the E-selectin sequence with the Entrez database No. A35046 and the Swiss-Prot entry, and the sequence of P-selectin with the Entrez database No. P16109 and the Swiss-Prot entry. There are a total of 1,691 hits for L-selectin, 2,711 hits for E-selectin, and 3,205 hits for P-selectins.

Julenius et al. (36) also use ANN to predict phosphorylation in O-GlcNAc proteins. The details of the ANN layers and the feature selection were not explained in their paper. Hansen et al. (43) evaluate ANN using binary encoding on a training set consisting of 2,329 samples, 264 positive and 1,065 negative samples, and two test sets containing 34 and 36 positive samples. When training ANNs using imbalanced data, negative samples are presented less frequently during the training.

3.4. Prediction Using Graph-Based Algorithms

Graph-based PTM site prediction methods use the nodes of the graphs to represent the peaks of the MS and the edges to denote the different types of peaks in the MS. The aim of PTM site prediction is to find the optimal combination of nodes which corresponds to an optimal path. The approaches are mainly as follows:

1. *Tree decomposition-based approaches.* By decomposing the graph into a tree with a small tree width, the approach partitions the graphs into trees that consist of tree bags (groups of closely related vertices).
2. *Problem formulation.* This approach gives the mathematical formula of the edge weights of the graph and the objectives to be achieved in the graph partition problem.
3. Dynamic programming is used to search for the optimal combination of the nodes.
4. Heuristic functions combined with a graph search to implement the path search for different sequence tags.

The key technique of graph-based methods is to partition the graph into a tree. However, partitioning the graph into a tree is a NP-hard problem. Many heuristic algorithms have been proposed to solve the problem.

Mark et al. (44) propose a web-based program using a method based on graph theory and a heuristic function. They treat PTM sites as a tree traversal of the MS. The tree is searched using a depth-first combined with a heuristic function. Fuzzy logic rule sets are constructed that have the advantage of being easily interpreted by experts. Liu et al. (23) develop a novel tree decomposition algorithm that can efficiently generate peptide sequence tags (PSTs) from an extended spectrum graph. They denote a mass peak of MS as a graph node and define three types of edges: B-ion, Y-ion, and noise type. Then they use a dynamic programming algorithm to partition the graph with the above-mentioned three types of edges. The algorithm is able to recognize the ion types of the MS peaks. Their experimental results show that the accuracy of identification is about 95%.

In light of what we have discussed above, machine learning approaches with mass spectrometry currently represent the most powerful techniques for PTM site prediction. Many challenges still exist (*see* **Notes 2** and **3**) and identification of PTM sites continues to be challenging. Each method of machine learning has internal merits and shortcomings (*see* **Note 2**).

4. Notes

1. Limitations of current PTM database developments are as follows: (1) Some of the amino acids have been modified under a single specific condition and return to the initial state when that condition changes. Such a static annotation can only indicate whether an amino acid has been modified and thus cannot fully reflect the actual biological activity. (2) The occurrence of PTMs as they relate to non-PTM sites. PTM events are highly associated with other biologically functional proteins. Integration of the interaction relationships with a PTM is not reflected in current databases.
2. ANNs are better for classification and regression because of the structure of the model. However, the process of the classification is a "black box" for users compared with other machine learning approaches. Another fatal problem of ANN is that they are easily trapped into a local minimum/maximum. The Bayesian neural network tries to solve such problems. Compared with ANNs, an SVM model does not have a local minimum/maximum problem.
3. Predicting PTM sites is time consuming and expensive, and has many limitations. With the discovery of known PTM sites, approaches that utilize the assistance of databases are promising. Statistical and machine learning methods are very popular in this research area. Although each method has good performance in some areas and novel characteristics for identifying peptide and proteins, both machine learning and statistically based methods continue to be weak and insufficient. Developing a simple, instructive, and general algorithm to identify the PTM sites is one of the urgent tasks for proteomic research. The probability model and statistical methods are especially useful in sequence alignment and scoring. Many statistical methods have been applied in this field, but the actual data distribution space cannot be accurately reflected using the present methods. The actual data space cannot be reflected sufficiently by any of the above. Machine leaning techniques such as ANN, SVM, and Bayesian networks have been applied to predict PTM sites and have shown good performance.

The challenge of PTM site prediction is also related to the quality of the data derived from the MS. On the one hand, large amounts of noise and missing mass values present in MS data directly affect the prediction results. On the other hand, imbalances between the negative and positive data can make the trained model insensitive to the noise and missing values in the data. To overcome these problems, improved, novel, and effective algorithms are urgently needed.

References

1. Jaeken J., Carchon H. (2001) Congenital disorders of glycosylation: the rapidly growing tip of the iceberg. *Curr Opin Neurol* 14, 811–815.
2. Martin P.T. (2005) The dystroglycanopathies: the new disorders of O-linked glycosylation. *Semin Pediatr Neurol* 12, 152–158.
3. Cohen, P. (2000) the regulation of protein function by multisite phosphorylation-a 25 year update. *Trends Biochem Sci* 25, 596–601.
4. Tyers, M., Jorgensen, P. (1989) Protein and carbohydrate structural analysis of a recombinant soluble CD4 receptor by mass spectrometry. *J Biol Chem* 264, 21286–21295.
5. Medzihradszky, K. F. (2008) Characterization of site-specific N-glycosylation. *Methods Mol Biol* 446, 293–316.
6. Ingrell, C. R., Miller, M. L., Jensen, O. N., Blom, N. (2007) NetPhosYeast: prediction of protein phosphorylation sites in yeast. *Bioinformatics* 23, 895–897.
7. Gupta, R. (2001) Prediction of glycosylation sites in proteomes: from post-translational modifications to protein function. Ph.D. thesis at CBS.
8. Kim, J. H., Lee, J., Oh, B., et al. (2004) Prediction of phosphorylation sites using SVMs. *Bioinformatics* 20, 3179–3184.
9. Plewczynski, D., Tkacz, A., Wyrwicz, L.S., Rychlewski, L. (2005) AutoMotif server: prediction of single residue post-translational modifications in proteins. *Bioinformatics* 21, 2525–2527.
10. Plewczynski, D., Tkacz, A., Wyrwicz, L. S., et al. (2008) AutoMotif Server for prediction of phosphorylation sites in proteins using support vector machine: 2007 update. *J Mol Model* 14, 69–76.
11. Wong, Y. H., Lee, T.Y., Liang, H. K., et al. (2007) KinasePhos 2.0: a web server for identifying protein kinase-specific phosphorylation sites based on sequences and coupling patterns. *Nucleic Acids Res* 35, W588–594.
12. Xue, Y., Li, A., Wang, L., Feng, H., Yao, X. (2006) PPSP: prediction of PK-specific phosphorylation site with Bayesian decision theory. *BMC Bioinformatics* 7, 163.
13. Yoo, P. D., Ho, Y. S., Zhou, B. B., Zomaya, A. Y. (2008) SiteSeek: posttranslational modification analysis using adaptive locality-effective kernel methods and new profiles. *BMC Bioinformatics* 9, 272.
14. Lee, T. Y., et al. (2006) dbPTM: an information repository of protein post-translational modification. *Nucleic Acids Res* 34, D622–D627.
15. Sigrist, C. J., Cerutti, L., Hulo, N., et al. (2002) PROSITE: A documented database using patterns and profiles as motif descriptors. *Brief Bioinfo* 3, 265–274.
16. Kiemer, L., Bendtsen, J. D., Blom, N. (2005) NetAcet: prediction of N-terminal acetylation sites. *Bioinformatics* 21, 1269–1270.
17. Johansen, M. B., Kiemer, L., Brunak, S. (2006) Analysis and prediction of mammalian protein glycation. *Glycobiology* 16, 844–853.
18. Hansen, J. E., Lund, O., Tolstrup, N., et al. (1998) NetOglyc: Prediction of mucin type O-glycosylation sites based on sequence context and surface accessibility. *Glycoconjugate J* 15, 115–130.
19. Blom, N., Gammeltoft, S., Brunak, S. (1999) Sequence and structure-based prediction of eukaryotic protein phosphorylation sites. *J Mol Biol* 294, 1351–1362.
20. Chang, W. C., Lee, T. Y., Shien DM, et al. (2009) Incorporating support vector machine for identifying protein tyrosine sulfation sites. *J Comput Chem* 30, 2526–2537.
21. http://ca.expasy.org/tools/. Accessed 18 August 2010.
22. Blom, N., Sicheritz-Pontén, T., Gupta, R., et al. (2004) Prediction of post-translational glycosylation and phosphorylation of proteins from the amino acid sequence. *Proteomics* 4, 1633–1649.
23. Liu, C. M., Blake, A., Burge, L., et al. (2006) The identification of ion types in tandem mass spectra based on a graph algorithm. *J Sci Practical Comput* 1, 46–60.
24. Jung, I., Matsuyama, A., Yoshida, M., Kim, D. (2010) PostMod: sequence based prediction of kinase-specific phosphorylation sites with indirect relationship. *BMC Bioinformatics* 11(Suppl1), S10.

25. Zhou, F. F., Xue, Y., Chen, G.L., Yao, X. (2004) GPS: a novel group-based phosphorylation predicting and scoring method. *Biochem Biophys Res Commun* 325(4), 1443–1448.
26. Na, S., Paek, E. (2009) Prediction of novel modifications by unrestrictive search of tandem mass spectra. *J Proteome Res* 8, 4418–4427.
27. Huang, H. D., Lee, T. Y., Tseng, S. W., Horng, J. T. (2005) KinasePhos: a web tool for identifying protein kinase-specific phosphorylation sites. *Nucleic Acids Res* 33, W226–229.
28. Zhou, C., Bowler, L. D., Feng, J. F. (2008) A machine learning approach to explore the spectra intensity pattern of peptides using tandem mass spectrometry data. *BMC Bioinformatics.* 9, 325.
29. Webb-Robertson, B. J., Cannon, W. R., Oehmen, C.S., et al. (2008) A support vector machine model for the prediction of proteotypic peptides for accurate mass and time proteomics. *Bioinformatics* 24, 1503–1509.
30. Blom, N., Sicheritz-Ponten, T., Gupta, R., et al. (2004) Prediction of post-translational glycosylation and phosphorylation of proteins from the amino acid sequence. *Proteomics* 4, 1633–1649.
31. Plewczynski, D., Tkacz, A., Wyrwicz, L. S., Rychlewski, L. (2005) AutoMotif server: prediction of single residue post-translational modifications in proteins. *Bioinformatics* 21, 2525–2527.
32. Lu, B., Ruse, C., Xu, T., et al. (2007) Automatic validation of phosphopeptide identifications from tandem mass spectra. *Anal Chem* 79, 1301–1310.
33. Wong, Y. H., Lee, T. Y., Liang, H. K., et al. (2007) KinasePhos 2.0: a web server for identifying protein kinase-specific phosphorylation sites based on sequences and coupling patterns. *Nucleic Acids Res* 35, W588–594.
34. Ahmad, I., Hoessli, D. C., Gupta, R., et al. (2007) In silico determination of intracellular glycosylation and phosphorylation sites in human selectins: implications for biological function. *J Cell Biochem* 100, 1558–1572.
35. Hansen, J. E., Lund, O., Tolstrup. N., et al. (1998) NetOGlyc: Prediction of mucin type O-glycosylation sites based on sequence context and surface accessibility. *Glycoconj J* 15, 115–130.
36. Julenius, K., Mølgaard, A., Gupta, R., Brunak, S. (2005) Prediction, conservation analysis and structural characterization of mammalian mucin-type O-glycosylation sites. *Glycobiology* 15, 153–164.
37. Gupta, R., Jung, E., Gooley, A. A., et al. (1999) Scanning the available *Dictyostelium discoideum* proteome for O-linked GlcNAc glycosylation sites using neural networks. *Glycobiology* 9, 1009–1022.
38. Hansen, J. E., Lund, O., Engelbrecht, J., et al. (1995) Prediction of O-glycosylation of mammalian proteins: specificity patterns of UDP-GalNAc: polypeptide *N*-acetylgalactosaminyltransferase. *Biochem J* 308, 801–813.
39. Julenius, K., Molgaard, A., Gupta, R., Brunak, S. (2005) Prediction, conservation analysis, and structural characterization of mammalian mucin-type O-glycosylation sites. *Glycobiology* 15, 153–164.
40. Torii, M., Liu, H., Hu, Z. (2009) Support vector machine-based mucin-type o-linked glycosylation site prediction using enhanced sequence feature encoding. *Proc AMIA Annu Symp* 14, 640–644.
41. Chen, K., Kurgan, L. A., Ruan, J. (2007) Prediction of flexible/rigid regions from protein sequences using k-spaced amino acid pairs. *BMC Struct Biol* 7, 25.
42. Hamby, S. E., Hirst, J. D. (2008) Prediction of glycosylation sites using random forests. *BMC Bioinformatics* 9, 500.
43. Hansen, J. F., Lund, O., Engelbrecht, J., et al. (1995) Prediction of O-glycosylation of mammalian proteins: specificity patterns of UDP-GalNAc:polypeptide N-acetylgalactosaminyltransferase. *Biochem J* t3, 801–813.
44. Mark, R., Holmes, M., C. (2004) Giddings prediction of posttranslational modifications using intact-protein mass spectrometric data. *Anal Chem* 76, 276–282.
45. Emanuelsson, O., Nielsen, H., von Heijne, G. (1999) a neural network-based method for predicting chloroplast transit peptides and their cleavage sites. *Protein Sci* 8, 978–984.
46. Puntervoll, P., Linding, R., Gemund, C., Chabanis, D.S. et al. (2003) ELM server: A new resource for investigating short functional sites in modular eukaryotic proteins. *Nucleic Acids Res* 31, 3625–3630.
47. Sigrist, C. J., Cerutti, L., Hulo, N., et al. (2002) PROSITE: A documented database using patterns and profiles as motif descriptors. *Brief Bioinfo* 3, 265–274.
48. Peri, S., Navarro, J., Amanchy, R., Kristiansen, T. et al. (2003) Development of human protein reference database as an initial platform for approaching systems biology in humans. *Genome Res* 13, 2363–2371.
49. Garavelli, J. (2003) The RESID Database of Protein Modifications: 2003 developments. *Nucleic Acids Res* 31, 499–501.

50. Obenauer, J.C., Cantley, L.C., Yaffe, M.B. (2003) Scansite 2.0: Proteome-wide prediction of cell signaling interactions using short sequence motifs. *Nucleic Acids Res* 31, 3635–3641.
51. Saunders, N.F., Brinkworth, R.I., Huber, T., et al. (2008) Predikin and PredikinDB: a computational framework for the prediction of protein kinase peptide specificity and an associated database of phosphorylation sites. *BMC Bioinformatics* 9, 245.
52. Blom, N., Gammeltoft, S., Brunak, S. (1999) P Sequence- and structure-based prediction of eukaryotic protein phosphorylation sites. *J Mol Biol* 294, 1351–1362.
53. Blom, N., Sicheritz-Ponten, T. Gupta, R. et al. (2004) Prediction of post-translational glycosylation and phosphorylation of proteins from the amino acid sequence. *Proteomics* 4, 1633–1649.
54. de Chiara, C., Menon, R.P., Strom, M., et al. (2009) Phosphorylation of S776 and 14-3-3 binding modulate ataxin-1 interaction with splicing factors. *PLoS ONE* 4, e8372.
55. Eisenhaber, B., Bork, P., Eisenhaber, F. (1998) Sequence properties of GPI-anchored proteins near the omega-site: constraints for the polypeptide binding site of the putative transamidase. *Protein Eng* 11, 1155–1161.
56. Cooper, C. A., Gasteiger, E., Packer, N. H. (2001) GlycoMod—a software tool for determining glycosylation compositions from mass spectrometric data. *Proteomics* 1, 340–349.
57. Julenius, K., Mlgaard, A., Gupta, R., Brunak, S. (2005) Prediction, conservation analysis and structural characterization of mammalian mucin-type O-glycosylation sites. *Glycobiology* 15, 153–164.
58. Gupta, R. Jung, E., Gooley, A.A., Williams, K.L., Brunak, S., Hansen, J. (1999) Scanning the available *Dictyostelium discoideum* proteome for O-linked GlcNAc glycosylation sites using neural networks. *Glycobiology* 9, 1009–1022.
59. Gupta, R., Brunak, S. (2002) Prediction of glycosylation across the human proteome and the correlation to protein function. *Pacific Symposium on Biocomputing* 7, 310–322.
60. Martinez, A., Traverso, J. A., Valot, B., Ferro, M., Espagne, C., Ephritikhine, G., Zivy, M., Giglione, C., Meinnel, T. (2008) Extent of N-terminal modifications in cytosolic proteins from eukaryotes. *Proteomics* 8, 2809–2831.
61. Duckert, P., Brunak, S., Blom, N. (2004) Prediction of proprotein convertase cleavage sites. *Protein Eng Design Sel* 17, 107–112.
62. Blom, N., Hansen, J., Blaas, D., Brunak, S. (1996) Cleavage site analysis in picornaviral polyproteins: discovering cellular targets by neural networks. *Protein Sci* 5, 2203–2216.
63. Bologna, G., Yvon, C., Duvaud, S., Veuthey, A. L. (2004) N-Terminal myristoylation predictions by ensembles of neural networks. *Proteomics* 4, 1626–1632.
64. Xue, Y., Ren, J., Gao, X., Jin, C., Wen, L., Yao, X. (2008) GPS 2.0, a tool to predict kinase-specific phosphorylation sites in hierarchy. *Mol Cell Proteomics* 7, 1598–1608.

Chapter 21

In Silico Protein Motif Discovery and Structural Analysis

Catherine Mooney, Norman Davey, Alberto J.M. Martin, Ian Walsh, Denis C. Shields, and Gianluca Pollastri

Abstract

A wealth of in silico tools is available for protein motif discovery and structural analysis. The aim of this chapter is to collect some of the most common and useful tools and to guide the biologist in their use. A detailed explanation is provided for the use of Distill, a suite of web servers for the prediction of protein structural features and the prediction of full-atom 3D models from a protein sequence. Besides this, we also provide pointers to many other tools available for motif discovery and secondary and tertiary structure prediction from a primary amino acid sequence. The prediction of protein intrinsic disorder and the prediction of functional sites and SLiMs are also briefly discussed. Given that user queries vary greatly in size, scope and character, the trade-offs in speed, accuracy and scale need to be considered when choosing which methods to adopt.

Key words: Protein structure prediction, secondary structure, disorder, functional sites, SLiMs.

1. Introduction

Compared with over 15 million known protein sequences (UniProtKB/TrEMBL (1)), as of May 2011, there are only 67,720 proteins of known structure deposited in the Protein Data Bank (PDB) (2). As experimental determination of a protein's structure is difficult, expensive and time consuming, the gap between sequence-known and structure-known proteins is continuing to grow rapidly. Currently the only feasible way to bridge this gap is computational modelling. This is especially important for analysis at a genomic or an inter-genomic level, where informative structural models need to be generated for thousands of gene products (or portions of them) in a reasonable amount of time.

B. Yu, M. Hinchcliffe (eds.), *In Silico Tools for Gene Discovery*, Methods in Molecular Biology 760,
DOI 10.1007/978-1-61779-176-5_21,

Computational modelling methods can be divided into two groups: those that use similarity to proteins of known structure to model all or part of the query protein (comparative or template-based modelling) and ab initio or de novo prediction methods where no similarity to a protein of known structure can be found. If a close homologue is found (e.g. a protein of known structure with a sequence identity greater than approximately 30% to the query), then a model can be produced with a high degree of confidence in its accuracy (3). However, many proteins share similar structures even though their sequences may share less than 15% sequence identity (4). Finding these remote homologues is a much more difficult task. As structural genomic (SG) projects worldwide gather momentum, the hope is to populate the protein fold space with a useful 3D model for all protein families using high-throughput protein structure determination methods (5). Providing more accurate templates for more proteins should lead to an increase in protein structure prediction accuracy for many proteins and move them out of the ab initio/de novo prediction category into the comparative/homology modelling category.

As the accuracy of predicted 3D protein models improves, they are becoming increasingly more useful in biomolecular and biomedical research. In the absence of an experimental structure, there are many applications for which a predicted structure may be of use to biologists. Moult (6) describes the uses of models at three levels of resolution. At the lowest level of resolution are models which have typically been produced by remote fold recognition relationships and are likely to have many errors; however, they may still be useful for domain boundary, super-family and approximate function identification. Medium-resolution models, built using less remote homologues, for instance, obtained from a carefully designed PSI-BLAST (7) search, may be used to identify possible protein–protein interaction sites, the likely role of disease-associated substitutions or the consequences of alternative splicing in protein function. Higher resolution models, where there is a known structure showing at least 30% sequence identity to the query sequence, may be useful for molecular replacement in solving a crystal structure and give insight into the impact of mutations in disease, the consequences of missense or nonsense mutations for protein structure and function, identification of orthologous functional relationships and aspects of molecular function which may not be possible from an experimental structure.

Due to space limitations, we cannot cover all web servers available for protein structural motif discovery and structure prediction but provide a useful overview of the area. Although we will provide a detailed description of our Distill suite of servers, we will also point the reader to other publicly available, up-to-date, accurate and use-to-use in silico tools which have the potential to predict structures, structural features or motifs at a genomic scale.

2. Materials

There are many freely available in silico tools to aid the active researcher which can not only save time but also, as many are constantly updated and improved upon, ensure that one's research is in keeping with or at the state of the art (*see* **Note 4**). Below we have listed those we have found to be most useful in our experience.

2.1. Protein Structural Feature Prediction

1. Distill (http://distill.ucd.ie/distill/)
2. PROTEUS (http://wks16338.biology.ualberta.ca/proteus/)
3. Scratch (SSpro and ACCpro) (http://scratch.proteomics.ics.uci.edu/)
4. Jpred 3 (http://www.compbio.dundee.ac.uk/www-jpred/)
5. PSIPRED (http://bioinf4.cs.ucl.ac.uk:3000/psipred/)
6. SABLE (http://sable.cchmc.org/)

2.2. Protein 3D Structure Prediction

1. 3Distill (http://distill.ucd.ie/distill/)
2. I-TASSER (http://zhanglab.ccmb.med.umich.edu/I-TASSER/)
3. HHpred (http://toolkit.tuebingen.mpg.de/hhpred/)
4. Robetta (http://robetta.bakerlab.org/)

2.3. Functional Site Prediction for Structured Proteins

1. SDPsite (http://bioinf.fbb.msu.ru/SDPsite/index.jsp)
2. ConSurf (http://consurf.tau.ac.il)
3. Evolutionary Trace (http://mammoth.bcm.tmc.edu/ETserver.html)
4. SITEHOUND (http://bsbbsinai.org/SHserver/SiteHound/)

2.4. Disorder Prediction

1. Spritz (http://distill.ucd.ie/spritz)
2. IUPred server (http://iupred.enzim.hu/)

2.5. SLiM Discovery, Rediscovery and Post-processing

1. The ELM server (http://elm.eu.org/)
2. Minimotif Miner (http://mnm.engr.uconn.edu/MNM/)
3. SIRW (http://sirw.embl.de/)
4. SLiMSearch, SLiMfinder and CompariMotif (http://bioware.ucd.ie/)

5. Dilimot (http://dilimot.embl.de/)
6. ANCHOR (http://anchor.enzim.hu/)
7. Conscore (http://conscore.embl.de)
8. PepSite (http://pepsite.russelllab.org/cgi-bin/pepsite/pepsite)

3. Methods

3.1. Prediction of Protein Structural Features

3.1.1. Distill: Protein Structure and Structural Feature Prediction Server

Distill (8) is a suite of web servers available to the public for protein structure and structural feature prediction. The Distill suite of servers currently contains nine predictors: six predictors of 1D features (i.e. properties which may be represented as a string of the same length as the amino acid sequence – secondary structure (9), contact density (10), local structural motifs (11), relative solvent accessibility (12), protein disorder (13) and protein domain boundary prediction (14)), a coarse contact map and protein topology predictor, a predictor of protein residue contact maps (15) and the predictor of full-atom 3D models and Cα traces (3Distill). The servers are based on large-scale ensembles of machine learning systems that include recursive neural networks, support vector machines and Monte Carlo simulations. They are trained on large, up-to-date, non-redundant subsets of the PDB (2).

Structural motifs (11) are identified by applying multidimensional scaling and clustering to pairwise angular distances between quadruplets of $\varphi - \psi$ dihedral angle pairs collected from high-resolution protein structures (16). Structural motif predictions are highly informative and provide a finer resolution picture of a protein backbone and may be used to improve traditional three-class secondary structure and for the identification of remote homologues (17). The definition and one-letter code for the 14 structural motifs are provided on the Distill help page.

Each of the servers takes as input a profile obtained from multiple sequence alignments of the protein sequence to its homologues in the UniRef90 database (18) to leverage evolutionary information. Until recently, predictors of 1D structural properties have generally been ab initio. However, it has been shown that evolutionary information from proteins of known structure can contribute to more accurate 1D prediction (12, 17, 19, 20). When available, this information, in the form of homologous structures from the PDB, is provided as a further input to all the servers, resulting in greatly improved reliability. For more information on the use of homology during the predictive process, see (12, 17).

In addition, 1D predictions augment the 2D and 3D predictions as follows: secondary structure and solvent accessibility are provided as additional input to the residue contact maps and coarse protein topology predictors; secondary structure, solvent accessibility and contact density are provided as additional input to the residue contact map predictor; secondary structure, solvent accessibility, structural motif, contact density, coarse and residue contact maps are provided as additional input to 3Distill (3D). For a more detailed description of the models and training algorithms, see (8–17).

All predictions are freely available through a simple joint web interface and the results are returned by email. In a single submission, a user can send protein sequences for over 32,000 residues to all or a selection of the servers. If a template is found in the PDB, the sequence identity between the query sequence and the best template is provided (*see* **Note 3**).

3.1.2. Other 1D Structural Feature Prediction Servers

Some other popular secondary structure (SS) and relative solvent accessibility (RSA) prediction servers are *PROTEUS* (19) and *Scratch* (SSpro and ACCpro) (20) which include homology to proteins of known structure in the PDB, if available, during the prediction process. *Jpred 3* (21) will notify the user if there is a homologous sequence available in the PDB prior to prediction but does not include this information in the prediction process. *PSIPRED* (22) and *SABLE* (23) are ab initio predictors (*see* **Note 2**). Methods of searching for and incorporating homology information into the prediction process vary between the different servers; see (17) for further discussion of some of the different methods for homology search and inclusion.

3.2. Three-Dimensional Protein Structure Prediction

3.2.1. 3D Prediction by Distill

3Distill (8) is a server for the prediction of full-atom 3D models of protein structures which accepts queries of up to 250 amino acids in length. 3Distill relies on a fast optimization algorithm guided by a potential based on secondary structure, solvent accessibility, structural motif, contact density, coarse contact maps and residue contact maps, all predicted by Distill. Note that, when available, homology information is provided to 3Distill which results in substantially improved predictions. 3Distill and the underlying servers have been tuned and generally improved in the lead-up to CASP9. Input into the servers is handled by the same two simple HTML forms for the submission of single and multiple queries as for 1D prediction. 3Distill's outputs come as attachments in PDB format. Five ranked models are returned in PDB file format, each one containing all atoms in the protein except hydrogen. When the query is longer than 250 residues, fold predictions by XStout are returned instead of full-atom models by 3Distill. An average sized protein takes less than 1 h to predict and no user expertise or intervention is required. 3Distill is free for academic use.

3.2.2. Other 3D Structure Prediction Servers

The critical assessment of techniques for protein structure prediction (CASP) experiment evaluates the current state of the art in protein structure prediction (24). There have been eight experiments to date taking place every 2 years since 1994. Participants predict the 3D structure, and other structural features, of a set of soon to be known structures; these predictions are then assessed by a panel of experts when the structures are known. Fully automated prediction by servers, has played an increasingly important role at CASP. Although most protein structure predictions are automated in some way, many still require human intervention by experts to get the most accurate results. Fully automated processes have the advantage of being available to the non-expert user and, in general being faster than human approaches, may be used at a genomic scale, something that is more of a requirement these days than just being desirable (*see* **Note 1**). The accuracy of server predictions has significantly increased over the last number of years with servers being ranked in the top five overall in CASP7 and CASP8. Some of the servers that have performed best at CASP are described below. For a detailed comparison and in-depth discussion of all methods that participated in CASP8, see the special edition of the journal *Proteins: Structure, Function, and Bioinformatics* (24) and look out for the results of CASP9 which took place in 2010.

I-TASSER (25) was ranked first in the server category of the CASP8 experiment. It is free for academic use, no expert knowledge is required and prediction from a protein sequence takes in the region of 24–48 h for full 3D structure and function prediction. The I-TASSER pipeline includes four general steps: template identification; structural reassembly; atomic model construction and final model selection. In cases where no appropriate template is identified, the whole structure is predicted ab initio. The success of I-TASSER is primarily due to the use of information from multiple templates.

HHpred (26) is primarily an interactive function and structure prediction server. For example, the user can search various databases, manually select templates or correct errors in the proposed target–template alignment. The prediction pipeline is as follows: build a multiple sequence alignment for the target sequence; search for homologous templates; re-rank the potential templates with a neural network; generate sets of multiple alignments with successively lower sequence diversities for the target sequence and the templates; rank target–template alignments of various alignment diversities with neural network; choose template(s); and run MODELLER (27). Some user expertise in the area of alignment/template selection is useful as users have the option to intervene at this step before the 3D model is built. Predictions are fast, taking less than 1 h for a protein of average size.

David Baker's *Robetta* (28) is one of the best known, consistently most accurate and popular of all protein structure prediction servers. The server parses protein chains into putative domains and predicts these domains either ab initio or by homology modelling. However, the popularity of the server and computational requirements result in long waiting times before the prediction process even starts, and public users are restricted to submitting one protein sequence at a time.

3.3. Functional Site Prediction for Structured Proteins

Predicting functionally important amino acids or active sites of proteins is a good starting point for structure-based function prediction. Most predictors use sequence conservation as an indication of functional importance with some newer predictors incorporating structural information. *SDPsite* (29) predicts functional sites using conserved positions and specificity-determining positions (SDP residues which are conserved within sub-groups of a protein family but differ between groups). The server takes as input a multiple sequence alignment and a phylogenetic tree of the proteins in the alignment.

The *ConSurf* server (30) takes as input a protein sequence, multiple sequence alignment or PDB file. The PDB file can be uploaded, in which case the functional site of a predicted protein model can be predicted, or if the structure is known, the PDB ID can be entered. If the input is a protein sequence or multiple sequence alignment, the output includes a sequence/multiple sequence alignment coloured according to the conservation scores and a phylogenetic tree. If a PDB structure is provided, the output is a PDB file with the predicted functionally important residues highlighted. ConSurf is free for academic use, easy to use, fast and requires no expert knowledge.

Evolutionary Trace (31) captures the extent of evolutionary pressure at a given position in a protein sequence and ranks the amino acids by their relative evolutionary importance. There are two tools available: the ET Viewer, which takes a PDB ID as input and displays a colour map of the structure showing the ranked residues, and the ET Report Maker, which takes either a PDB ID or a UniProt accession number as input and returns a detailed report which includes information about protein sequence, structure, suggested mutations and substitutions for selective functional site knockout. The Evolutionary Trace server is free for academic use.

SITEHOUND (32) takes as input a protein structure in PDB format and identifies regions corresponding to putative ligand-binding sites. These sites are characterized by favourable noncovalent interactions with a chemical probe. The selection of different chemical probes results in the identification of different types of binding site. Currently, carbon and phosphate probes are available to identify binding sites for drug-like molecules and phosphorylated ligands, respectively. The output is a list of residues which correspond to the putative binding sites.

3.4. Disorder Prediction

Many proteins or protein regions fail to fold into fixed tertiary structures. Over the last 10 years, these intrinsically unstructured (IU)/disordered proteins have been shown to be important functionally, leading to an alternative view of protein function to the traditional sequence–structure–function paradigm (33). *Spritz* (13) is a web server for the prediction of intrinsically disordered regions in protein sequences. Spritz is available as part of the Distill suite of servers described above and predicts ordered/disordered residues using two specialized binary classifiers both implemented with probabilistic soft-margin support vector machines or C-SVM. The SVM-LD (LD, long disorder) classifier is trained on a subset of non-redundant sequences known to contain only long disordered protein fragments ($\geq$30 AA). The SVM-SD (SD, short disorder) classifier is trained instead on a subset of non-redundant sequences with only short disordered fragments.

The *IUPred* server (34) predicts disorder based on the difference between estimates of the pairwise energy content for globular proteins which have the potential to form a large number of favourable interactions compared with disordered proteins which do not form sufficiently favourable interactions to adopt a stable structure due to their amino acid composition. For a comprehensive list of other disorder predictors, see http://www.disprot.org/predictors.php.

3.5. Short Linear Motifs (SLiMs)

Short linear motifs (SLiMs) are abundant protein microdomains that play a central role in cell regulation. SLiMs, also referred to as linear motifs, minimotifs or eukaryotic linear motifs (ELMs, in eukaryotes) typically act as protein ligands and mediate many biological processes including cell signalling, post-translational modification (PTM) and trafficking target proteins to specific subcellular localizations (numerous excellent reviews of motif biology are available (35–37)). Several organizations, such as the eukaryotic linear motif (ELM) resource (38, 39) and Minimotif Miner (MnM) (40, 41), are actively curating the available SLiM literature and currently 200 classes of motifs are known, yet without a doubt many more remain to be discovered. SLiMs are defined by a conduciveness to convergently evolve, their preferential occurrence in disordered regions and their short length. Each of these attributes contributes to the difficulty of motif discovery, both experimentally and computationally; however, despite the challenges, several useful motif discovery tools are available.

3.5.1. Motif Rediscovery

The *ELM server* (38, 39) searches the ELM database for regular expression matches and discovers putatively functional novel instances of known SLiMs. Returned motifs are filtered to exclude motifs occurring in globular regions of proteins using information from Pfam (42, 43), SMART (44) and the PDB when available. *Minimotif Miner* (40, 41) searches an input protein for matches to the MnM dataset, scoring motifs based on surface accessibility, conservation and fold enrichment (based on the ratio of observed motifs to expected motifs). *SIRW* is a web server that calculates motif enrichment, using the Fisher's exact test, in a set of proteins with a particular keyword or gene ontology (GO) (45) terms (*see* **Chapter 9** for gene ontology resources). Similarly, *SLiMSearch* uses the masking and statistical methods of the SLiMfinder tool (46) to search for motifs in an input dataset.

3.5.2. De Novo Motif Discovery

Dilimot (47) and *SLiMfinder* (46), using motif over-representation, attempt de novo computational discovery of SLiMs in datasets of proteins. Dilimot masks globular regions and enriches convergently evolved motifs by removing all but one representative homologous region. Returned motifs are scored using a binomial scoring scheme. Finally, conservation of the motif in several species is incorporated into a final combined score. SLiMfinder excludes under-conserved residues, non-disordered regions predicted using IUPred (34) and UniProt (1) annotated features such as domains. Motifs are scored using an extension of binomial statistics allowing the consideration of homologous motif instances and correction for multiple testing. *ANCHOR* (48) attempts the difficult task of de novo motif discovery from primary sequence by predicting disordered binding regions. These are regions that undergo a disorder-to-order transition on binding to a structured partner. ANCHOR uses the same pairwise energy estimation approach as IUPred to identify protein segments that reside in disordered regions but are unable to form enough favourable intra-chain interactions to fold on their own and therefore are likely to require an interaction with a globular protein partner to gain stabilizing energy.

3.5.3. Post-processing

After discovery of a novel motif, there are multiple steps that can help increase confidence of functionality. *CompariMotif* (49) searches for matches to known functional motifs. Novel motifs are compared against motif databases using shared information content, allowing the best matches to be easily identified in large comparisons. Currently, the ELM (38, 39) and MnM (40, 41) databases, as well as several other specialized datasets, are available to search. Conservation is one of the strongest classifiers of novel motif functionality and several tools are available to score the conservation of motif occurrences. For example, *Conscore* (50) uses an information content-based scoring scheme which incorporates phylogeny information to weight sequences and Dinkel and Sticht (51) introduced an average conservation score.

PepSite (52) can be used to scan known interactors for binding sites for a discovered motif. Using spatial position-specific scoring matrices (PSSMs) created from known 3D structures of motif/protein complexes, PepSite scores the surface of the target and suggests potential binding site and rough orientation of the motif.

3.5.4. Biological Uses

Several examples of experimentally validated motifs discovered by in silico methods are available. Neduva et al. (47) applied Dilimot to discover and verify a protein phosphatase 1 binding motif (DxxDxxxD) and a motif that binds Translin (VxxxRxYS). Keyword enrichment has been used to discover novel KEN box (53), KEPE (54) and EH1 motifs (55) (*see* **Chapter 8** for in silico knowledge and content tracking). Two 14-3-3 motifs in EFF-1 were discovered using MnM and subsequently experimentally validated (40, 41). For more on SLiM discovery, see the review by Davey et al. (56).

4. Notes

1. The number of protein sequences is growing at an ever increasing pace and many in silico methods are available for the efficient annotation of these sequences. Given that user queries vary greatly in size, scope and character, when choosing which methods to adopt the speed, accuracy and scale of the method need to be considered. As a first approximation, especially in the case of structure prediction, the greater the accuracy, the slower the processing time. The larger the scale of a query (e.g. when genomic-scale predictions are necessary), the harder it will be to obtain the most accurate answers available, unless one has access to a large amount of computational resources and has the time to download and set up one of the methods that are available for local installation.
2. When deciding which prediction method to use, the main consideration to make is whether there is a homologue for the query in the PDB. If so, methods incorporating homology are usually significantly more accurate. Another consideration is the scale of predictions to be performed. All servers handle predictions at a small scale (tens of queries), some (e.g. Distill) facilitate predictions at a larger scale (hundreds of queries). If genomic or especially multi-genomic-scale predictions are needed, it may be necessary to resort to one of the methods that can be downloaded and run locally. When possible consensus predictions are desirable, that is

polling multiple methods for the same query and comparing the results. Where methods agree generally predictions are to be considered more reliable.

3. Greater confidence can be placed in the accuracy of structure predictions if there is high sequence similarity between the query sequence and a protein of known structure which can act as a template. However, it is worth remembering that even with little or no sequence similarity, proteins may share the same structure and therefore a low sequence identity template does not imply that the prediction is inaccurate. In Distill we find templates via the SAMD program (17), which may yield informative templates even for very low sequence identity.
4. During our research experiences, we have often encountered resistance from some experimental researchers in exploiting all the computational tools that are available to simplify their jobs. Even in the absence of resistance, countless times we have observed ageing and outdated tools being adopted when far better ones were freely available and ready to use. Within the limits of this chapter, we hope we have made a small step toward solving this problem and bringing the power of novel predicting methods to its full fruition.

Acknowledgements

C.M. is supported by Science Foundation Ireland (SFI) grant 08/IN.1/B1864. ND is supported by an EMBL Interdisciplinary Postdoc (EIPOD) fellowship. CM, GP, IW and AJMM were partly supported by SFI grant 05/RFP/CMS0029, grant RP/2005/219 from the Health Research Board of Ireland, a UCD President's Award 2004 and UCD Seed Funding 2009 award SF371.

References

1. The UniProt Consortium (2008) The Universal Protein Resource (UniProt). *Nucleic Acids Res* 36, D190–D195.
2. Berman, H., Westbrook, J., Feng, Z., et al. (2000) The Protein Data Bank. *Nucleic Acids Res* 28, 235–242.
3. Aloy, P., Pichaud, M., Russell, R. (2005) Protein complexes: structure prediction challenges for the 21st century. *Curr Opin Struct Biol* 15, 15–22.
4. Chothia, C., Lesk, A. (1986) The relation between the divergence of sequence and structure in proteins. *EMBO J* 5, 823–826.
5. Chandonia, J., Brenner, S. (2006) The impact of structural genomics: expectations and outcomes. *Science* 311, 347.
6. Moult, J. (2008) Comparative modeling in structural genomics. *Structure* 16, 14–16.
7. Altschul, S., Madden, T., Schaffer, A., et al. (1997) Gapped BLAST and PSI-BLAST: a new generation of protein database search programs. *Nucleic Acids Res* 25, 3389.
8. Baù D, Martin, A., Mooney, C., et al. (2006) Distill: a suite of web servers for the prediction of one-, two- and three-dimensional

structural features of proteins. *BMC Bioinformatics* 7, 402.
9. Pollastri, G., McLysaght, A. (2005) Porter: a new, accurate server for protein secondary structure prediction. *Bioinformatics* 21, 1719–1720.
10. Vullo, A., Walsh, I., Pollastri, G. (2006) A two-stage approach for improved prediction of residue contact maps. *BMC Bioinformatics* 7, 180.
11. Mooney, C., Vullo, A., Pollastri, G. (2006) Protein structural motif prediction in multidimensional phi–psi space leads to improved secondary structure prediction. *J Comput Biol* 13, 1489–1502.
12. Pollastri, G., Martin, A., Mooney, C., Vullo, A. (2007) Accurate prediction of protein secondary structure and solvent accessibility by consensus combiners of sequence and structure information. *BMC Bioinformatics* 8, 201.
13. Vullo, A., Bortolami, O., Pollastri, G., Tosatto, S. (2006) Spritz: a server for the prediction of intrinsically disordered regions in protein sequences using kernel machines. *Nucleic Acids Res* 34, W164.
14. Walsh, I., Martin, A., Mooney, C., et al. (2009) Ab initio and homology based prediction of protein domains by recursive neural networks. *BMC Bioinformatics* 10, 195.
15. Walsh, I., Baù, D., Martin, A., et al. (2009) Ab initio and template-based prediction of multi-class distance maps by two-dimensional recursive neural networks. *BMC Struct Biol* 9, 5.
16. Sims, G., Choi, I., Kim, S. (2005) Protein conformational space in higher order $\psi-\varphi$ maps. *Proc Natl Acad Sci USA* 18, 618–621.
17. Mooney, C., Pollastri, G. (2009) Beyond the Twilight Zone: automated prediction of structural properties of proteins by recursive neural networks and remote homology information. *Proteins* 77, 181–190.
18. Suzek, B., Huang, H., McGarvey, P., et al. (2007) UniRef: comprehensive and non-redundant UniProt reference clusters. *Bioinformatics* 23, 1282.
19. Montgomerie, S., Sundararaj, S., Gallin, W., Wishart, D. (2006) Improving the accuracy of protein secondary structure prediction using structural alignment. *BMC Bioinformatics* 7, 301.
20. Cheng, J., Randall, A., Sweredoski, M., Baldi, P. (2005) SCRATCH: a protein structure and structural feature prediction server. *Nucleic Acids Res* 33, W72.
21. Cole, C., Barber, J., Barton, G. (2008) The Jpred 3 secondary structure prediction server. *Nucleic Acids Res* 36, W197–W201.
22. Jones, D. (1999) Protein secondary structure prediction based on position-specific scoring matrices. *J Mol Biol* 292, 195–202.
23. Adamczak, R., Porollo, A., Meller, J. (2005) Combining prediction of secondary structure and solvent accessibility in proteins. *Proteins* 59, 467–475.
24. Moult, J., Fidelis, K., Kryshtafovych, A., et al. (2009) Critical assessment of methods of protein structure prediction – Round VIII. *Proteins* 77, 1–4.
25. Zhang, Y. (2009) I-TASSER: Fully automated protein structure prediction in CASP8. *Proteins* 77, 100.
26. Hildebrand, A., Remmert, M., Biegert, A., Söding, J. (2009) Fast and accurate automatic structure prediction with HHpred. *Proteins* 77, 128–132.
27. Eswar, N., Webb, B., Marti-Renom, M., et al. (2007) Comparative protein structure modeling using Modeller. *Curr Protoc Protein Sci* 50:2.9.1–2.9.31.
28. Raman, S., Vernon, R., Thompson, J., et al. (2009) Structure prediction for CASP8 with all-atom refinement using Rosetta. *Proteins* 77, 89–99.
29. Kalinina, O., Gelfand, M., Russell, R. (2009) Combining specificity determining and conserved residues improves functional site prediction. *BMC Bioinformatics* 10, 174.
30. Landau, M., Mayrose, I., Rosenberg, Y., et al. (2005) ConSurf 2005: the projection of evolutionary conservation scores of residues on protein structures. *Nucleic Acids Res* 33, W299.
31. Morgan, D., Kristensen, D., Mittelman, D., Lichtarge, O. (2006) ET viewer: an application for predicting and visualizing functional sites in protein structures. *Bioinformatics* 22, 2049.
32. Hernandez, M., Ghersi, D., Sanchez, R. (2009) SITEHOUND-web: a server for ligand binding site identification in protein structures. *Nucleic Acids Res* 37, W413–W416.
33. Dyson, H., Wright, P. (2005) Intrinsically unstructured proteins and their functions. *Nat Rev Mol Cell Biol* 6, 197–208.
34. Dosztanyi, Z., Csizmok, V., Tompa, P., Simon, I. (2005) IUPred: web server for the prediction of intrinsically unstructured regions of proteins based on estimated energy content. *Bioinformatics* 21, 3433.
35. Diella, F., Haslam, N., Chica, C., et al. (2008) Understanding eukaryotic linear motifs and their role in cell signaling and regulation. *Front Biosci* 13, 6580–6603.

36. Neduva, V., Russell, R. (2006) Peptides mediating interaction networks: new leads at last. *Curr Opin Biotechnol* 17, 465–471.
37. Neduva, V., Russell, R. (2005) Linear motifs: evolutionary interaction switches. *FEBS Lett* 579, 3342–3345.
38. Puntervoll, P., Linding, R., Gemund, C., et al. (2003) ELM server: a new resource for investigating short functional sites in modular eukaryotic proteins. *Nucleic Acids Res* 31, 3625.
39. Gould, C., Diella, F., Via, A., et al. (2010) ELM: the status of the 2010 eukaryotic linear motif resource. *Nucleic Acids Res* 38, D167.
40. Balla, S., Thapar, V., Verma, S., et al. (2006) Minimotif Miner: a tool for investigating protein function. *Nat Methods* 3, 175–177.
41. Rajasekaran, S., Balla, S., Gradie, P., et al. (2009) Minimotif miner 2nd release: a database and web system for motif search. *Nucleic Acids Res* 37, D185.
42. Bateman, A., Birney, E., Cerruti, L., et al. (2002) The Pfam protein families database. *Nucleic Acids Res* 30, 276.
43. Finn, R., Mistry, J., Tate, J., et al. (2009) The Pfam protein families database. *Nucleic Acids Res* 36, 281–288.
44. Letunic, I., Doerks, T., Bork, P. (2008) SMART 6: recent updates and new developments. *Nucleic Acids Res* 1, 4.
45. Ashburner, M., Ball, C., Blake, J., et al. (2000) Gene Ontology: tool for the unification of biology. *Nat Genet* 25, 25–29.
46. Edwards, R., Davey, N., Shields, D. (2007) SLiMFinder: a probabilistic method for identifying over-represented, convergently evolved, short linear motifs in proteins. *PloS One* 2, e967.
47. Neduva, V., Linding, R., Su-Angrand, I., et al. (2005) Systematic discovery of new recognition peptides mediating protein interaction networks. *PLoS Biol* 3, 2090.
48. Mészáros B, Simon, I., Dosztányi Z (2009) Prediction of protein binding regions in disordered proteins. *PLoS Comput Biol* 5, 5.
49. Edwards, R., Davey, N., Shields, D. (2008) CompariMotif: quick and easy comparisons of sequence motifs. *Bioinformatics* 24, 1307.
50. Chica, C., Labarga, A., Gould, C., et al. (2008) A tree-based conservation scoring method for short linear motifs in multiple alignments of protein sequences. *BMC Bioinformatics* 9, 229.
51. Dinkel, H., Sticht, H. (2007) A computational strategy for the prediction of functional linear peptide motifs in proteins. *Bioinformatics* 23, 3297.
52. Petsalaki, E., Stark, A., García-Urdiales, E., Russell, R. (2009) Accurate prediction of peptide binding sites on protein surfaces. *PLoS Comput Biol* 5, e1000335.
53. Michael, S., Trave, G., Ramu, C., et al. (2008) Discovery of candidate KEN-box motifs using cell cycle keyword enrichment combined with native disorder prediction and motif conservation. *Bioinformatics* 24, 453.
54. Diella, F., Chabanis, S., Luck, K., et al. (2009) KEPE—a motif frequently superimposed on sumoylation sites in metazoan chromatin proteins and transcription factors. *Bioinformatics* 25, 1.
55. Copley, R. (2005) The EH 1 motif in metazoan transcription factors. *BMC Genomics* 6, 169.
56. Davey, N., Edwards, R., Shields, D. (2010) Computational identification and analysis of protein short linear motifs. *Front Biosci* 15, 801–825.

INDEX

Note: The letters 'f' and 't' following the locators refer to figures and tables respectively.

B. Yu, M. Hinchcliffe (eds.), *In Silico Tools for Gene Discovery*, Methods in Molecular Biology 760,
DOI 10.1007/978-1-61779-176-5, © Springer Science+Business Media, LLC 2011

E

MIX
Papier aus verantwortungsvollen Quellen
Paper from responsible sources
FSC® C105338

If you have any concerns about our products,
you can contact us on
ProductSafety@springernature.com

In case Publisher is established outside the EU,
the EU authorized representative is:
Springer Nature Customer Service Center GmbH
Europaplatz 3, 69115 Heidelberg, Germany

Printed by Libri Plureos GmbH
in Hamburg, Germany